Obstructive Sleep Apnea

Editors

SHIRLEY F. JONES
JAMES A. BARKER

SLEEP MEDICINE CLINICS

www.sleep.theclinics.com

December 2013 • Volume 8 • Number 4

ELSEVIER

1600 John F. Kennedy Boulevard • Suite 1800 • Philadelphia, Pennsylvania, 19103-2899

http://www.theclinics.com

SLEEP MEDICINE CLINICS Volume 8, Number 4
December 2013, ISSN 1556-407X, ISBN-13: 978-0-323-26128-9

Editor: Katie Saunders
Developmental Editor: Stephanie Carter

Sleep Medicine Clinics (ISSN 1556-407X) is published quarterly by Elsevier Inc., 360 Park Avenue South, New York, NY 10010-1710. Months of issue are March, June, September and December. Business and Editorial Offices: 1600 John F. Kennedy Blvd., Ste. 1800, Philadelphia, PA 19103-2899. Customer Service Office: 3251 Riverport Lane, Maryland Heights, MO 63043. Periodicals postage paid at New York, NY and additional mailing offices. Subscription prices are $195.00 per year (US individuals), $95.00 (US residents), $406.00 (US institutions), $235.00 (Canadian and foreign individuals), $135.00 (Canadian and foreign residents) and $452.00 (Canadian and foreign institutions). Foreign air speed delivery is included in all *Clinics* subscription prices. All prices are subject to change without notice. **POSTMASTER:** Send change of address to *Sleep Medicine Clinics*, Elsevier Health Sciences Division, Subscription Customer Service, 3251 Riverport Lane, Maryland Heights, MO 63043. Customer Service: **Tel: 1-800-654-2452 (U.S. and Canada); 314-447-8871 (outside U.S. and Canada). Fax: 314-447-8029. E-mail: journalscustomerservice-usa@elsevier.com (for print support); journalsonlinesupport-usa@elsevier.com (for online support).**

Reprints. For copies of 100 or more of articles in this publication, please contact the Commercial Reprints Department, Elsevier Inc., 360 Park Avenue South, New York, NY 10010-1710. Tel.: 212-633-3874; Fax: 212-633-3820; E-mail: reprints@elsevier.com.

Printed and bound by CPI Group (UK) Ltd, Croydon, CR0 4YY

Transferred to digital print 2012

PROGRAM OBJECTIVE

The goal of *Sleep Clinics of North America* is to keep practicing physicians up to date with current clinical practice by providing timely articles reviewing the state of the art in patient care.

TARGET AUDIENCE

All practicing physicians and other healthcare professionals.

LEARNING OBJECTIVES

Upon completion of this activity, participants will be able to:

1. Discuss therapies for obstructive sleep apnea including weight loss management, pharmacological therapy, surgical treatment, and alternative therapies.
2. Identify complex sleep apnea.
3. Describe the upper airway anatomy and pathophysiology of obstructive sleep apnea.

ACCREDITATION

The Elsevier Office of Continuing Medical Education (EOCME) is accredited by the Accreditation Council for Continuing Medical Education (ACCME) to provide continuing medical education for physicians.

The EOCME designates this enduring material for a maximum of 15 *AMA PRA Category 1 Credit*(s)™. Physicians should claim only the credit commensurate with the extent of their participation in the activity.

All other health care professionals requesting continuing education credit for this enduring material will be issued a certificate of participation.

DISCLOSURE OF CONFLICTS OF INTEREST

The EOCME assesses conflict of interest with its instructors, faculty, planners, and other individuals who are in a position to control the content of CME activities. All relevant conflicts of interest that are identified are thoroughly vetted by EOCME for fair balance, scientific objectivity, and patient care recommendations. EOCME is committed to providing its learners with CME activities that promote improvements or quality in healthcare and not a specific proprietary business or a commercial interest.

The planning committee, staff, authors and editors listed below have identified no financial relationships or relationships to products or devices they or their spouse/life partner have with commercial interest related to the content of this CME activity:
Vivien C. Abad, MD, MBA, FAASM; Mary J. Aigner, PhD, RN, FNP-BC; Anas Al-Sadi, MD; Archana Banerjee, RPh; James A. Barker, MD, CPE, FACP, FCCP, FAASM; Carl Boethel, MD, FCCP, FAASM, DABSM; Macario Camacho, MD; Richard J. Castriotta, MD; Ahmad Chebbo, MD; Christopher Cielo, DO; Nancy Collop, MD; Nicole Congleton; Leopoldo P. Correa, BDS, MS; Shekhar Ghamande, MD, FCCP, FAASM; Katie Hartner; Brynne Hunter; Richard L. Jacobson, DMD, MS; Shirley F. Jones, MD, FCCP, FAASM; Sophia H. Kim, MD; Jorge R. Kizer, MD, MSc, FACC; Vidya Krishnan, MD, MHS; Sandy Lavery; Ruckshanda Majid, MD; Amit Mann, MD; Jill McNair; Mahalakshmi Narayan; Susheel P. Patil, MD, PhD; Stephen A. Schendel, MD, DDS, FACS; Neomi Shah, MD, MPH; Pawan Sikka, MD, FACP, FAASM, CBSM; Amer Tfaili, MD; Harneet K. Walia, MD; Leslie D. Wilke, DO; H. Klar Yaggi, MD, MPH.

The planning committee, staff, authors and editors listed below have identified financial relationships or relationships to products or devices they or their spouse/life partner have with commercial interest related to the content of this CME activity:
Lee J. Brooks, MD has stock ownership in various health-related companies; none specified.
Teofilo Lee-Chiong Jr, MD is a consultant/advisor for CareCore National and Elsevier; has employment affiliation, has stock ownership in, and receives a research grant from Phillips Respironics; has royalties/patents with Elsevier.
Reena Mehra, MD, MS serves on the Medical Advisory Board for Care Core National; has received funding from the National Institutes of Health for research; has received positive airway devices from Philips Respironics for research for which she is the Principal Investigator.

UNAPPROVED/OFF-LABEL USE DISCLOSURE

The EOCME requires CME faculty to disclose to the participants:

1. When products or procedures being discussed are off-label, unlabelled, experimental, and/or investigational (not US Food and Drug Administration (FDA) approved); and
2. Any limitations on the information presented, such as data that are preliminary or that represent ongoing research, interim analyses, and/or unsupported opinions. Faculty may discuss information about pharmaceutical agents that is outside of FDA-approved labelling. This information is intended solely for CME and is not intended to promote off-label use of these medications. If you have any questions, contact the medical affairs department of the manufacturer for the most recent prescribing information.

TO ENROLL

To enroll in the Sleep Medicines Clinic Continuing Medical Education program, call customer service at 1-800-654-2452 or sign up online at http://www.theclinics.com/home/cme. The CME program is available to subscribers for an additional annual fee of USD $126.

METHOD OF PARTICIPATION

In order to claim credit, participants must complete the following:

1. Complete enrolment as indicated above.
2. Read the activity.
3. Complete the CME Test and Evaluation. Participants must achieve a score of 70% on the test. All CME Tests and Evaluations must be completed online.

CME INQUIRIES/SPECIAL NEEDS

For all CME inquiries or special needs, please contact elsevierCME@elsevier.com.

SLEEP MEDICINE CLINICS

FORTHCOMING ISSUES

March 2014
Central Sleep Apnea
Peter Gay, *Editor*

June 2014
Evaluation of Sleep Complaints
Clete Kushida, *Editor*

September 2014
Behavioral Aspects of Sleep Problems in Childhood and Adolescence
Judith Owens, *Editor*

RECENT ISSUES

September 2013
Insomnia
Jack D. Edinger, *Editor*

June 2013
Fatigue
Max Hirshkowitz, and
Amir Sharafkhaneh, *Editors*

March 2013
Sleep and Anesthesia
Frances Chung, *Editor*

RELATED INTEREST

Medical Clinics of North America, 2010 (Vol. 94, Issue 3)
Sleep Medicine
Christian Guilleminault, MD, *Editor*

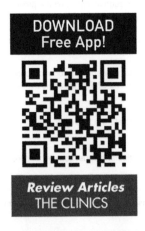

Contributors

CONSULTING EDITOR

TEOFILO LEE-CHIONG Jr, MD
Professor of Medicine, Division of Pulmonary,
Critical Care and Sleep Medicine, Department
of Medicine, National Jewish Health, University
of Colorado, Denver, Colorado; Chief Medical
Liaison, Philips Respironics, Pennsylvania

EDITORS

SHIRLEY F. JONES, MD, FCCP, FAASM
Senior Staff, Pulmonary and Sleep Medicine,
Scott and White Healthcare, Assistant
Professor of Medicine, Texas A&M HSC COM,
Temple, Texas

**JAMES A. BARKER, MD, CPE, FACP, FCCP,
FAASM**
Senior Staff, Pulmonary, Critical Care, and
Sleep Disorders, Pulmonary and Sleep
Medicine, Medical Director for Fragile
Populations, Scott and White Health Plan, Scott
and White Healthcare, Professor of Medicine,
Texas A&M HSC COM, Temple, Texas

AUTHORS

VIVIEN C. ABAD, MD, MBA, FAASM
Adjunct Clinical Assistant Professor,
Division of Sleep Medicine, Department of
Psychiatry and Behavioral Science, Stanford
Sleep Medicine Center, Redwood City,
California

MARY AIGNER, PhD, RN, FNP-BC
Nurse Practitioner, Pulmonary Sleep Medicine,
Central Texas Veterans Health Care System,
Temple, Texas

ANAS AL-SADI, MD
Department of Medicine, Scott and White
Healthcare, Temple, Texas

ARCHANA BANERJEE, RPh
Clinical Pharmacy Specialist, Department of
Pharmacy, Central Texas Veterans Health Care
System, Temple, Texas

**JAMES A. BARKER, MD, CPE, FACP, FCCP,
FAASM**
Senior Staff, Pulmonary, Critical Care, and
Sleep Disorders, Pulmonary and Sleep

Medicine, Medical Director for Fragile
Populations, Scott and White Health Plan,
Scott and White Healthcare, Professor of
Medicine, Texas A&M HSC COM, Temple,
Texas

**CARL D. BOETHEL, MD, FCCP, FAASM,
DABSM**
Division of Pulmonary, Critical Care, and
Sleep Medicine, Interim Division Director,
Medical Director, Scott and White Sleep
Institute, Scott and White Healthcare;
Assistant Professor of Medicine, Texas A&M
Health Science Center College of Medicine,
Temple, Texas

LEE J. BROOKS, MD
Professor of Pediatrics, Division of Pulmonary
Medicine, Attending Physician, Sleep Center,
The Children's Hospital of Philadelphia,
University of Pennsylvania, Philadelphia,
Pennsylvania

MACARIO CAMACHO, MD
Consulting Assistant Professor, Sleep Division, Department of Otolaryngology-Head and Neck Surgery, Stanford University, Stanford, California

RICHARD J. CASTRIOTTA, MD
Professor of Medicine and Director, Division of Pulmonary and Sleep Medicine, University of Texas Medical School at Houston; Medical Director, Sleep Disorders Center, Memorial Hermann Hospital – Texas Medical Center, University of Texas Medical School at Houston, Houston, Texas

AHMAD CHEBBO, MD
Physician, Department of Pulmonary and Critical Care Medicine, Maricopa Integrated Health System, Phoenix, Arizona

CHRISTOPHER CIELO, DO
Fellow, Sleep Medicine and Pulmonary Medicine, Division of Pulmonary Medicine, The Children's Hospital of Philadelphia, Philadelphia, Pennsylvania

NANCY COLLOP, MD
Professor of Medicine and Neurology, Director, Emory Sleep Center, Emory University, Atlanta, Georgia

LEOPOLDO P. CORREA, BDS, MS
Diplomate, American Board of Dental Sleep Medicine; Associate Professor and Division Head, Dental Sleep Medicine, Department of Oral and Maxillofacial Pathology, Oral Medicine and Craniofacial Pain, Tufts University School of Dental Medicine, Boston, Massachusetts

SHEKHAR GHAMANDE, MD, FCCP, FAASM
Assistant Professor, Department of Medicine, Division of Pulmonary, Critical Care, and Sleep Medicine, Scott and White Memorial Hospital, Texas A&M Health and Science Center, Texas A&M University, Temple, Texas

RICHARD L. JACOBSON, DMD, MS
Clinical Instructor, Department of Orthodontics, School of Dentistry, University of California, Los Angeles, California

SHIRLEY F. JONES, MD, FCCP, FAASM
Senior Staff, Pulmonary and Sleep Medicine, Scott and White Healthcare, Assistant Professor of Medicine, Texas A&M HSC COM, Temple, Texas

SOPHIA H. KIM, MD
Fellow in Sleep Medicine, Emory Sleep Center, Emory University, Atlanta, Georgia

JORGE R. KIZER, MD, MSc, FACC
Director of Clinical Cardiovascular Research, Associate Professor of Medicine, Associate Professor of Epidemiology and Population Health, Department of Medicine, Department of Epidemiology and Population Health, Montefiore Medical Center, Albert Einstein College of Medicine, Bronx, New York

VIDYA KRISHNAN, MD, MHS
Assistant Professor of Medicine, Case Western Reserve University, MetroHealth Medical Center, Division of Pulmonary, Critical Care, and Sleep Medicine, Cleveland, Ohio

RUCKSHANDA MAJID, MD
Assistant Professor of Medicine, Division of Pulmonary and Sleep Medicine, University of Texas Medical School at Houston; Co-Medical Director, Harris Health Sleep Disorders Center, Quentin Meese Community Hospital, Houston, Texas

AMIT MANN, MD
Fellow, Pulmonary and Critical Care, Texas A&M University, Temple, Texas

REENA MEHRA, MD, MS
Associate Professor of Medicine, Cleveland Clinic Lerner College of Medicine of Case Western Reserve University; Director, Sleep Disorders Research, Center of Sleep Medicine, Neurologic Institute, Cleveland Clinic; Adjunct Staff, Molecular Cardiology Department, Lerner Research Institute, Heart and Vascular Institute, Respiratory Institute, Cleveland, Ohio

SUSHEEL P. PATIL, MD, PhD
Assistant Professor of Medicine, Johns Hopkins School of Medicine, Division of Pulmonary and Critical Care Medicine, Johns Hopkins Sleep Disorders Center, Baltimore, Maryland

STEPHEN A. SCHENDEL, MD, DDS, FACS
Professor Emeritus, Department of Plastic Surgery, Stanford University, Stanford, California

NEOMI SHAH, MD, MPH
Associate Director, Pulmonary Sleep Lab, Department of Medicine, Montefiore Medical Center, Assistant Professor of Medicine, Assistant Professor of Epidemiology and Population Health, Albert Einstein College of Medicine, Bronx, New York

PAWAN SIKKA, MD, FACP, FAASM, CBSM
Chief, Pulmonary, Critical Care and Sleep Medicine, Central Texas Veterans Health Care System, Temple, Texas

AMER TFAILI, MD
Fellow, Division of Pulmonary and Critical Care and Sleep Medicine, Department of Medicine, Scott and White Healthcare, Texas A&M Health Science Center, Temple, Texas; Intensivist at Aurora St. Luke's Medical Center in Milwaukee, Milwaukee; Aurora Medical Center in Grafton, Grafton, Wisconsin

HARNEET K. WALIA, MD
Sleep Disorders Center, Neurologic Institute, Cleveland Clinic; Assistant Professor of Family Medicine, Cleveland Clinic Lerner College of Medicine of Case Western Reserve University, Cleveland, Ohio

LESLIE D. WILKE, DO
Department of Medicine, Division of Pulmonary, Critical Care, and Sleep Medicine, Scott and White Memorial Hospital, Texas A&M Health and Science Center, Temple, Texas

H. KLAR YAGGI, MD, MPH
Director, Program in Sleep Medicine, Director of Sleep Research, Section of Pulmonary, Critical Care, and Sleep Medicine, VA Clinical Epidemiology Research Center, Associate Professor, Yale University School of Medicine, New Haven, CT

Contents

Upper airway anatomy influences the pathophysiology of obstructive sleep apnea (OSA). Understanding this anatomy helps dissect the pathophysiologic factors involved in OSA. During sleep, the complex interaction among pharyngeal dilator tone, upper airway narrowing, changes in lung volume, arousal threshold, and respiratory control instability plays an important role in OSA and leads to considerable heterogeneity in the mechanism of OSA. This complexity also helps to explain the known risk factors for OSA, such as obesity, sex, and age.

The metabolic syndrome is a term characterized by a clustering of independent cardiovascular risk factors. A wealth of epidemiologic and experimental data have implicated obstructive sleep apnea (OSA) as a key pathophysiologic factor in the evolution of metabolic dysfunction and as a culprit in increasing cardiovascular risk. Conceptual frameworks are emerging with respect to the mechanistic underpinnings of OSA that contribute to the various facets of metabolic dysfunction, which are elaborated in this article. The effect of the reversal of the adverse accompanying pathophysiologic effects of OSA on metabolic outcomes is also reviewed.

This article reviews current evidence on the impact of treatment of obstructive sleep apnea with continuous positive airway pressure on specific cardiovascular outcomes, namely, subclinical atherosclerosis (endothelial dysfunction), coronary heart disease, cardiac arrhythmias, and stroke. The scope of this article is restricted to studies that involve obstructive sleep apnea. The database PubMed was searched from 1990 to February 2013 for all relevant articles pertaining to these cardiovascular conditions and a critical review of each article was conducted. Articles with the most scientific impact are discussed.

Complex sleep apnea entails the combination of obstructive and central sleep apnea during the same polysomnographic study. Treatment-emergent central sleep apnea during administration of positive airway pressure for obstructive sleep apnea is the most common form of complex sleep apnea. In most cases of treatment-emergent complex sleep apnea without cardiovascular comorbidity or opioid use, the central component may resolve with use of continuous positive airway pressure sufficient to eliminate the obstructive component. Effective treatment of persistent complex sleep apnea can be achieved with the use of adaptive servoventilation.

weight loss strategies including surgical, pharmacologic, dietary, exercise and their impacts on weight management and OSA. The effects of CPAP on weight management will be discussed.

Obstructive sleep apnea (OSA) is a major health hazard that affects approximately 12 million Americans. Positive airway pressure therapy remains the gold standard, although the use of an oral appliance and surgical modalities are alternatives. Pharmacotherapy remains in an adjunctive role. This article reviews the pharmacologic treatment of OSA: stimulant therapy to address residual sleepiness, medications that address the ventilatory control of breathing, treatment of comorbid diseases and associated conditions, and special issues, such as residual pediatric OSA, drugs to avoid, anesthetic precautions, and possible future targets.

Patients are interested in alternative therapies and a common disorder such as obstructive sleep apnea (OSA) is approached by many as an opportunity to pursue these. The search for an alternative to continuous positive airway pressure (CPAP) has produced some promising results. Some of these alternatives are effective in certain categories of OSA, although further tailoring and refining are required. These alternatives should be entertained in selected patients with OSA who are intolerant of CPAP because CPAP is likely to remain first-line therapy in the near future. We predict that alternatives to CPAP will become mainstream within 20 years.

Obstructive sleep apnea is a common disease, often unrecognized, with potential health ramifications. It is also a chronic condition often present in patients with other comorbidities. Studies have clearly shown both quality of life and health benefits from treatment and possibly mortality reduction. In the studies that have examined cost-benefit ratio, treatment advantages far outweigh the costs of diagnosis for most.

There is evidence that patients with obstructive sleep apnea (OSA) can have residual excessive daytime sleepiness (EDS), possibly related to other underlying sleep disorders. Further areas of study concerning patients treated adequately for OSA include looking for a biomarker that can easily measure alertness or sleepiness. Radiological modalities may offer another means of assessing patients with EDS. A modality that can provide data without costing too much is needed for clinical management. Some patients continue to have sleepiness after adequate treatment with continuous positive airway pressure, and until these patients can be better classified, it will be difficult to outline better treatment options.

> Hypersomnia, or excessive daytime sleepiness, is common with obstructive sleep apnea (OSA) but normally improves with use of continuous positive airway pressure (CPAP) therapy. OSA is well known for breathing disturbances associated with variations in heart rate, arousals, and resulting sleepiness in the daytime. Some people continue to experience hypersomnia despite routine use of CPAP therapy. Assessment of OSA patients who continue to complain of excessive sleepiness despite CPAP use must include an initial assessment of therapy compliance. If other potential causes of hypersomnia are not found or thought to be the issue, then treatment with medication is warranted.

> Obstructive sleep apnea (OSA) is associated with an increased risk of accidents related to driving or mass transportation. In this article, the mechanisms for neurocognitive deficits and common subjective and objective testing for determining alertness-related impairments are reviewed. The basis of legal culpability for sleep-related accidents and the role of the clinician or sleep physician are discussed. Education of the patient and public on the risk of OSA on driving ability is a critical role of the clinician. General laws and regulations regarding OSA and driving are reviewed. Physicians are responsible for familiarizing themselves with policies that govern their jurisdiction.

Preface
Treatment of Obstructive Sleep Apnea

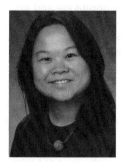 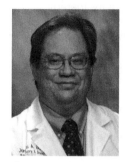

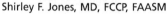

Shirley F. Jones, MD, FCCP, FAASM   James A. Barker, MD, CPE, FACP, FCCP, FAASM

Editors

Sleep Medicine is no longer in its infancy as a specialty. Rather, we are now in our adolescence! The first descriptions of sleep apnea were in the 1970s and Sullivan's invention of CPAP (continuous positive airway pressure) was just in 1981. We took great pleasure in planning and then editing this issue of *Sleep Medicine Clinics*. Our focus has been on "What is currently known in this field?" and "What would we (and you the readers) like to know more about?" These two questions then are the guiding principles for this issue.

We start with the basics: Drs Chebbo and Ghamande elegantly describe the anatomy and physiology of the upper airway in obstructive sleep apnea. We learned great information in reading this article and you will also. Following this, we took editorial license and did not devote a single article to PAP (positive airway pressure, including CPAP, BIPAP, and ASV). Rather PAP therapy is discussed in detail within the context of each pertinent article. PAP therapy issues are complex and we felt a robust approach was needed in a focused way. See if you agree.

Much attention is now focused on outcomes. In other words, does treating a disease or a syndrome actually change results for the patient? Thus we have two excellent articles that follow: "OSA Therapy and Metabolic Outcomes" by H.K. Walia and R. Mehra from Cleveland Clinic and "Effects of OSA Therapy on Cardiovascular Disease" by Drs Shah, Kizer, and Yaggi. Again, the data here are up to date and enlightening.

Complex sleep apnea has been considered an enigma. Do we need to treat Cheyne Stokes breathing and central apnea? Is the development of central apnea in a PAP titration a harbinger of complex apnea or just a function of brain stem reset? Drs Castriotta and Majid answer these questions and more in their coverage of this emerging topic.

Leslie Wilke, DO and Shekhar Ghamande, MD next cover mask interfaces. We feel this is an often overlooked but very important topic. There is no adherence to PAP therapy if the mask is uncomfortable or leaks.

Drs Cielo and Brooks from CHOP (Children's Hospital of Philadelphia and University of Pennsylvania School of Medicine) give an excellent detailed outline of the state of art for therapy of childhood OSA. Tonsillectomy is more complex than many of us know. Likewise, they comprehensively cover other therapeutic choices as well as common chronic diseases with overlap.

There is much more available than just PAP therapy for our adult patients as well. Drs Camacho, Jacobson, and Schendel nicely cover the gamut of surgical options for patients. The oral appliance article, written by Dr Correa of Tufts University School of Dental Medicine, is particularly rich and informative. More patients seem to be opting for this therapy rather than CPAP. We tell all our patients to lose weight. What is the evidence that it makes a difference? How many actually do it? Drs Shirley Jones and Ahmad

Sleep Med Clin 8 (2013) xiii–xiv
http://dx.doi.org/10.1016/j.jsmc.2013.08.003
1556-407X/13/$ – see front matter © 2013 Published by Elsevier Inc.

Chebbo answer these questions and more in detail. The answers are surprising! Dr Vivien Abad updates us on potential pharmacologic therapy for both weight loss and apnea. In addition, molecular signature techniques for planning therapy are the coming future. We know that our patients use alternative or complementary therapy very often. Tfaili and coauthors comprehensively review the available evidence on everything from nasal resistive devices and body positioning to acupuncture. Keep this article handy for that certain group of patients who are soon to come in for a clinic visit.

The cost of testing and of therapy is on everyone's mind at present. As the cost of health care eats more and more into the gross domestic product, can we afford to treat OSA? Or, is it more expensive to leave it untested and untreated? Drs Kim and Collop do a great job of explaining the state of the art of cost modeling and the likelihood scenarios as applied to our apnea patients. Dr Collop is a former president of the American Academy of Sleep Medicine.

The final three articles deal with the all important issues of residual sleepiness. What causes it? Is it all noncompliance with PAP therapy? Do I need to search for other disorders? Do stimulant medications play a role? Drs Boethel and Sikka along with coauthors, answer these questions in their respective articles. And how do medical legal issues affect our work and our care of these patients? Drs Krishnan and Patil detail the role of the clinician in sleep-related accidents. Read on, this will not disappoint!

Many thanks to Dr Teofilo Lee-Chiong for inviting us to work on this labor of love. We have made new friends and learned much. Finally, we express our most sincere gratitude and appreciation to our families (Matt, Steven, and Abigail Jones) and (Karen Barker and Taylor W.), whose love and encouragement have strengthened and enriched our lives.

Shirley F. Jones, MD, FCCP, FAASM
Division of Pulmonary, Critical Care and
Sleep Medicine
Scott & White Healthcare
Texas A&M HSC COM
2401 South 31st Street
Temple, TX 76508, USA

James A. Barker, MD, CPE, FACP, FCCP, FAASM
Pulmonary and Sleep Medicine
Scott & White Healthcare
Fragile Populations, SW Health Plan
Texas A&M HSC COM
2401 South 31st Street
Temple, TX 76508, USA

E-mail addresses:
shjones@sw.org (S.F. Jones)
jabarker@sw.org (J.A. Barker)

Anatomy and Physiology of Obstructive Sleep Apnea

Ahmad Chebbo, MD[a], Amer Tfaili, MD[b],
Shekhar Ghamande, MD[b,*]

KEYWORDS

- Obstructive sleep apnea • Pathophysiology • Anatomy • Hypoglossal nerve • Pcrit
- Ventilator control • Pharyngeal • Risk factors

KEY POINTS

- The oropharynx is the most common site of airway collapse in obstructive sleep apnea (OSA), and enlarged parapharyngeal fat pad, thicker lateral pharyngeal walls, and increased tongue volume play key roles.
- Pharyngeal closing pressure is influenced by craniofacial abnormalities, soft tissue crowding from obesity, caudal traction, and lung volumes.
- Reversible heightened arousal threshold in apneic patients combined with high loop gain ventilator response to arousals contribute to ventilatory instability.
- Obesity, sex, and age are pathophysiologic factors that promote OSA.

ANATOMY

This article reviews how the upper airway anatomy influences the pathophysiology of obstructive sleep apnea (OSA), and the pertinent anatomy.

The upper airway is a common passageway for digestive, respiratory and phonatory systems. Traditionally it is divided to 3 sections: the nasopharynx, oropharynx, and hypopharynx.

The nasopharynx extends from the posterior margin of the nasal turbinates; it sits above the soft palate and continues inferiorly with the oropharynx. The posterior wall is occupied by adenoids, which when inflamed can partially obstruct the upper airway. The soft palate, a nearly vertical flap, extends from the posterior edge of hard palate and terminates in the uvula. All the muscles of the soft palate are innervated by the pharyngeal branch of vagus nerve except the tensor veli palatini, which is innervated by the medial pterygoid nerve. A posterior elevation of the soft palate toward the posterior pharyngeal wall can cause enlargement of the oral cavity during swallowing and produce narrowing of the nasopharynx. Adenotonsillar disease can lead to sleep-disordered breathing. Polysomnography in children with allergic rhinitis and adenoidal hypertrophy found that 66% have mild apnea.[1] In fact in children, tonsillectomy and/or adenoidectomy is the first therapeutic modality to be considered for the treatment of OSA.[2]

Humans naturally breathe through the nose, particularly during sleep, when the daily oral fraction of breathing, estimated at 7%, drops to 4% during sleep.[3] Although during wakefulness both nasal and oral resistances are equal, nasal resistance is lower than the oral at night,[4] but increases in the supine position.[5] Hippocrates[6] first mentioned the connection between the nose and breathing in sleep when he described a role of

a Department of Pulmonary and Critical Care Medicine, Maricopa Integrated Health System, 2601 East Roosevelt Street, Phoenix, AZ 85008, USA; b Department of Medicine, Division of Pulmonary & Critical Care Medicine, Scott & White Memorial Hospital, 2401 South 31st Street, Temple, TX 76508, USA
* Corresponding author. Department of Medicine, Texas A&M University, Temple, TX.
E-mail address: sghamande@sw.org

Sleep Med Clin 8 (2013) 425–431
http://dx.doi.org/10.1016/j.jsmc.2013.07.016
1556-407X/13/$ – see front matter © 2013 Elsevier Inc. All rights reserved.

nasal polyps in restless sleep. Nasal obstruction can occur secondary to deviated septum, chronic rhinosinusitis, and nasal polyps. Nasal congestion has been associated with a 3-fold increase in the incidence of snoring and daytime sleepiness.[7] Earlier studies indicate that acute nasal obstruction could increase the apnea-hypopnea index (AHI), prolong rapid eye movement (REM) latency, and increase non-REM (NREM) sleep.[8] However, nasal obstruction alone is not thought to cause any moderate or severe OSA.[6,9]

The hard and the soft palate form the roof of the oral cavity, and the lingual mucosa covers the floor. The lateral part of the oral cavity is covered by buccal mucosa and anterior pillars of palatine tonsils, which define the junction with oropharynx. The tongue, which occupies the major part of the oral cavity, has both extrinsic and intrinsic muscle groups. The 4 extrinsic tongue muscles are the genioglossus, hyoglossus, palatoglossus, and styloglossus. The genioglossus is the largest and most-studied pharyngeal dilator muscle. All of these muscles are innervated by the hypoglossal nerve except the palatoglossus, which is innervated by the vagus nerve. The intrinsic muscles of the tongue (superior and inferior longitudinal, transverse, and vertical muscles) are confined to the tongue. The anterior two-thirds of the tongue is innervated by the facial nerve, whereas the posterior one-third is innervated by cranial nerve IX. The size of the tongue is an important risk factor for OSA.[10]

An increase in the size of type II muscle fibers is seen in OSA compared with normal subjects, which could represent a response to vibratory strain or perhaps neuronal activity.[11,12]

The hypoglossal nerve is a critical component in the motor control of upper airway dilatation. The muscle fibers in the posterior part of the tongue are fatigue-resistant, thereby sustaining the forward tongue position and preventing its collapse into the retroglossal area. Using this mechanism, the therapeutic effect of proximal hypoglossal nerve stimulation can be used to treat OSA.[13]

The oropharynx extends from the soft palate to the epiglottis. The anterior part of oropharynx is formed by the posterior part of the tongue and the soft palate, whereas the posterior part is formed by the pharyngeal constrictor muscles. The lateral pharyngeal walls are formed by the pharyngeal constrictors, muscles of the extrinsic tongue, muscles of the soft palate, and the larynx. Other structures that contribute to upper airway lumen, located in the retropalatal area, are the palatine tonsils and parapharyngeal fat pads.

A magnetic resonance imaging (MRI) study revealed a smaller minimum airway area in patients with OSA in the retropalatal region, and particularly in the lateral dimension, compared with individuals with normal breathing.[14] The volume of the tongue and lateral walls have been shown to independently increase the risk of OSA.[15]

The oropharynx is the most common site of airway collapse in patients with OSA,[16] which is more likely to occur during REM sleep.[17] A recent study evaluating the role of parapharyngeal fat in the predisposition to OSA used MRI to examine pharyngeal anatomy. Patients with retropalatal airway closure had a higher percentage of parapharyngeal and soft palate fat, whereas patients with retroglossal airway closure had an increased volume of the tongue and parapharyngeal fat pad (**Fig. 1**).[18]

The caudal portion of the upper airway is the hypopharynx, which extends from the superior border of the epiglottis to the inferior border of the cricoid cartilage. It is formed anteriorly by the base of the tongue and the epiglottis, and

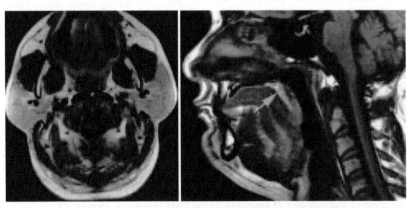

Fig. 1. Parapharyngeal fat pad and fat tissues in the soft palate (*green arrow*). (*From* Li Y, Lin N, Ye J, et al. Upper airway fat tissue distribution in subjects with obstructive sleep apnea and its effect on retropalatal mechanical loads. Respir Care 2012;57(7):1100; with permission.)

postero-laterally by the inferior pharyngeal constrictor. Obstruction at the level of the hypopharynx is less common than at the oropharynx. The structures in the hypopharynx, such as the lingual tonsils, can have a potential role in OSA.[19] In children with tonsillar hypertrophy, tonsillectomy is an effective treatment for snoring and OSA.[20] Epiglottic prolapse during inspiration has been described as a cause of OSA, with a partial laser epiglottidectomy reported as a cure.[21]

PATHOPHYSIOLOGY

The pathophysiology of OSA is multifactorial, with much individual variability. The complex interaction among pharyngeal dilator tone, arousal threshold, respiratory control instability, and changes in lung volume during sleep plays an important role in OSA. Considerable heterogeneity exists in the mechanism of OSA in patients.[22] This section focuses on how these and other factors interact to cause obstruction of the upper airway during sleep, but does not dwell on the pathophysiologic consequences of OSA on the body.

Upper Airway Collapsibility

The vulnerable airway extends from the hard palate to the larynx, and can collapse during sleep. This collapse can occur because of variations in transmural pressure, such as decreased intraluminal pressure or increased external tissue pressure, or a reduction in the longitudinal tension on the pharynx. MRI studies indicate that the apneic airway is different from the normal airway because of thicker lateral pharyngeal walls with an anterior-posterior elliptical configuration, unlike the horizontal configuration in the normal airway. This thickened anatomy seems to be more important than the enlargement of parapharyngeal fat pads in causing airway narrowing in apneic patients.[14] The minimal airway area is also smaller in apneic patients, contributing to the airway collapse. The threshold pressure required to maintain patency of the upper airway is called the pharyngeal closing pressure (Pcrit). Pcrit has been shown to correlate with OSA severity.[23]

When the principles of a Starling resistor are applied, the pharyngeal airway can be conceptualized as a collapsible tube surrounded by tissue within a bony box.[24] The luminal size is determined by the properties of the tube and the transmural pressure, which is the difference between pressures inside and outside the tube. Increase in the outside tissue pressure will promote luminal narrowing. Pcrit will increase as tissue pressure increases, which could occur from a reduction in size of the bony box from micrognathia, a high arched palate, or mid-face hypoplasia, or from soft tissue crowding caused by macroglossia, adenotonsillar hypertrophy, and central adiposity.[25] Obesity acts synergistically with narrowing of the bony box. The receded mandibles in apneic patients contribute to increased tissue pressure[26] and, consequently, pharyngeal collapse. Conversely, weight loss has been shown to reduce Pcrit,[27] and the resolution of sleep-disordered breathing depends on the degree of Pcrit reduction. Similarly, a stepwise advancement of the mandible in apneic patients leads to dose-dependent reductions in Pcrit.[28]

Effect of Lung Volumes

Caudal traction and elongation of the airway reduces Pcrit through stiffening the airway and mitigating the surrounding tissue pressures.[29,30] The supine position reduces lung volumes in apneic patients, which decreases caudal traction on the airway. An increase in end-expiratory lung volume using continuous positive airway pressure (CPAP) has been shown to substantially reduce apnea severity and improve sleep architecture.[31] Improvement in caudal traction on the trachea is one mechanism involving in achieving this goal. Apnea severity has also been shown to improve with sleeping in the semi-recumbent position, which would occur through improved caudal traction.[32]

Upper Airway Dilator Muscle Activity

Collapsing forces related to tissue pressure and intraluminal negative pressure are offset by pharyngeal dilator muscle activity. The genioglossus is the largest and most extensively studied pharyngeal dilator.[33] Upper airway dilator tone is high during wakefulness, and this maintains an open airway. With sleep onset, a decrease in the tone of the genioglossus muscle occurs. In apneic patients who are relying on a heightened genioglossus tone to support the airway, this leads to airway instability.[34] The degree to which this occurs also depends on the sleep stage. Slow-wave sleep has been associated with heightened genioglossus tone, which might be protective against OSA.[35] During REM sleep, a reduction in tonic genioglossus activity occurs, which potentiates further apneas.[36] Local reflexes generated by negative pharyngeal pressure during sleep modulate an increase in both genioglossus and tensor palatine tone, especially in the supine position.[37,38] Genioglossus activity increases during inspiration but decreases during expiration.[33] More recently, a secondary suppression phase after an initial excitatory phase was shown in the genioglossus, but not the tensor palatine, in response to negative pharyngeal pressure. Thus, the genioglossus has both excitatory and inhibitory responses to airway collapse, but the response is variable.[39]

Arousal Response in OSA

Most episodes of apneas are followed by arousals, which are thought to be mediated via negative intrathoracic pressure generation.[40] However, apnea termination can occur without arousals through the accumulation of stimuli, such as chemical drive and negative intrapharyngeal pressures.[41–43] OSA impairs the arousal threshold, and therefore apneic patients need greater inspiratory efforts to trigger an arousal.[44] This function likely represents an acquired response, and means that apneic patients experience prolonged event duration because of the heightened length of inspiratory effort required to trigger an arousal. Treatment with CPAP has been shown to reduce the heightened arousal threshold in apneic patients.[45] Slow-wave sleep may stabilize the breathing in apneic patients via the arousal threshold. Ratnavadivel and colleagues[46] showed that the arousal threshold is further increased in slow-wave sleep compared with N2 sleep, but they did not find evidence supporting increased ventilatory drive or increased upper airway responses during slow-wave sleep compared with N2 sleep.

Ventilatory Control Stability

Ventilatory control stability contributes to OSA pathogenesis but is incompletely understood.[22] The feedback loop that controls the respiratory response to airway collapsibility and arousal can be conceptualized as "loop gain," which refers to the magnitude of the response relative to the intensity of the input.[47] Apneic patients have an elevated loop gain, particularly those with severe OSA,[48,49] which translates into an overshoot of the ventilator response to apneas and arousal, leading to disproportionately lowered carbon dioxide (CO_2). In a recent study, Yuan and colleagues[50] found that obese adolescents with OSA had a higher sensitivity to CO_2 during wakefulness compared with the lean control group. However, in other studies, the ventilator response during wakefulness in OSA has been inconsistent.[51] Importantly, the sensitivity decreased during sleep in the apneic adolescents. This blunting would lead to prolonged obstructive events. However, the magnitude of the ventilatory response to spontaneous arousal may promote driving the CO_2 below the apneic threshold, leading to further sleep-disordered breathing.[50] In a novel study,

Edwards and colleagues[52] showed that acetazolamide reduced the ventilator response to spontaneous arousal in patients with OSA treated with CPAP, and improved this ventilatory instability. They found that the ventilator response to spontaneous arousals correlated with the severity of OSA, further increasing the evidence regarding the role of post-arousal ventilatory instability in perpetuating OSA.

Pharyngeal Neuropathy

Pharyngeal neuropathy has been described in patients with OSA.[53–55] A selective impairment of the ability to detect mechanical stimuli in the upper airway of patients with OSA and snorers has been shown using 2-point discrimination and vibratory tests.[53] Abnormal laryngeal sensation has been shown in patients with OSA using air pressure pulses during endoscopy.[54] Inflammation and denervation affect the oral mucosa and upper airway muscles in patients with OSA.[55] Whether it is the vibratory strain[56] or intermittent hypoxia[57] that plays a major role in promoting the pharyngeal neuropathy remains unclear. A recent study found neurogenic changes in the genioglossus.[58] Using measurements of motor unit potentials, Saboisky and colleagues[58] reported evidence of collateral sprouting and reinnervation in the genioglossus, which correlated with lowest oxygen desaturation in patients with OSA. How this neuropathy affects upper airway function during sleep remains to be determined.

EFFECT OF RISK FACTORS ON OSA
Obesity

Obese patients with OSA have increased fat deposits in the soft tissue surrounding the upper airway, including in the soft palate.[59,60] Schwab and colleagues[14] indicated that fat deposits along the lateral pharyngeal wall and posterior tongue play an important role in OSA. Furthermore, the difference in upper airway soft tissue volumes between obese patients with OSA and nonobese controls was small (30 cm^3) compared with differences in body mass index.[14] This finding of a small increase in upper airway soft tissue volume in apneic patients compared with normal controls was confirmed in Japanese patients.[61] Furthermore, a small decrease of 17 cm^3 in upper airway volume from overall weight loss (average of 7.8 kg) led to a 31% decrease in the apnea-hypopnea index.[62] A reduction in functional residual capacity (FRC) is seen in obese individuals,[63] and decreased upper airway patency from low FRC is an additional mechanism contributing to OSA in obese patients.[64] Consequently, weight loss and improvement in FRC would augment upper airway patency.

Male Sex

The upper airway was found to be longer in patients with OSA, and the length correlates with the severity.[65] An increase in pharyngeal airway length and soft palate area may explain the higher predisposition to pharyngeal collapsibility in men.[66] Arousals from sleep in men are associated with a greater ventilatory response and with hypoventilation on falling back asleep compared with women. This heightened propensity for ventilatory instability on arousal in men was shown to be further exaggerated in supine position.[67]

Age

The prevalence of OSA increases with age, with a plateau after 65 years of age.[68,69] In fact, the increased tendency for OSA has been observed even in otherwise healthy nonobese men older than 50 years.[70,71] Increased parapharyngeal fat and upper airway narrowing has been observed in elderly patients.[72,73] Whether age predisposes to increased upper airway collapsibility is unclear, but studies indicate that patients have an increased vulnerability from longer airways with age.[74,75]

SUMMARY

Understanding of the pathogenesis of OSA is evolving. Airway obstruction can occur at several sites in the upper airway, with the oropharynx the most common. The hypoglossal nerve is a key player in upper airway dilator function. Retrognathia, adenotonsillar hypertrophy, enlarged tongue, lateral pharyngeal wall thickening, and parapharyngeal fat pads are important anatomic risk factors. The arousal response is heightened in apneic patients. Elevated loop gain leads to an overshoot of ventilator response in OSA, contributing to ventilator instability. The role of pharyngeal neuropathy in the pathophysiology of OSA is being investigated.

REFERENCES

1. Ramos RT, Da Cunha Daltro CH, Gregório PB, et al. OSAS in children: clinical and polysomnographic respiratory profile. Braz J Otorhinolaryngol 2006; 72(3):355–61.
2. Marcus CL, Brooks LJ, Ward SD, et al. Diagnosis and management of childhood obstructive sleep apnea syndrome. Pediatrics 2012;130(3): e714–55.
3. Fitzpatrick MF, Driver HS, Chatha N, et al. Partitioning of inhaled ventilation between the nasal and oral routes during sleep in normal subjects. J Appl Physiol 2003;94(3):883–90.
4. Fitzpatrick MF, McLean H, Urton AM, et al. Effect of nasal or oral breathing route on upper airway resistance during sleep. Eur Respir J 2003; 22(5):827–32.
5. Duggan CJ, Watson RA, Pride NB. Postural changes in nasal and pulmonary resistance in subjects with asthma. J Asthma 2004;41(7):701–7.
6. Georgalas C. The role of the nose in snoring and obstructive sleep apnoea: an update. Eur Arch Otorhinolaryngol 2011;268(9):1365–73.
7. Young T, Finn L, Palta M. Chronic nasal congestion at night is a risk factor for snoring in a population-based cohort study. Arch Intern Med 2001;161(12): 1514–9.
8. Olsen KD, Kern EB, Westbrook PR. Sleep and breathing disturbance secondary to nasal obstruction. Otolaryngol Head Neck Surg 1981; 89(5):804–10.
9. McNicholas WT. The nose and OSA: variable nasal obstruction may be more important in pathophysiology than fixed obstruction. Eur Respir J 2008; 32(1):3–8.
10. Schwab RJ, Pasirstein M, Pierson R, et al. Identification of upper airway anatomic risk factors for obstructive sleep apnea with volumetric magnetic resonance imaging. Am J Respir Crit Care Med 2003;168(5):522–30.
11. Series F, Cote C, Simoneau JA, et al. Physiologic, metabolic, and muscle fiber type characteristics of musculus uvulae in sleep apnea hypopnea syndrome and in snorers. J Clin Invest 1995;95: 20–5.
12. Lindman R, Stal PS. Abnormal palatopharyngeal muscle morphology in sleep-disordered breathing. J Neurol Sci 2002;195:11–23.
13. Zaidi FN, Meadows P, Jacobowitz O, et al. Tongue anatomy and physiology, the scientific basis for a novel targeted neurostimulation system designed for the treatment of obstructive sleep apnea. Neuromodulation 2012. http://dx.doi.org/10.1111/j. 1525-1403.2012.00514.x.
14. Schwab RJ, Gupta KB, Gefter WB, et al. Upper airway and soft tissue anatomy in normal subjects and patients with sleep-disordered breathing. Significance of the lateral pharyngeal walls. Am J Respir Crit Care Med 1995;152:1673–89.
15. Katsantonis GP, Moss K, Miyazaki S, et al. Determining the site of airway collapse in obstructive sleep apnea with airway pressure monitoring. Laryngoscope 1993;103(10):1126–31.
16. Schwab RJ, Gefter WB, Hoffman EA, et al. Dynamic upper airway imaging during awake respiration in normal subjects and patients with sleep

disordered breathing. Am Rev Respir Dis 1993;
148(5):1385–400.

17. Boudewyns AN, Van de Heyning PH, De Backer WA. Site of upper airway obstruction in obstructive apnoea and influence of sleep stage. Eur Respir J 1997;10(11):2566–72.

18. Li Y, Lin N, Ye J, et al. Upper airway fat tissue distribution in subjects with obstructive sleep apnea and its effect on retropalatal mechanical loads. Respir Care 2012;57(7):1098–105.

19. Suzuki K, Kawakatsu K, Hattori C, et al. Application of lingual tonsillectomy to sleep apnea syndrome involving lingual tonsils. Acta Otolaryngol Suppl 2003;550:65–71.

20. Abdel-Aziz M, Ibrahim N, Ahmed A, et al. Lingual tonsils hypertrophy; a cause of obstructive sleep apnea in children after adenotonsillectomy: operative problems and management. Int J Pediatr Otorhinolaryngol 2011;75(9):1127–31.

21. Catalfumo FJ, Golz A, Westerman ST, et al. The epiglottis and obstructive sleep apnoea syndrome. J Laryngol Otol 1998;112(10):940–3.

22. Eckert DJ, Malhotra A. Pathophysiology of adult obstructive sleep apnea. Proc Am Thorac Soc 2008;5:144–53.

23. Issa FG, Sullivan CE. Upper airway closing pressures in obstructive sleep apnea. J Appl Physiol 1984;57:520–7.

24. Smith PL, Wise RA, Gold AR, et al. Upper airway pressure-flow relationships in obstructive sleep apnea. J Appl Physiol 1988;64(2):789–95.

25. Schwartz AR, Smith PL, Schneider H, et al. Invited editorial on "Lung volume and upper airway collapsibility: what does it tell us about pathogenic mechanisms?". J Appl Physiol 2012;113:689–90.

26. Watanabe T, Isono S, Tanaka A, et al. Contribution of body habitus and craniofacial characteristics to segmental closing pressures of the passive pharynx in patients with sleep-disordered breathing. Am J Respir Crit Care Med 2002;165: 260–5.

27. Schwartz AR, Gold AR, Schubert N, et al. Effect of weight loss on upper airway collapsibility in obstructive sleep apnea. Am Rev Respir Dis 1991;144:494–8.

28. Kato J, Isono S, Tanaka A, et al. Dose-dependent effects of mandibular advancement on pharyngeal mechanics and nocturnal oxygenation in patients with sleep-disordered breathing. Chest 2000;117: 1065–72.

29. Thut DC, Schwartz AR, Roach D, et al. Tracheal and neck position influence upper airway airflow dynamics by altering airway length. J Appl Physiol 1993;75:2084–90.

30. Kairaitis K, Byth K, Parikh R, et al. Tracheal traction effects on upper airway patency in rabbits: the role of tissue pressure. Sleep 2007;30:179–86.

31. Heinzer RC, Stanchina ML, Malhotra A, et al. Effect of increased lung volume on sleep disordered breathing in patients with sleep apnoea. Thorax 2006;61:435–9.

32. McEvoy RD, Sharp DJ, Thornton AT. The effects of posture on obstructive sleep apnea. Am Rev Respir Dis 1986;133:662–6.

33. Jordan AS, White DP. Pharyngeal motor control and the pathogenesis of obstructive sleep apnea. Respir Physiol Neurobiol 2008;160:1–7.

34. Mezzanotte WS, Tangel DJ, White DP. Influence of sleep onset on upper-airway muscle activity in apnea patients versus normal controls. Am J Respir Crit Care Med 1996;153:1880–7.

35. Basner RC, Ringler J, Schwartzstein RM, et al. Phasic electromyographic activity of the genioglossus increases in normals during slow-wave sleep. Respir Physiol 1991;83:189–200.

36. Jordan AS, White DP, Lo YL, et al. Airway dilator muscle activity and lung volume during stable breathing in obstructive sleep apnea. Sleep 2009; 32(3):361–8.

37. Malhotra A, Trinder J, Fogel R, et al. Postural effects on pharyngeal protective reflex mechanisms. Sleep 2004;27:1105–12.

38. Wheatley JR, Tangel DJ, Mezzanotte WS, et al. Influence of sleep on response to negative airway pressure of tensor palatini muscle and retropalatal airway. J Appl Physiol 1993;75:2117–24.

39. Eckert DJ, Saboisky JP, Jordan AS, et al. A secondary reflex suppression phase is present in genioglossus but not tensor palatini in response to negative upper airway pressure. J Appl Physiol 2010;108(6):1619–24.

40. Gleeson K, Zwillich CW, White DP. The influence of increasing ventilatory effort on arousal from sleep. Am Rev Respir Dis 1990;142:295–300.

41. Younes M. Role of arousals in the pathogenesis of obstructive sleep apnea. Am J Respir Crit Care Med 2004;169:623–33.

42. Lo YL, Jordan AS, Malhotra A, et al. Genioglossal muscle response to CO2 stimulation during NREM sleep. Sleep 2006;29:470–7.

43. Horner RL, Innes JA, Murphy K, et al. Evidence for reflex upper airway dilator muscle activation by sudden negative airway pressure in man. J Physiol 1991;436:15–29.

44. Berry RB, Kouchi KG, Der DE, et al. Sleep apnea impairs the arousal response to airway occlusion. Chest 1996;109:1490–6.

45. Haba-Rubio J, Sforza E, Weiss T, et al. Effect of CPAP treatment on inspiratory arousal threshold during NREM sleep in OSAS. Sleep Breath 2005;9:12–9.

46. Ratnavadivel R, Stadler D, Windler S, et al. Upper airway function and arousability to ventilatory challenge in slow wave versus stage 2 sleep in obstructive sleep apnoea. Thorax 2010;65:107–12.

47. Khoo MC, Kronauer RE, Strohl KP, et al. Factors inducing periodic breathing in humans: a general model. J Appl Physiol 1982;53:644–59.
48. Ryan CM, Bradley TD. Pathogenesis of obstructive sleep apnea. J Appl Physiol 2005;99:2440–50.
49. Younes M, Ostrowski M, Thompson W, et al. Chemical control stability in patients with obstructive sleep apnea. Am J Respir Crit Care Med 2001; 163:1181–90.
50. Yuan H, Pinto SJ, Huang J, et al. Ventilatory responses to hypercapnia during wakefulness and sleep in obese adolescents with and without obstructive sleep apnea syndrome. Sleep 2012; 35(9):1257–67.
51. Foster GE, Hanly PJ, Ostrowski M, et al. Ventilatory and cerebrovascular responses to hypercapnia in patients with obstructive sleep apnoea: effect of CPAP therapy. Respir Physiol Neurobiol 2009;165: 73–81.
52. Edwards BA, Connolly JG, Campana LM, et al. Acetazolamide attenuates the ventilatory response to arousal in patients with obstructive sleep apnea. Sleep 2013;36(2):281–5.
53. Kimoff RJ, Sforza E, Champagne V, et al. Upper airway sensation in snoring and obstructive sleep apnea. Am J Respir Crit Care Med 2001;164: 250–5.
54. Nguyen AT, Jobin V, Payne R, et al. Laryngeal and velopharyngeal sensory impairment in obstructive sleep apnea. Sleep 2005;28:585–93.
55. Boyd JH, Petrof BJ, Hamid Q, et al. Upper airway muscle inflammation and denervation changes in obstructive sleep apnea. Am J Respir Crit Care Med 2004;170:541–6.
56. Friberg D, Ansved T, Borg K, et al. Histological indications of a progressive snorers disease in an upper airway muscle. Am J Respir Crit Care Med 1998;157:586–93.
57. Mayer P, Dematteis M, Pepin JL, et al. Peripheral neuropathy in sleep apnea: a tissue marker of the severity of nocturnal desaturation. Am J Respir Crit Care Med 1999;159:213–9.
58. Saboisky JP, Stashuk DW, Hamilton-Wright A, et al. Neurogenic changes in the upper airway of patients with obstructive sleep apnea. Am J Respir Crit Care Med 2012;185(3):322–9.
59. Shelton KE, Woodson H, Gay S, et al. Pharyngeal fat in obstructive sleep apnea. Am Rev Respir Dis 1993;148:462–6.
60. Horner RL, Mohiaddin RH, Lowell DG, et al. Sites and sizes of fat deposits around the pharynx in obese patients with obstructive sleep apnoea and weight matched controls. Eur Respir J 1989;2: 613–22.
61. Saigusa H, Suzuki M, Higurashi N, et al. Three-dimensional morphological analyses of positional dependence in patients with obstructive sleep apnea syndrome. Anesthesiology 2009;110:885–90.
62. Sutherland K, Lee RW, Phillips CL, et al. Effect of weight loss on upper airway size and facial fat in men with obstructive sleep apnoea. Thorax 2011; 66:797–803.
63. Jones RL, Nzekwu MM. The effects of body mass index on lung volumes. Chest 2006;130:827–33.
64. Hoffstein V, Zamel N, Phillipson EA. Lung volume dependence of pharyngeal cross-sectional area in patients with obstructive sleep apnea. Am Rev Respir Dis 1984;130:175–8.
65. Susarla SM, Abramson ZR, Dodson TB, et al. Cephalometric measurement of upper airway length correlates with the presence and severity of obstructive sleep apnea. J Oral Maxillofac Surg 2010;68:2846–55.
66. Malhotra A, Huang Y, Fogel RB, et al. The male predisposition to pharyngeal collapse: importance of airway length. Am J Respir Crit Care Med 2002; 166:1388–95.
67. Jordan AS, Eckert DJ, Catcheside PG, et al. Ventilatory response to brief arousal from non-rapid eye movement sleep is greater in men than in women. Am J Respir Crit Care Med 2003;168:1512–9.
68. Bixler EO, Vgontzas AN, Ten Have T, et al. Effects of age on sleep apnea in men: I, prevalence and severity. Am J Respir Crit Care Med 1998;157:144–8.
69. Young T, Shahar E, Nieto FJ, et al. Predictors of sleep-disordered breathing in community-dwelling adults. Arch Intern Med 2002;162:893–900.
70. Pavlova MK, Duffy JF, Shea SA. Polysomnographic respiratory abnormalities in asymptomatic individuals. Sleep 2008;31:241–8.
71. Hoch CC, Reynolds CF III, Monk TH, et al. Comparison of sleep-disordered breathing among healthy elderly in the seventh, eighth, and ninth decades of life. Sleep 1990;13:502–11.
72. Malhotra A, Huang Y, Fogel R, et al. Aging influences on pharyngeal anatomy and physiology: the predisposition to pharyngeal collapse. Am J Med 2006;119:72.e9–14.
73. Martin SE, Mathur R, Marshall I, et al. The effect of age, sex, obesity and posture on upper airway size. Eur Respir J 1997;10:2087–90.
74. Edwards BA, O'Driscoll DM, Ali A, et al. Aging and sleep: physiology and pathophysiology. Semin Respir Crit Care Med 2010;31(5):618–33.
75. Huang Y, White DP, Malhotra A. Use of computational modeling to predict responses to upper airway surgery in obstructive sleep apnea. Laryngoscope 2007;117:648–53.

Obstructive Sleep Apnea Therapy and Metabolic Outcomes

Harneet K. Walia, MD[a,b,*], Reena Mehra, MD, MS[b,c,d]

KEYWORDS

- Obstructive sleep apnea • Metabolic syndrome • Obesity • Hypertension
- Continuous positive airway pressure

KEY POINTS

- There are both epidemiologic and experimental data implicating obstructive sleep apnea (OSA) as a key pathophysiologic factor in the evolution of metabolic dysfunction and as a culprit in increasing cardiovascular risk.
- The metabolic syndrome consists of a constellation of clinical risk factors encompassing truncal obesity, atherogenic dyslipidemia, elevated blood pressure, low glucose tolerance, and hyperinsulinemia, which in aggregate set the stage for the development of diabetes mellitus and cardiovascular disease.
- Conceptual frameworks are emerging with respect to the mechanistic underpinnings of OSA including intermittent hypoxia, sleep fragmentation, systemic inflammation and oxidative stress that contribute to the various facets of metabolic dysfunction.
- Reversal of the adverse accompanying pathophysiologic effects of OSA can have an impact on metabolic outcomes.
- The data suggests that treatment of OSA may ameliorate some of the metabolic parameters of metabolic syndrome.

INTRODUCTION

Aligned with the obesity epidemic, metabolic dysfunction has evolved into a highly prevalent condition with pervasive, far-reaching public health implications. The metabolic syndrome, a term characterized by a clustering of independent cardiovascular risk factors, has a current estimated prevalence of 30% in the United States population, with projections for a continued increase in frequency slated to reach levels in the epidemic realm.[1] The metabolic syndrome consists of a constellation of clinical risk factors encompassing truncal obesity, atherogenic dyslipidemia (high levels of triglyceride and low levels of high-density lipoprotein [HDL] cholesterol), elevated blood pressure (BP), low glucose tolerance, and hyperinsulinemia in the context of a prothrombotic

Conflicts of Interest Declaration: R. Mehra serves on the Medical Advisory Board for Care Core National, has received funding from the National Institutes of Health for research, and her institution has received positive airway devices from Philips Respironics for research for which she is the Principal Investigator. H. Walia has no conflicts of interest to disclose.
R. Mehra was partially supported through funding by the NIH NHLBI 1R01HL109493 and R21HL108226.

[a] Center for Sleep Disorders, Neurologic Institute, Cleveland Clinic, 11203 Stokes Boulevard, 2nd Floor, Cleveland, Ohio 44104, USA; [b] Cleveland Clinic Lerner College of Medicine of Case Western Reserve University, 9500 Euclid Avenue, Cleveland, Ohio 44195, USA; [c] Sleep Disorders Research, Center of Sleep Medicine, Neurologic Institute, Cleveland Clinic, 9500 Euclid Avenue, Cleveland, Ohio 44195, USA; [d] Molecular Cardiology Department, Lerner Research Institute, Heart and Vascular Institute, Respiratory Institute, 9500 Euclid Avenue, Cleveland, Ohio, 44195, USA
* Corresponding author.
E-mail address: WALIAH@ccf.org

Sleep Med Clin 8 (2013) 433–452
http://dx.doi.org/10.1016/j.jsmc.2013.07.009
1556-407X/13/$ – see front matter © 2013 Elsevier Inc. All rights reserved.

state and upregulation of systemic inflammation, which in aggregate set the stage for the development of diabetes mellitus and cardiovascular disease.[1,2] These risk factors result in serious adverse health effects by interacting synergistically to increase cardiovascular morbidity and mortality by 2- to 3-fold.[1,2] Diagnostic evaluation and targeted intervention coupled with identification of critical contributors of metabolic syndrome are paramount in the paradigm of cardiovascular risk reduction. Reduction of cardiovascular risk is of the utmost importance from the standpoint of public health imperatives as well as in targeting reduction of the high economic costs associated with cardiovascular disease, namely, estimated direct and indirect costs of $500 billion in 2010 with $150 billion resulting from loss of productivity related to disability and death.[3]

A wealth of both epidemiologic and experimental data have implicated obstructive sleep apnea (OSA) as a key pathophysiologic factor in the evolution of metabolic dysfunction and as a culprit in increasing cardiovascular risk. A singular challenge in investigating the interrelationships of obesity, metabolic syndrome, and OSA has been to effectively take into consideration and dissect the influence of OSA on metabolic syndrome independent of the effect of obesity. OSA is a highly prevalent disorder affecting approximately 15% of adults, characterized by reduction in upper airway muscle tone during sleep resulting in repetitive complete (resulting apnea) or partial (resulting in hypopnea) upper airway closure in the presence of continued thoracoabdominal effort and, often, paradox. OSA results in accompanying physiologic perturbations including intermittent hypoxia, ventilatory overshoot hyperoxia, intrathoracic pressure alterations, autonomic instability, and sleep fragmentation. These effects then lead to further adverse effects including increased systemic inflammation and elevated oxidative stress. The apnea-hypopnea index (AHI) is considered as the disease-defining metric for OSA, and is defined by the number of apneas and hypopneas per hour of sleep. Other measures used to ascertain the severity of OSA include the oxygen desaturation index and percentage of sleep time spent in hypoxia. Conceptual frameworks are emerging with respect to the mechanistic underpinnings of OSA that contribute to the various facets of metabolic dysfunction, which are elaborated in this article. Furthermore, the effect of the reversal of the adverse accompanying pathophysiologic effects of OSA on metabolic outcomes is reviewed herein. These areas of investigation are of paramount importance in achieving the goal of effective treatment of metabolic parameters to mitigate cardiovascular risk, particularly in light of data demonstrating synergism of OSA and metabolic syndrome in increasing cardiovascular risk.[4]

EPIDEMIOLOGY AND INTERRELATIONSHIPS OF OBSTRUCTIVE SLEEP APNEA, METABOLIC SYNDROME, AND OBESITY

Identified relationships of OSA and metabolic syndrome are not unanticipated given the overlap of established associated factors including obesity, diabetes mellitus, and cardiovascular disease. The co-occurrence of metabolic risk factors for both type 2 diabetes and cardiovascular disease (abdominal obesity, hyperglycemia, dyslipidemia, and hypertension) suggested the existence of a "metabolic syndrome," also known as insulin resistance syndrome. According to criteria proposed by the National Cholesterol Education Program (NCEP) Adult Treatment Panel III, the metabolic syndrome is defined by the presence of 3 or more of the following: (1) abdominal obesity with waist circumference greater than 40 inches (102 cm) in men and 35 inches (88 cm) in women, (2) serum triglycerides of 150 mg/dL, (3) HDL cholesterol less than 40 mg/dL in men and less than 50 mg/dL in women, (4) BP greater than 130/85 mm Hg or drug treatment for hypertension, and (5) fasting glucose level greater than 110 mg/dL.[5] The prevalence of metabolic syndrome as defined by NCEP criteria as per National Health and Nutrition Examination Survey (NHANES) data has undergone a substantive increase from 22% in NHANES 1988 to 1994 to 34.5% in NHANES 1999 to 2002.[6] Along these lines, as expected, an age-dependent increase in the prevalence of metabolic syndrome was also observed. Corroborating data from a large epidemiologic cohort, the Framingham Heart Study involving 3500 participants without diabetes or cardiovascular disease at baseline, demonstrated an increase in prevalence of metabolic syndrome of 26.8% in men and 16.6% in women at baseline, and an almost doubling of prevalence of the metabolic syndrome in both men and women after an 8-year follow-up period.[7] A likely contributing factor to the noted dramatic increase in prevalence of metabolic syndrome is the concordant obesity epidemic, which has been observed across of range of ethnicities.[8]

OSA is also a highly prevalent disorder with prevalence estimates of 9% to 24%,[9] with a distinct risk-factor profile characterized by increased risk in men; positive linear relationships with increasing age; and augmented risk related to obesity, owing to mechanical effects on the upper airway predisposing to collapsibility, as well as neurohumoral effects of adipokines and craniofacial structural alterations resulting in compromise of upper airway caliber and function.[10] Adverse effects of OSA, including intermittent hypoxia and autonomic nervous system fluctuations, contribute to the increased risk of intermediate cardiovascular factors comprising metabolic syndrome, as well as a wealth of data supporting relationships between OSA and increased cardiovascular morbidity and mortality.[11,12] Although obesity can be posited as the culprit connecting OSA and metabolic syndrome, mounting data indicate that this is not entirely the case. Metabolic syndrome has been noted to be significantly associated with moderate to severe OSA in a comparison with obese controls, suggesting that obesity-independent OSA pathophysiologic pathways are contributing to the evolution of metabolic syndrome.[13] Amassing evidence also demonstrates a relative synergism of the presence of OSA and metabolic syndrome, such that the burden of cardiovascular disease is far greater with both of these factors compared with either alone.[14] It has been posited that OSA, given its coaggregation and synergism with metabolic syndrome, may represent a salient component of metabolic syndrome constituting a cluster that has been termed Syndrome Z.[15] The co-occurrence of OSA and metabolic syndrome, Syndrome Z,[15] recently has been identified to be associated with a significantly greater atherogenic burden and higher prevalence of calcified carotid artery atheromas when compared with OSA alone in the absence of metabolic syndrome,[16] and is also correlated with intracoronary stenosis detected by multislice computed tomography.[17] Syndrome Z also appears to be related to alterations in cardiac morphology, specifically left ventricular hypertrophy and diastolic dysfunction.[18] Epidemiologic data from the Wisconsin Sleep Cohort support strong associations between OSA and metabolic syndrome. Age-adjusted and sex-adjusted associations resulted in a 4-fold increased odds of metabolic syndrome in those with moderate to severe OSA, which persisted after adjustment for markers of sympathetic or neuroendocrine activation (urinary norepinephrine, cortisol, heart-rate variability); after further adjustment for obesity this was mitigated to a 2.5-fold increased odds of metabolic syndrome, although it remained significant.[19] Furthermore, in a hospital-based urban northern Indian population, those with OSA were 4 times more likely to have metabolic syndrome than those without OSA, supporting the notion of consistent relationships across different ethnic groups.[20] The strong magnitude of association between OSA and metabolic syndrome was further substantiated by data from a British study showing a 9-fold increased likelihood of metabolic syndrome in men with OSA even after consideration of obesity.[13] Taken together, accumulating evidence points to a steadily increasing prevalence of metabolic syndrome and a high prevalence of OSA, with risk-factor profiles derived from a "common soil," and relationships that are strong in magnitude seemingly demonstrating a consistent pattern of independence from obesity.[13]

PHYSIOLOGIC AND BIOLOGICAL MECHANISMS OF ALTERED METABOLIC REGULATION IN OBSTRUCTIVE SLEEP APNEA

The mechanisms linking OSA and alterations in metabolic regulation are likely to be multifactorial. OSA via repetitive upper airway collapse results in bouts of intermittent hypoxia, hyperoxia, hypercapnia, sympathetic nervous system activation, and sleep disruption/fragmentation, which may be detrimental to glucose and lipid metabolism via intermediate mechanisms that include upregulation of pathways of systemic inflammation and oxidative stress and abnormalities of the hypothalamic-pituitary axis. This section focuses primarily on the impact of OSA-related intermittent hypoxia, sleep fragmentation, and increased systemic inflammation on metabolic function, as gaining a firm understanding of these concepts not only is crucial in setting the stage for the examination of interventional trial data targeting reversal of OSA pathophysiology on metabolic outcomes, but also is instrumental in the interpretation of these data.

Impact of Hypoxemia on Metabolic Function

Experiments in animal models have shown that intermittent hypoxia can decrease insulin sensitivity and induce glucose intolerance.[21,22] Some of these effects may occur via the sympathetic nervous system and altered autonomic function, the latter of which is impaired in OSA and also in prediabetic persons with impaired glucose metabolism.[23] Catecholamines also inhibit insulin secretion by activating α2-adrenoreceptors in β cells.[24] Exposure to intermittent hypoxia in young healthy adults has been shown to impair insulin sensitivity with a lack of compensatory hyperinsulinemia, suggesting a concordant suppression of β-cell function.[25]

Independently of autonomic nervous system activation, in animal models intermittent hypoxia contributes to decreased glucose utilization in oxidative muscle fibers.[26] Furthermore, intermittent hypoxia contributes to increased β-cell proliferation and cell death, the latter secondary to oxidative stress.[27] Increased oxidative stress, increased lipid peroxidation, and upregulation of nuclear factor κB (NF-κB) and hypoxia-inducible factor 1 are likely the main mechanisms of insulin resistance induced by hypoxia.[28]

Similar relationships have been confirmed in human studies examining the effects of intermittent hypoxia on metabolic regulation. Specifically, a study randomizing participants to 5 hours of intermittent hypoxia versus normoxia during wakefulness supported the notion that hypoxic stress in OSA may increase the predisposition for metabolic dysfunction by impairing insulin sensitivity, glucose effectiveness, and insulin secretion.[25] Moreover, in a large, prospective Japanese study involving about 4000 middle-aged individuals, nocturnal intermittent hypoxia (3% oxygen saturation dips $\geq$15/h on pulse oximetry at baseline) was established as a risk factor for development of type 2 diabetes mellitus after a 3-year median follow-up period (1.7-fold risk of incidental diabetes mellitus compared with those without significant hypoxia) after adjustment for multiple confounders.[29] In the Cleveland Family study, measures of hypoxic stress (time spent with <90% O_2 saturation) were the strongest polysomnographic index associated with glucose intolerance.[30]

Relationship of Sleep Fragmentation with Metabolic Regulation

Although sleep fragmentation may occur in various sleep disorders, it is a cardinal feature of OSA and results in alterations in glucose metabolism independent of sleep duration. Both human and animal experimental data support the notion of sleep fragmentation representing an allostatic load on the endocrine and autonomic systems, potentially resulting in development of metabolic dysregulation.[31] For instance, it is recognized that the initiation of slow-wave sleep coincides with hormonal changes that affect glucose homeostasis.[32] As such, all-night selective suppression of slow-wave sleep for 3 consecutive nights has been shown to result in an approximately 25% reduction in insulin sensitivity without adequate compensatory increase in insulin secretion, thereby leading to reduced glucose tolerance and increased risk of developing diabetes.[32] Moreover, 2 days of enforced sleep fragmentation resulting in poor sleep quality and reduced slow-wave sleep yielded similar results.[32] Nonselective fragmentation of sleep induced by auditory and mechanical stimuli across all stages for 2 nights is also associated with a decrease in insulin sensitivity and non–insulin-dependent glucose disposal, the latter referring to glucose mobilization independent of an insulin

response.[33] Of note, fasting intravenous glucose tolerance testing was used in this study, a technique considered to be the gold standard in the assessment of glucose regulation.[33] Sleep fragmentation also led to an increase in morning cortisol levels and a shift in sympathovagal balance toward an increase in sympathetic nervous system modulation and reduction in parasympathetic activity, hence shedding light on potential mechanistic underpinnings.[33] Moreover, chronic sleep loss related to sleep-disordered breathing is likely to worsen the metabolic disturbances and may predispose to insulin resistance.[34] Experimental animal studies using intravenous glucose tolerance testing before and after an 8-day period of sleep restriction and disturbance, in the absence of sleep curtailment, resulted in hyperglycemia and decreased insulin levels, further corroborating the results from human studies.[35] More recent experimental data further support this premise, and extend the length of sleep fragmentation to 14 days using a sleep interruption model intended to minimize stressful stimulation to the animal. Findings in the latter work demonstrated not only an impact on peripheral glucose metabolism but also on appetite, with evidence of hyperphagia in the absence of weight gain suggesting alterations in the metabolic rate as a potential culprit.[36]

Systemic Inflammation and Oxidative Stress in Obstructive Sleep Apnea as Instigators of Altered Metabolic Function

Inflammation has been proposed as a putative mechanism of cardiovascular risk in patients with OSA, and it may also impair insulin action in peripheral tissues. Intermittent hypoxia and sleep fragmentation in OSA are postulated to be triggers of the cascade of inflammation in the adipose tissue and vascular compartment, and thus an array of inflammatory products may be released.[37] Multiple inflammatory markers and mediators, including NF-κB, C-reactive protein, tumor necrosis factor α, and interleukin-6, are elevated in patients with OSA,[38] and these markers have been noted to be culprits in inducing insulin resistance.[39] The authors' group has shown relationships between markers of systemic inflammation (including soluble interleukin-6 receptor) and increasing severity of OSA, independent of confounding by obesity and apparent diurnal patterns such that morning levels were more closely tied to OSA severity, potentially signifying a reflection of overnight OSA-related physiologic stress.[40] The presence of these markers of inflammation in metabolic syndrome[41] support that OSA may play a role in development of metabolic syndrome. Furthermore, the adipokines, including leptin, ghrelin, and adiponectin, are altered in patients with OSA and can promote metabolic syndrome.[38] Because of the close association between inflammation and insulin resistance, it has been suggested that visceral obesity is a potential pathogenic factor in promoting inflammation and leading to insulin resistance and sleep apnea.[42] Elevated oxidative stress is emerging as a central player in the pathogenesis of metabolic syndrome, and may represent a unifying factor in progression of disease. In particular, oxidative stress has been identified as a major mechanism underlying the microvascular and macrovascular complications in metabolic syndrome.[43] OSA has been recognized as providing the ideal milieu for oxidative stress to occur, given the repetitive intermittent bouts of hypoxemia and subsequent episodes of reoxygenation, which may lead to generation of free radicals and a state of enhanced oxidative stress. This resultant state of augmented oxidative stress may thus lead to the metabolic insults seen in the representative components of metabolic syndrome.

EFFECT OF OBSTRUCTIVE SLEEP APNEA TREATMENT WITH CONTINUOUS POSITIVE AIRWAY PRESSURE ON LIPID BIOLOGY AND VISCERAL ADIPOSITY

It has been hypothesized that continuous positive airway pressure (CPAP) via amelioration of breathing disturbances during sleep can improve the lipid profile, such as total cholesterol, low-density lipoprotein (LDL) cholesterol, HDL cholesterol, triglycerides, and apolipoproteins A, B, and C. However, despite mechanistic studies consistently demonstrating relationships between OSA and lipid biosynthesis and regulation, the effect of CPAP on lipids has revealed conflicting results. Several studies have shown that CPAP treatment is beneficial for improving the lipid profile of OSA patients. A meta-analysis of 2 randomized, placebo-controlled trials in OSA patients compared the effect of therapeutic and subtherapeutic CPAP treatment on cholesterol and triglycerides. There was a significant reduction in total cholesterol levels among patients receiving therapeutic CPAP for a short treatment duration of 1 month compared with those receiving subtherapeutic CPAP, and no significant changes were observed in serum triglycerides in either group.[44] A large study of OSA patients showed a small but statistically significant increase in HDL cholesterol after 6 months of CPAP therapy. Significant improvements in serum levels of HDL cholesterol, LDL cholesterol, total cholesterol, and triglycerides in OSA patients with baseline

abnormal lipid/lipoprotein serum levels were also noted.[45] Data from a smaller randomized trial showed an improvement in postprandial triglycerides and total cholesterol levels in patients with moderate to severe OSA with CPAP therapy.[46] A significant improvement in the ratio of HDL to total cholesterol and levels of total cholesterol, triglycerides, and LDL and non-HDL cholesterol with autoadjusting positive airway pressure (PAP) was noted in a randomized controlled trial, with a significant increase in HDL cholesterol noted only in more adherent patients.[47] It remains unclear, however, whether the improvement in lipid profiles may be secondary to concomitant reduction in body mass index, or secondary to direct reversal of OSA adverse physiologic effects with PAP. On the other hand, data from several studies have suggested that CPAP treatment does not improve serum lipid levels. In a randomized, controlled, crossover trial, obese Caucasians with symptoms of OSA underwent intervention with 6 weeks of therapeutic versus sham CPAP without an appreciable change in lipids. In the therapeutic CPAP group, there was no significant change in cholesterol triglycerides, HDL cholesterol, and LDL cholesterol after CPAP treatment.[48] Similarly, in a double-blind, randomized controlled trial of therapeutic and sham CPAP for 3 months in men with type 2 diabetes and OSA, no significant reduction in total cholesterol, HDL cholesterol, or triglycerides was observed before and after treatment.[49]

Visceral adipose mass is considered to be a more accurate measure of dysfunctional adipose tissue than body mass index when considering facets of metabolic syndrome. Quantitative radiologic measures of visceral adiposity using standard computed tomography (CT) scans have been reported as the gold-standard method for assessing visceral adiposity, given its ability to precisely and reliably measure abdominal fat compartments.[50] In a randomized crossover trial involving those with moderate to severe OSA, a significant reduction in visceral fat in addition to subcutaneous fat was noted,[47] which is contrary to the findings of another randomized trial that failed to demonstrate reduction in visceral abdominal fat over a 12-week period and did not show improvement at 6 months during an uncontrolled portion of the study.[51] Two other recent trials performed over an 8-week period did not show reduction in visceral abdominal fat with CPAP treatment of OSA.[52,53]

Overall, the effect of CPAP on visceral abdominal fat has been inconsistent, with some studies showing improvement in the amount of visceral fat. This finding may be attributable to the relatively limited duration of OSA treatment implemented in these trials.[54,55]

OBSTRUCTIVE SLEEP APNEA TREATMENT AND HYPERTENSION

OSA has been linked with hypertension (HTN), an increased prevalence of a nondipping BP pattern, and increased risk of resistant HTN. Apnea-related arousals and/or hypoxemia can result in sympathetic nervous system activation, leading to elevated nocturnal or daytime BP. The guidelines on HTN detection and treatment recommend evaluation of OSA as a cause of difficult-to-treat HTN.[56] Numerous studies, ranging from uncontrolled studies through clinical observational to randomized double-blind trials, have investigated the effect of CPAP on HTN (**Table 1**). However, the effect of CPAP treatment on BP was highly variable, and some individuals do not show any antihypertensive benefit other than having manifested a very high BP response. This variability in response can be explained by multiple reasons: most studies were of small sample size; most studies were performed in a single center; the methods used for measuring BP such as the 24-hour ambulatory BP monitoring or office BP measurement varied widely between the studies; and studies included patients with and without hypertension, as well as different types of hypertension and treatment interventions. Furthermore, the method used to diagnose OSA varied; the studies had different designs, such as crossover or parallel; studies used different interventions such as sham CPAP, subtherapeutic CPAP, drug therapy, or conservative treatment in control participants; and the duration of intervention varied between different studies. Even the meta-analyses of randomized trials are limited by the trials they included, and many of the trials did not involve the patients most likely to benefit, which may explain the variability of the results. Use of CPAP has generally shown a consistent, albeit modest, antihypertensive benefit. Patients who are most likely to benefit include those with more severe OSA, and higher baseline pretreatment BP levels, and patients more compliant with CPAP use.

Two large, randomized controlled trials evaluating the role of CPAP in HTN were recently published.[57,58] The first was randomized, multicenter, double-blind, placebo-controlled trial of 340 patients, primarily men (81%), which showed a statistically significant decline in 24-hour arterial BP, systolic BP (SBP), and diastolic BP (DBP) by 1.5, 2.1, and 1.3 mm Hg, respectively. Mean nocturnal BP decreased by 2.0 mm Hg after 3 months of treatment in patients with newly diagnosed HTN.[57] This observed reduction was smaller than

anticipated and did not achieve the 3-mm Hg drop in mean 24-hour ambulatory BP that the trial was powered to detect. In the second study, the Spanish Sleep and Breathing Group trial of more than 350 asymptomatic individuals with severe OSA in which one arm was treated with CPAP, at 1-year follow-up the group treated with CPAP had a significant reduction in SBP and DBP of 1.9 mm Hg and 2.2 mm Hg, respectively. The most significant reduction in BP was seen in patients who used CPAP for more than 5.6 hours per night.[58]

Several meta-analyses suggest that the beneficial effects of CPAP on BP are detectable in the first few weeks of treatment, this being counterintuitive to what one may expect, as the vascular remodeling and other structural cardiovascular changes are not expected to be evident in short-term trials of CPAP treatment, and longer treatment may be needed to obtain greater reductions in BP. However, results from randomized trials have found significant reductions in BP within a few weeks of CPAP treatment.[59-61]

A 2007 meta-analysis of 10 randomized controlled trials did not show any difference in SBP or DBP between the PAP and the control group using ambulatory BP monitoring and office BP measurements combined.[62] In another meta-analysis including 16 trials conducted between 1996 and 2006 and a total of 818 patients, a small but statistically significant mean net change in SBP of 2.5 mm Hg and DBP of 1.8 mm Hg was observed. Net reductions in BP were not statistically different between daytime and nighttime. This meta-analysis included predominantly obese middle-aged men and comprised studies that were not blinded.[63]

In one of the prospective observational studies with a longer follow-up of 55 patients, a significant decrease was shown only for DBP (−2.2 mm Hg) but not SBP or 24-hour mean arterial BP. Subgroup analyses, however, showed that 24-hour mean BP did decrease significantly in patients with uncontrolled HTN at entry (−4.4 mm Hg, $P = .01$) as well as in those with high CPAP compliance (−5.3 mm Hg, $P = .01$).[64]

A significant decrease in BP was reported by Pepperell and colleagues[61] in 118 patients, with the largest effect on BP observed with CPAP in severe OSA (oxygen desaturation index >33/h, decrease in BP of 5.1 mm Hg), Moreover, use of therapeutic CPAP for more than 5 hours per night showed a greater trend toward decreased BP. Becker and colleagues[65] showed the largest reduction in BP of about 10 mm Hg SBP, mean arterial BP, and DBP in a 9-week double-blind trial in patients with moderate to severe sleep apnea.

This drop in BP was seen in patients with therapeutic CPAP treatment with an approximately 95% reduction in AHI. Despite the reduction in AHI by 50%, in the subtherapeutic control group there was no significant reduction in BP. Coughlin and colleagues[48] showed a reduction in mean SBP and DBP of 6.7 mm Hg and 4.9 mm Hg, respectively, with CPAP in obese individuals, and there were no changes in metabolic parameters.

In another randomized study that used ambulatory BP measurements in patients with OSA, a 12-week CPAP regimen resulted in a reduction in 24-hour mean BP and DBP by 3.8 and 3.5 mm Hg, respectively. In this study, the majority of subjects were not sleepy based on the Epworth Sleepiness Scale (ESS) score.[66] Whereas some of the trials have shown improvement in BP with CPAP in hypersomnolent patients,[59] Robinson and colleagues[67] showed no significant improvement in BP with CPAP in nonhypersomnolent patients, suggesting a role of hypersomnolence in the pathogenesis of HTN caused by OSA. There have been other randomized trials reinforcing the improvement of various BP measurements with CPAP.[68]

The effect on BP by CPAP withdrawal has also been measured, which showed an increase in morning SBP and DBP and morning heart rate, along with increases in other clinical features and inflammatory markers of OSA.[69] In 2011, Drager and colleagues[70] showed the impact of CPAP on a novel group of patients with pre-HTN and or masked HTN. Thirty-six male patients randomized to no treatment and CPAP for 3 months showed a significant reduction of pre-HTN (from 94% to 55%) and masked HTN (from 39% to 5%). This finding is important from clinical standpoint, as most patients with pre-HTN develop HTN later. This study is the first to evaluate the effect of BP in pre-HTN patients. Overall, CPAP has been shown to have a modest effect in reducing BP, which also is important from the clinical viewpoint because it can have a significant effect in reducing comorbidity.

Most results available on the effect on BP of an oral appliance are based on observational data. Most studies showed a significant improvement in BP in mild to moderate sleep apnea with use of an oral appliance.[71,72] A Chinese study of 46 patients compared a group wearing an oral appliance monitored by ambulatory BP with a nontolerated oral appliance treatment group.[73] There was a significant improvement in SBP, DBP, 24-hour and diurnal SBP, and mean arterial pressure in the oral appliance group in comparison with the other group after 12 weeks of treatment. Another observational study involving 161 patients showed improvement in SBP, DBP, and mean arterial

BP.[74] A small study involving only 11 subjects with an oral appliance showed improvement in ambulatory BP monitoring after titration.[75] A randomized, controlled, crossover trial of 61 patients showed significant reduction in mean 24-hour DBP and awake BP; however, no reduction was seen in SBP.[76] Andren and colleagues[77] conducted a long-term follow-up study of patients with mild OSA, and showed that a reduction in SBP and DBP was maintained after 3 years of use of a mandibular advancement oral appliance. A meta-analysis indicated the pooled estimate of mean changes and the corresponding 95% confidence interval (CI) for SBP, DBP, and mean arterial BP, respectively, from each trial were: -2.7 mm Hg (95% CI: -0.8 to -4.6); -2.7 mm Hg (95% CI: -0.9 to -4.6); and -2.40 mm Hg (95% CI: -4.01 to -0.80).

The clinical significance of SBP and DBP reductions of 2 to 4 mm Hg can be put into perspective by data showing a 15% and 42% reduction in the risk of coronary artery disease and stroke, respectively, with a reduction in BP of 5 mm Hg.[78] With respect to the effect of OSA treatment on BP reduction, there is a clinically significant cardiovascular benefit to OSA treatment in potentially reducing adverse cardiovascular outcomes, for which hypertension represents a firm risk factor. Areas of future work should focus on better understanding the relationships of OSA and nondipping BP profiles, in particular to examine the potential benefits of chronotherapy for antihypertensive medication in OSA patients. Use of supplemental oxygen as a treatment of OSA-related intermittent hypoxia may also serve to blunt sympathetic nervous system surges and reduce BP; therefore interventional trials examining this effect are desired. Along these lines, results of a multicenter, randomized controlled trial involving patients from cardiology clinics with moderate to severe OSA randomized to CPAP, supplemental oxygen, or a healthy lifestyle are forthcoming. Moreover, OSA as a culprit of resistant hypertension and nondipping BP patterns needs to be addressed from the standpoint of ascertaining improvement in BP profiles in this high-risk group.

EFFECT OF POSITIVE AIRWAY PRESSURE AND NON–POSITIVE AIRWAY PRESSURE MODALITIES OF OBSTRUCTIVE SLEEP APNEA THERAPY ON COMPONENTS OF METABOLIC SYNDROME
Uncontrolled Trials

Several uncontrolled trials have focused on the effect of CPAP therapy on OSA and its impact on metabolic syndrome. These studies have been

Table 1
Studies investigating the effect of CPAP on blood pressure

Authors,[Ref.] Year	Type	N	Male (%)	Age (y)	Intervention	Duration	OSA	BP	Effect of Treatment on BP Parameters
Duran-Cantolla et al,[57] 2010	Randomized controlled double-blind trial	340	81	53.2, 51.7	CPAP and sham CPAP (<1 cm H_2O)	3 mo	AHI >15	History of HTN or on antihypertensive medications	↓ in ABP by 1.5 mm Hg ↓ SBP 2.1 mm Hg, ↓DBP 1.3 mm Hg
Becker et al,[65] 2003	Randomized controlled trial	32	60	54.4, 52.3	CPAP and subtherapeutic PAP	9 wk	AHI ≥5, ESS 10	None	↓ 9.9 mm Hg, MBP and SBP and DBP ↓ by 10 mm Hg
Pepperell et al,[61] 2002	Randomized controlled parallel-group trial	118	100	51	Therapeutic and subtherapeutic CPAP (1 cm H_2O)	1 mo	ESS >9, ODI (4%) >10	None	↓ MAP by 2.5 mm Hg Effect more pronounced in severe OSA
Robinson et al,[67] 2006	Randomized controlled crossover trial	35	31	54	Auto PAP and subtherapeutic CPAP	1 mo	ODI (4%) >10	Excluded BP <140/90 or not on antihypertensive	No significant difference in mean 24-h BP in nonhypersomnolent patients
Hui et al,[66] 2006	Randomized controlled parallel-group trial	28	22/6, 21/7	50.3, 51.2	Therapeutic (10.7 cm H_2O) CPAP and subtherapeutic CPAP (4 cm H_2O)	12 wk	AHI >5 with symptoms of OSA	None	↓ in 24-h mean BP by 3.8 mm Hg and DBP by 3.5 mm Hg
Coughlin et al,[48] 2007	Randomized controlled crossover trial	34	100	49.0 ± 8.3	CPAP and sham CPAP	6 wk	AHI >15	Excluded BP >180/110	↓ in SBP and DBP by 6.7 and 4.9 mm Hg, no change in metabolic parameters

Study	Design				Intervention	Duration	AHI/ODI	BP criteria	Outcomes
Kohler et al,[69] 2011	Randomized controlled trial	41	19/1, 21/0	63.6, 61.8	CPAP or withdrawal CPAP (subtherapeutic CPAP)	2 wk	ODI (4%) ≥10	Excluded inadequately controlled HTN	CPAP withdrawal was associated with increase in morning office SBP (8.5 mm Hg), morning DBP (6.9 mm Hg)
Drager et al,[70] 2011	Randomized controlled trial	36	100	43 CPAP 44 control	No treatment or CPAP treatment (based on PSG)	3 mo	AHI >30	Pre-HTN (SBP 120–139, DBP 80–89), masked HTN (AABP 135>85)	CPAP (from 126 ± 5 to 121 ± 7 mm Hg; $P = .001$) and a trend DBP (from 75 ± 7 to 73 ± 8 mm Hg; $P = .08$). Significant reduction in frequency of pre-HTN (from 94% to 55%; $P = .02$) and masked HTN (from 39% to 5%; $P = .04$) only in the CPAP group
Barbe et al,[58] 2010	Randomized controlled trial	359	100	56 ± 10	CPAP or conservative treatment	1 y	AHI >19, ESS <11	SBP >140 or DBP >90	Reduction of in SBP and DBP of 1.9 mm Hg and 2.2 mm Hg, respectively. Most significant reduction in BP seen in patients who used CPAP for more than 5.6 h per night
Facenda et al,[59] 2001	Randomized controlled crossover trial	68	81	50	CPAP or oral placebo	4 wk	AHI >15	24 h BP	1.5 mm Hg reduction in DBP

Abbreviations: ABP, ambulatory blood pressure (mm Hg); AHI, apnea-hypopnea index; BP, blood pressure (mm Hg); CPAP, continuous positive airway pressure; DBP, diastolic blood pressure (mm Hg); HTN, hypertension; MAP, mean arterial blood pressure (mm Hg); ODI, oxygen desaturation index; OSA, obstructive sleep apnea; PSG, polysomnography; SBP, systolic blood pressure (mm Hg).

limited by their small sample size, uncontrolled nature, and varying consideration of primary and secondary outcomes. One of the first studies reporting the effect of OSA treatment with CPAP on metabolic syndrome assessed this effect on insulin resistance as ascertained by the insulin sensitivity index gleaned from the gold-standard hyperinsulinemic euglycemic clamp studies, which were performed in 40 patients over a 3-month period.[79] The degree of apnea was moderate to severe (AHI >20) and the investigators observed a significant increase in insulin sensitivity after 2 days of CPAP treatment, which persisted at 3 months and appeared to be most pronounced in the nonobese individuals (ie, those with a body mass index <30 kg/m^2). These effects were noted in the absence of significant changes in body mass index. The investigators surmised that the early improvement in insulin sensitivity may be secondary to reversal of sympathetic nervous system surges related to OSA, and that the preferential benefit noted in the nonobese may reflect primarily an obesity-driven source of insulin resistance in obese individuals with a lesser extent of OSA influence in this setting. Limitations of this study included the involvement of only men, with results generalizable as such, and also that only a small proportion of individuals had impaired glucose tolerance.[79]

Another clinic-based study of primarily men who were morbidly obese (mean body mass index of 43 ± 8.7 kg/m^2) showed an improvement in postprandial glucose values as well as a reduction in hemoglobin A$_{1c}$ (HbA1c) levels in those with a baseline HbA1c level of greater than 7%. Furthermore, there was a relationship of improved glucose handling relative to PAP usage such that in those individuals using CPAP for greater than 4 hours per day, the reduction in HbA1c level correlated with the days of CPAP usage; this finding was not observed in those less adherent with therapy.[80] Similarly, findings from another study with a small sample size demonstrated a correlation of hypoxemia in patients with OSA and HbA1c levels in a group ranging from normal to prediabetic and diabetic. Individuals with optimal adherence after 3 to 5 months of CPAP therapy showed a significant reduction in HbA1c levels.[81]

Two months of CPAP therapy in a small study showed improvement in cardiovascular risk profiles of patients with severe OSA and concurrent metabolic syndrome, resulting in reductions in BP, total cholesterol levels, insulin resistance measured by Homeostatic Model Assessment— Insulin Resistance (HOMA-IR), tumor necrosis factor α, and oxidative stress markers. Similar to other data, these beneficial effects of therapy were observed in those who used CPAP for more than 4 hours per day.[82] A few studies have assessed metabolic parameters of individuals undergoing treatment for OSA over a more prolonged period of time. Specifically, another study involving a small sample size but following patients with OSA and on CPAP for a 1-year period, demonstrated a 45% reduction in prevalence of metabolic syndrome and an improvement in HDL cholesterol as well as waist circumference and body mass index; however, no improvement was noted in fasting blood glucose, triglyceride, or BP levels.[83] A 6-month study of male patients with moderate to severe OSA treated with autoadjusting CPAP showed that treatment resulted in a reduction in prevalence of metabolic syndrome from 63.5% to 47.3%, primarily attributable to reductions in BP and triglycerides.[84]

In summary, results from uncontrolled interventional studies appear to be somewhat consistent in demonstrating improvements in metabolic parameters, albeit showing discrepancies regarding which specific components of metabolic syndrome show improvement. Data suggest that early improvements are noted (as soon as 2 days after therapy) and that effects may be more pronounced in the nonobese. The degree of improvement in metabolic function also appears to be related to the level of CPAP adherence. The results seem to be generalizable to primarily men. Of note, some of the studies showed improvement in body mass index during follow-up, precluding one's ability to effectively ascertain whether improvements in metabolic function were related to direct treatment of OSA or indirect improvement in anthropometrics. Overall these studies were limited by smaller sample sizes, mostly shorter duration of therapy, limited generalizability, and few gold-standard techniques used to assess insulin resistance.

Randomized Controlled Interventional Trials

There have been 6 randomized controlled trials that have evaluated the role of CPAP in reversing metabolic abnormalities in patients with OSA (Table 2). These trials have examined populations with different ethnic backgrounds and differing background characteristics of subjects, and have used varying study designs and eligibility criteria as well as different durations of therapy.

The largest and, likely, most appropriately powered trial to examine the effects of PAP on metabolic function was a randomized, crossover, double-blinded, controlled trial based in India involving 86 participants, with the goal of assessing the reversal of metabolic syndrome with

Table 2
Controlled trials evaluating the role of CPAP in reversing metabolic abnormalities in patients with OSA

Authors,[Ref.] Year	Age (y)	Gender	Body Mass Index (kg/m²)	Number	Power Calculations	Study Design	OSA Definition	Predefined Outcome	Duration	Type of Treatment	Findings
Weinstock et al,[85] 2012	54 Range: 18–75	42% males with baseline impaired glucose tolerance, USA	39	50, n = 1 lost to follow-up	80% power to detect difference in glucose tolerance status (anticipating 20%–35% CPAP and 10%–15% of sham improved to normal)	Randomized, crossover, double-blind trial with 1 mo washout and 2 wk run-in period, the latter to assess adherence	AHI >15	Primary: Normalization of mean 2 h oral glucose tolerance testing Secondary: Improvement in ISI (0, 120)	8 wk of CPAP or sham CPAP followed by alternative therapy after 1 mo washout	CPAP vs sham CPAP, CPAP adherence 4.8 h/d	13.3% improvement in ISI and 28.7% reduction in 2 h insulin level in CPAP group in severe OSA (AHI >30) Impaired glucose tolerance normalized after CPAP with moderate OSA and obesity Each hour of active CPAP associated with improvement in insulin sensitivity (0, 120) A subset of participants underwent CPAP treatment for 12 wk without improvement in insulin sensitivity

(continued on next page)

Table 2
(continued)

Authors,[Ref.] Year	Age (y)	Gender	Body Mass Index (kg/m²)	Number	Power Calculations	Study Design	OSA Definition	Predefined Outcome	Duration	Type of Treatment	Findings
Hoyos et al,[51] 2012	49 ± 12	100% males, Australia	31.3 ± 5.2	65, 13 withdrawals post randomization		Randomized parallel-design controlled trial	AHI ≥20	Primary: Change in visceral abdominal fat Secondary: Change in insulin sensitivity index and liver fat, body composition and metabolic markers	12 wk	CPAP vs sham CPAP followed by 12 wk of CPAP for both groups, mean CPAP adherence 3.6 h	No significant improvement in metabolic outcomes including visceral abdominal fat At 24 wk, improvement of insulin sensitivity was noted
Sharma et al,[47] 2011	45 Range: 30–65	84% males in CPAP first group vs 95% males in sham CPAP first group ESS 14.8 ± 3.7 in CPAP group vs 14.1 ± 3.5 in sham group India	33.8	86	80% power to detect a 15% reduction in metabolic syndrome	Randomized, crossover double-blind trial with 1 mo washout period	AHI ≥15	Primary: 15% reduction in metabolic syndrome	12 wk	Auto PAP vs sham CPAP, CPAP adherence 4.8 ± 1.4 h	11% of the CPAP group vs 1% of the sham group had reversal of the metabolic syndrome ($P = .003$). Decrease in systolic and diastolic BP, total cholesterol, non-HDL, triglycerides, and glycated hemoglobin. Decrease in BMI, visceral and subcutaneous fat

Study	Age	Population	BMI	N	Power	Design	Inclusion	Outcomes	Duration	Intervention	Results
Lam et al,[86] 2010	46.3 ± 10.2	100% males, China	27.5 ± 3.7	61, n = 1 lost to follow-up	90% power to detect difference in insulin tolerance test (Kitt) 1.7 ± 1.5 mmol/min	Randomized parallel-design controlled trial	AHI ≥15	Primary: Change in short insulin tolerance test	1 wk followed by 11 wk of open study	Auto CPAP for 1 wk and fixed PAP for 11 wk vs sham CPAP	Early improvement in insulin sensitivity ($P = .022$) which was not sustained at 12 wk, improvement in insulin sensitivity in subgroup with BMI >25 kg/m²
Coughlin et al,[48] 2007	49 ± 8.3	All males, Caucasian, no diabetes mellitus, ESS ≥10, UK	36.1 ± 7.6	34, 1 withdrawal	90% power to detect 20% reduction of metabolic syndrome	Randomized, controlled, blinded crossover trial	AHI >15	Primary: Metabolic syndrome, HOMA, Change in waking BP or glucose, baroreceptor sensitivity	6 wk	CPAP vs sham CPAP, mean CPAP adherence 3.9 h (range 0-7.4)	No change in HOMA-IR, or lipids, mean systolic and diastolic BP decreased by 6.7 and 4.9 mm Hg, respectively
West et al,[49] 2007	Range: 18-75	All males with diabetes mellitus and sleepiness (ESS ≥9), UK	CPAP: 36.6 ± 4.9 Sham: 36.8 ± 4.6	42, n = 2 lost to follow-up	90% power to detect 0.8 difference in HbA1c	Randomized parallel-design double-blind trial	>10 oxygen saturation dips of >4%/h	Primary: HbA1c; also examined were HOMA and euglycemic hyperinsulinemic clamp	12 wk	Auto CPAP vs placebo CPAP, mean usage of CPAP 3.6 ± 2.8 h	No change in glycemic index and insulin resistance (HbA1c, euglycemic clamp, HOMA, adipoonectin)

Abbreviations: AHI, apnea-hypopnea index; BMI, body mass index; CPAP, continuous positive airway pressure; ESS, Epworth Sleepiness Scale; HbA1c, hemoglobin A₁c; HDL, high-density lipoprotein cholesterol; HOMA (-IR), Homeostasis Model Assessment (Insulin Resistance); ISI, Insulin Sensitivity Index; OGTT, oral glucose tolerance test; OSA, obstructive sleep apnea.

3 months of autoadjusting PAP followed by 3 months of sham PAP (or vice versa) separated by a 1-month washout period to minimize carryover effects.[47] The study involved predominantly obese, middle-aged men with moderate to severe OSA (overall mean AHI of 48) and excessive daytime sleepiness, but without diabetes mellitus. The sample had a high degree of sleepiness, with an ESS score of 14.8 ± 3.7 in the PAP-first group versus 14.1 ± 3.4 in the sham-first group. The PAP adherence noted in this trial was higher than that of other studies, namely 4.8 ± 1.4 hours of daily usage. Autoadjusting PAP treatment compared with sham PAP was associated with a significant reduction in glycated hemoglobin, triglycerides, and total cholesterol, as well as a significant increase in HDL cholesterol to total cholesterol ratio. The reversal of metabolic syndrome (primary outcome) was observed in 13% of participants using autoadjusting PAP therapy, compared with 1% with sham PAP. Concomitant significant reductions in body mass index, visceral fat, and subcutaneous fat were seen in treatment with autoadjusting PAP in comparison with the control period. In subgroup analyses, significant improvement in carotid intima-media thickness was noted among the more adherent patients, suggesting a potential role for PAP therapy in reversing endothelial damage caused by OSA and metabolic syndrome.[47]

Another recent study using a crossover design involved 50 obese, middle-aged individuals with moderate to severe OSA (AHI 44 ± 27 in the CPAP-first group and 32 ± 20 in the sham CPAP group) and impaired glucose tolerance who were randomized to 8 weeks of CPAP followed by sham CPAP (or vice versa) after a 1-month washout period.[85] Education on healthy lifestyle behavior was provided to all participants. Adherence to CPAP was similar to that of the India-based study, at average 4.8 hours of daily usage. Overall, there was no improvement in the primary outcome, insulin sensitivity, in those on CPAP versus sham CPAP; however, in subgroup analyses those with severe OSA had 13% improvement noted in the Insulin Sensitivity Index (0, 120) and a 28% reduction in the 2-hour insulin level after CPAP in comparison with those on sham CPAP. Moreover, each additional hour of active CPAP usage was associated with a significant improvement in the Insulin Sensitivity Index, and this improvement was more pronounced in sleepier participants. This study demonstrated a dose-response effect for both the severity of disease and adherence to treatment.[85] Contrary to the study based in India, there was no reduction in CT-based ascertainment of visceral abdominal

fat with CPAP versus sham CPAP, suggesting that the reduction in adiposity as a result of CPAP may have been driving the improvement in metabolic parameters in the study by Sharma and colleagues,[47] and could potentially account for the differences in the study results. Alternatively, the reduction in visceral fat may have been a result of differential behavioral or lifestyle habits rather than a direct effect of CPAP; however, there was no evidence of this, based on the social and lifestyle habits collected.

The goal of a parallel-group randomized controlled trial involving 61 middle-aged, overweight, Chinese men with moderate to severe OSA was to examine the effect of 1 week of autotitrating CPAP versus sham CPAP on short insulin tolerance test (SITT) results and then to perform an extended investigation of effects of 12 weeks of CPAP.[86] Insulin sensitivity, measured by the SITT, was shown to be significantly improved after 1 week of CPAP, and the effect was sustained at 12 weeks in only a subgroup of overweight/obese individuals (body mass index>25 kg/m^2). The results are consistent with the observation of early improvement of insulin sensitivity in response to CPAP noted in uncontrolled trial data; however, the lack of sustained effects may be due to lack of a control comparison arm. Interestingly, the sustained metabolic improvement in those who were overweight/obese counters the existing uncontrolled data.[86]

Two randomized controlled trials based in the United Kingdom examined the effect of moderate to severe OSA treatment on components of metabolic syndrome in men.[48,49] The first involved middle-aged, obese men without diabetes mellitus participating in a randomized crossover study, with results consistent with lack of reversal of metabolic syndrome with 6 weeks of CPAP versus sham CPAP (mean CPAP adherence 3.9 hours). Although reductions in SBP and DBP were noted, there was no change in the HOMA-IR (measure of insulin sensitivity) nor was there improvement in the lipid profile. Of note, lack of use of a washout period to minimize the potential carryover effect of CPAP is a methodologic flaw of this study, and an important aspect to bear in mind when interpreting results.[48] The other randomized, parallel-design United Kingdom-based study involving middle-aged, obese men with diabetes mellitus failed to show evidence of reduction in HbA1c with 12 weeks of autoadjusting CPAP versus sham CPAP. Although the euglycemic hyperinsulinemic clamp technique was used in this study, the small sample size and lower CPAP adherence, which were also issues with the other United Kingdom study, may have precluded ascertainment of significant findings.[49] Subgroup analyses were performed in both of these studies with respect to good versus poor CPAP adherence, with consistency in findings of lack of improvement in metabolic parameters.[48,49]

Contrary to other studies, the parallel-design randomized controlled trial involving middle-aged, obese Australian men with moderate to severe OSA considered visceral abdominal fat as a primary outcome after 12 weeks of CPAP versus sham CPAP.[51] No differences were observed in insulin sensitivity, visceral abdominal fat, and liver fat at 12 weeks. At 24 weeks, after an additional 12 weeks of treatment for the entire group (those randomized to CPAP and sham CPAP), insulin sensitivity, but not visceral abdominal fat or liver fat, were improved over baseline. These findings suggest that a longer duration of OSA treatment may be required to observe substantive improvements in metabolic function.[51]

Two recent meta-analyses have explored the relationship of CPAP with its effect on metabolic outcomes. The first meta-analysis examined 3 parallel-group trials, 2 crossover, randomized controlled trials, and 1 randomized trial of 296 subjects. This meta-analysis did not show any influence of CPAP on plasma insulin or HOMA-IR, adiponectin levels, or HbA1c values.[87] The second meta-analysis evaluated the impact of CPAP on glycated hemoglobin. This meta-analysis included 9 observational studies and randomized trials of 151 subjects, and treatment durations ranging from 41 days to 6 months. The analysis concluded that CPAP usage in the short term did not show a reduction in HbA1c.[88]

Effect of Non–Positive Airway Pressure Modalities of Obstructive Sleep Apnea Therapy on Components of Metabolic Syndrome

There are limited data on the direct effect of bariatric surgery as treatment of OSA on metabolic parameters. Based on a recent systematic review involving 69 studies and 13,900 patients, one can surmise that irrespective of the type bariatric surgery (ie, Roux-en-Y gastric bypass, laparoscopic sleeve gastrectomy, or biliopancreatic diversion), improvement in OSA severity ensued after the bariatric intervention.[89] Data have also been amassed from numerous studies highlighting remission of type 2 diabetes after the bariatric procedures.[90] Furthermore, in a recent single-center, randomized controlled trial comparing intensive medical therapy with surgical treatment involving gastric bypass or sleeve gastrectomy as a means to improve glycemic control in obese patients with uncontrolled type 2 diabetes (and a high prevalence of metabolic syndrome), 12 months of medical therapy plus bariatric surgery achieved glycemic control in significantly more patients than did medical therapy alone.[91] Similar to evaluating PAP trials in OSA on metabolic function, it is unclear whether an improvement in metabolic regulation in treated OSA is a function of direct effects of reversing OSA pathophysiology versus reduction in body fat, or as a direct or indirect result of OSA treatment. A recently published randomized trial helps to shed light on the answer to this question.[92] The trial involved obese patients with moderate to severe OSA randomized to conventional weight loss versus laparoscopic adjustable gastric banding, and examined the AHI as well as changes in anthropometrics and metabolic variables. Despite major differences in weight loss, there was no statistically significant reduction in AHI between the 2 groups, nor was there significant improvement in metabolic syndrome, lipid profile, or glycemic control. These findings imply that despite weight reduction, if OSA is not adequately ameliorated by intervention (in this case bariatric surgery), achieving improvement in metabolic parameters does not occur. These data suggest that addressing OSA pathophysiology in the face of weight loss is likely a key factor in improving metabolic function.[92] Regarding investigation of the effects of other non-PAP therapies for OSA on metabolic function such as oral appliances and upper airway surgery, there are virtually no data that investigate the effects on glucose homeostasis or lipid profiles, underscoring the need for future research in these areas.

SUMMARY

In summary, these uncontrolled and controlled studies across a vast array of different ethnicities and racial backgrounds show that the effects of OSA treatment on metabolic outcomes have been discrepant, despite adequate biological plausibility to support the notion of anticipated benefits of therapeutic interventions for OSA on metabolic regulation. The external validity of existing studies applies primarily to middle-aged, obese men. Although the data from the PAP randomized controlled trials have been inconsistent, 3 of the 6 trials conducted to date that demonstrated improvements in metabolic function, either overall or in subgroup analyses, involved larger sample sizes and were likely more appropriately powered to detect changes in metabolic outcomes.[47,85,86] Moreover, 2 of the 3 trials that showed significant metabolic improvements used crossover designs, which are inherently more efficient and allow for enhanced power given a similar number of participants enrolled in a parallel-design trial.[47,85] The randomized trial studies involved predominantly obese, sleepy, middle-aged participants, and all except 1 involved primarily male participants, thereby limiting the associated generalizability, and highlighting the need to focus future investigations on the metabolic function of nonobese individuals or women. Although 2 of the uncontrolled studies involved a follow-up period of 6 to 12 months, the randomized controlled trials involved follow-up periods of 6 to 12 weeks, time frames that may be too short to appreciate metabolic improvements. Differences in the usage of static versus autoadjusting CPAP also characterize these studies and may also lead to differences in results. For example, if a certain subset of participants was more likely to have positional or rapid eye movement sleep–related OSA, perhaps more benefit may have been gleaned with autoadjusting than with static CPAP. Varying approaches were used in assessing insulin resistance in the randomized clinical trials, with only 1 study using the gold-standard euglycemic hyperinsulinemic clamp technique to characterize insulin resistance. Of interest, the results of the latter study were not consistent with beneficial effects of CPAP on metabolic parameters; however, the study was limited by a smaller sample size and potentially suboptimal adherence.[49] There appears to be some evidence to suggest that CPAP results in improvement in metabolic syndrome and some of its components. It is worthwhile noting that data from the largest study to date did show reversal of metabolic syndrome with OSA treatment using autotitrating PAP. It is unclear whether this is a reflection of enhanced ability to detect differences because of better power, superior CPAP adherence, the use of autoadjusting PAP, consideration of a group with pronounced daytime sleepiness and severe OSA, and/or improvements in visceral adiposity, thereby translating into metabolic improvements.[47] Another factor to consider is differential ethnicity–oriented OSA treatment effects on metabolic regulation, based on genetic susceptibility in this specific group of Indian participants.[47]

However, it is still not unambiguous that CPAP treatment of OSA decreases insulin resistance and/or improves glucose intolerance. Larger-scale randomized controlled trials with assessments of insulin sensitivity and glucose tolerance are needed to estimate the effects of CPAP in OSA patients on metabolic outcomes, perhaps with a focus on those with more severe OSA burden. Although data from bariatric intervention

in OSA reflect lack of improvement in metabolic parameters despite weight loss in the setting of nonsignificant reversal of OSA, thereby suggesting weight-independent effects of OSA treatment on metabolic regulation, adequately powered studies should be focused on addressing and better understanding the impact of weight changes on metabolic function in OSA treatment. The interplay of excessive daytime sleepiness should also be investigated, as it seems that sleepier individuals with OSA may potentially derive more metabolic benefit from OSA treatment. Questions regarding optimal duration and the amount of CPAP still remain unanswered, and will need to be addressed in future studies. Future interventional studies should also focus on populations that have not been examined closely thus far, including women, nonobese individuals, and those with severe OSA, as the latter group may in particular derive treatment benefit from a metabolic standpoint based on preliminary subgroup analyses of existing trial data. Such interventional studies are essential to delineate the causes of OSA and alterations in glucose metabolism, and the treatment effects of CPAP intervention in this patient population.

REFERENCES

1. Alberti KG, Eckel RH, Grundy SM, et al. Harmonizing the metabolic syndrome: a joint interim statement of the International Diabetes Federation Task Force on Epidemiology and Prevention; National Heart, Lung, and Blood Institute; American Heart Association; World Heart Federation; International Atherosclerosis Society; and International Association for the Study of Obesity. Circulation 2009;120: 1640–5.
2. Duvnjak L, Duvnjak M. The metabolic syndrome—an ongoing story. J Physiol Pharmacol 2009; 60(Suppl 7):19–24.
3. Lloyd-Jones D, Adams RJ, Brown TM, et al. Executive summary: heart disease and stroke statistics—2010 update: a report from the American Heart Association. Circulation 2010;121:948–54.
4. Goodson BL, Wung SF, Archbold KH. Obstructive sleep apnea hypopnea syndrome and metabolic syndrome: a synergistic cardiovascular risk factor. J Am Acad Nurse Pract 2012;24:695–703.
5. Third Report of the National Cholesterol Education Program (NCEP) Expert Panel on Detection, Evaluation, and Treatment of High Blood Cholesterol in Adults (Adult Treatment Panel III) final report. Circulation 2002;106:3143–421.
6. Mozumdar A, Liguori G. Persistent increase of prevalence of metabolic syndrome among U.S.

adults: NHANES III to NHANES 1999-2006. Diabetes Care 2011;34:216–9.

7. Wilson PW, D'Agostino RB, Parise H, et al. Metabolic syndrome as a precursor of cardiovascular disease and type 2 diabetes mellitus. Circulation 2005;112:3066–72.

8. Cameron AJ, Shaw JE, Zimmet PZ. The metabolic syndrome: prevalence in worldwide populations. Endocrinol Metab Clin North Am 2004;33:351–75 [table of contents].

9. Young T, Palta M, Dempsey J, et al. The occurrence of sleep-disordered breathing among middle-aged adults. N Engl J Med 1993;328:1230–5.

10. Young T, Peppard PE, Gottlieb DJ. Epidemiology of obstructive sleep apnea: a population health perspective. Am J Respir Crit Care Med 2002;165:1217–39.

11. Punjabi NM, Caffo BS, Goodwin JL, et al. Sleep-disordered breathing and mortality: a prospective cohort study. PLoS Med 2009;6:e1000132.

12. Young T, Finn L, Peppard PE, et al. Sleep disordered breathing and mortality: eighteen-year follow-up of the Wisconsin sleep cohort. Sleep 2008;31:1071–8.

13. Coughlin SR, Mawdsley L, Mugarza JA, et al. Obstructive sleep apnoea is independently associated with an increased prevalence of metabolic syndrome. Eur Heart J 2004;25:735–41.

14. Drager LF, Bortolotto LA, Maki-Nunes C, et al. The incremental role of obstructive sleep apnoea on markers of atherosclerosis in patients with metabolic syndrome. Atherosclerosis 2010;208:490–5.

15. Nock NL, Li L, Larkin EK, et al. Empirical evidence for "syndrome Z": a hierarchical 5-factor model of the metabolic syndrome incorporating sleep disturbance measures. Sleep 2009;32:615–22.

16. Chang TI, Tanner JM, Harada ND, et al. Prevalence of calcified carotid artery atheromas on the panoramic images of patients with syndrome Z, coexisting obstructive sleep apnea, and metabolic syndrome. Oral Surg Oral Med Oral Pathol Oral Radiol 2012;113:134–41.

17. Nakanishi-Minami T, Kishida K, Nakagawa Y, et al. Metabolic syndrome correlates intracoronary stenosis detected by multislice computed tomography in male subjects with sleep-disordered breathing. Diabetol Metab Syndr 2012;4:6.

18. Usui Y, Takata Y, Inoue Y, et al. Coexistence of obstructive sleep apnoea and metabolic syndrome is independently associated with left ventricular hypertrophy and diastolic dysfunction. Sleep Breath 2012;16:677–84.

19. Nieto FJ, Peppard PE, Young TB. Sleep disordered breathing and metabolic syndrome. WMJ 2009;108:263–5.

20. Agrawal S, Sharma SK, Sreenivas V, et al. Prevalence of metabolic syndrome in a north Indian hospital-based population with obstructive sleep apnoea. Indian J Med Res 2011;134:639–44.

21. Polotsky VY, Li J, Punjabi NM, et al. Intermittent hypoxia increases insulin resistance in genetically obese mice. J Physiol 2003;552:253–64.

22. Yokoe T, Alonso LC, Romano LC, et al. Intermittent hypoxia reverses the diurnal glucose rhythm and causes pancreatic beta-cell replication in mice. J Physiol 2008;586:899–911.

23. Wang W, Redline S, Khoo MC. Autonomic markers of impaired glucose metabolism: effects of sleep-disordered breathing. J Diabetes Sci Technol 2012;6:1159–71.

24. Chan SL, Perrett CW, Morgan NG. Differential expression of alpha 2-adrenoceptor subtypes in purified rat pancreatic islet A- and B-cells. Cell Signal 1997;9:71–8.

25. Louis M, Punjabi NM. Effects of acute intermittent hypoxia on glucose metabolism in awake healthy volunteers. J Appl Physiol 2009;106:1538–44.

26. Iiyori N, Alonso LC, Li J, et al. Intermittent hypoxia causes insulin resistance in lean mice independent of autonomic activity. Am J Respir Crit Care Med 2007;175:851–7.

27. Xu J, Long YS, Gozal D, et al. Beta-cell death and proliferation after intermittent hypoxia: role of oxidative stress. Free Radic Biol Med 2009;46:783–90.

28. Furukawa S, Fujita T, Shimabukuro M, et al. Increased oxidative stress in obesity and its impact on metabolic syndrome. J Clin Invest 2004;114:1752–61.

29. Muraki I, Tanigawa T, Yamagishi K, et al. Nocturnal intermittent hypoxia and metabolic syndrome; the effect of being overweight: the CIRCS study. J Atheroscler Thromb 2010;17:369–77.

30. Sulit L, Storfer-Isser A, Kirchner HL, et al. Differences in polysomnography predictors for hypertension and impaired glucose tolerance. Sleep 2006;29:777–83.

31. Deurveilher S, Rusak B, Semba K. Time-of-day modulation of homeostatic and allostatic sleep responses to chronic sleep restriction in rats. Am J Physiol Regul Integr Comp Physiol 2012;302:R1411–25.

32. Tasali E, Leproult R, Ehrmann DA, et al. Slow-wave sleep and the risk of type 2 diabetes in humans. Proc Natl Acad Sci U S A 2008;105:1044–9.

33. Stamatakis KA, Punjabi NM. Effects of sleep fragmentation on glucose metabolism in normal subjects. Chest 2010;137:95–101.

34. Spiegel K, Knutson K, Leproult R, et al. Sleep loss: a novel risk factor for insulin resistance and Type 2 diabetes. J Appl Physiol 2005;99:2008–19.

35. Barf RP, Meerlo P, Scheurink AJ. Chronic sleep disturbance impairs glucose homeostasis in rats. Int J Endocrinol 2010;2010:819414.

36. Baud MO, Magistretti PJ, Petit JM. Sustained sleep fragmentation affects brain temperature, food intake and glucose tolerance in mice. J Sleep Res 2013;22:3–12.

37. Kent BD, Ryan S, McNicholas WT. Obstructive sleep apnea and inflammation: relationship to cardiovascular co-morbidity. Respir Physiol Neurobiol 2011;178:475–81.

38. Calvin AD, Albuquerque FN, Lopez-Jimenez F, et al. Obstructive sleep apnea, inflammation, and the metabolic syndrome. Metab Syndr Relat Disord 2009;7:271–8.

39. Tsigos C, Papanicolaou DA, Kyrou I, et al. Dose-dependent effects of recombinant human interleukin-6 on glucose regulation. J Clin Endocrinol Metab 1997;82:4167–70.

40. Mehra R, Storfer-Isser A, Kirchner HL, et al. Soluble interleukin 6 receptor: a novel marker of moderate to severe sleep-related breathing disorder. Arch Intern Med 2006;166:1725–31.

41. Pradhan AD, Manson JE, Rifai N, et al. C-reactive protein, interleukin 6, and risk of developing type 2 diabetes mellitus. JAMA 2001;286:327–34.

42. Trakada G, Chrousos G, Pejovic S, et al. Sleep apnea and its association with the stress system, inflammation, insulin resistance and visceral obesity. Sleep Med Clin 2007;2:251–61.

43. Hutcheson R, Rocic P. The metabolic syndrome, oxidative stress, environment, and cardiovascular disease: the great exploration. Exp Diabetes Res 2012;2012:271028.

44. Robinson GV, Pepperell JC, Segal HC, et al. Circulating cardiovascular risk factors in obstructive sleep apnoea: data from randomised controlled trials. Thorax 2004;59:777–82.

45. Borgel J, Sanner BM, Bittlinsky A, et al. Obstructive sleep apnoea and its therapy influence high-density lipoprotein cholesterol serum levels. Eur Respir J 2006;27:121–7.

46. Phillips CL, Yee BJ, Marshall NS, et al. Continuous positive airway pressure reduces postprandial lipidemia in obstructive sleep apnea: a randomized, placebo-controlled crossover trial. Am J Respir Crit Care Med 2011;184:355–61.

47. Sharma SK, Agrawal S, Damodaran D, et al. CPAP for the metabolic syndrome in patients with obstructive sleep apnea. N Engl J Med 2011;365:2277–86.

48. Coughlin SR, Mawdsley L, Mugarza JA, et al. Cardiovascular and metabolic effects of CPAP in obese males with OSA. Eur Respir J 2007;29:720–7.

49. West SD, Nicoll DJ, Wallace TM, et al. Effect of CPAP on insulin resistance and HbA1c in men with obstructive sleep apnoea and type 2 diabetes. Thorax 2007;62:969–74.

50. Gradmark AM, Rydh A, Renstrom F, et al. Computed tomography-based validation of abdominal adiposity measurements from ultrasonography, dual-energy X-ray absorptiometry and anthropometry. Br J Nutr 2010;104:582–8.

51. Hoyos CM, Killick R, Yee BJ, et al. Cardiometabolic changes after continuous positive airway pressure for obstructive sleep apnoea: a randomised sham-controlled study. Thorax 2012;67:1081–9.

52. Kritikou I, Basta M, Tappouni R, et al. Sleep apnoea and visceral adiposity in middle-aged male and female subjects. Eur Respir J 2013;41:601–9.

53. Sivam S, Phillips CL, Trenell MI, et al. Effects of 8 weeks of continuous positive airway pressure on abdominal adiposity in obstructive sleep apnoea. Eur Respir J 2012;40:913–8.

54. Chin K, Shimizu K, Nakamura T, et al. Changes in intra-abdominal visceral fat and serum leptin levels in patients with obstructive sleep apnea syndrome following nasal continuous positive airway pressure therapy. Circulation 1999;100:706–12.

55. Munzer T, Hegglin A, Stannek T, et al. Effects of long-term continuous positive airway pressure on body composition and IGF1. Eur J Endocrinol 2010;162:695–704.

56. Chobanian AV, Bakris GL, Black HR, et al. The Seventh Report of the Joint National Committee on prevention, detection, evaluation, and treatment of high blood pressure: the JNC 7 report. JAMA 2003;289:2560–72.

57. Duran-Cantolla J, Aizpuru F, Montserrat JM, et al. Continuous positive airway pressure as treatment for systemic hypertension in people with obstructive sleep apnoea: randomised controlled trial. BMJ 2010;341:c5991.

58. Barbe F, Duran-Cantolla J, Capote F, et al. Long-term effect of continuous positive airway pressure in hypertensive patients with sleep apnea. Am J Respir Crit Care Med 2010;181:718–26.

59. Faccenda JF, Mackay TW, Boon NA, et al. Randomized placebo-controlled trial of continuous positive airway pressure on blood pressure in the sleep apnea-hypopnea syndrome. Am J Respir Crit Care Med 2001;163:344–8.

60. Norman D, Loredo JS, Nelesen RA, et al. Effects of continuous positive airway pressure versus supplemental oxygen on 24-hour ambulatory blood pressure. Hypertension 2006;47:840–5.

61. Pepperell JC, Ramdassingh-Dow S, Crosthwaite N, et al. Ambulatory blood pressure after therapeutic and subtherapeutic nasal continuous positive airway pressure for obstructive sleep apnoea: a randomised parallel trial. Lancet 2002;359:204–10.

62. Alajmi M, Mulgrew AT, Fox J, et al. Impact of continuous positive airway pressure therapy on blood pressure in patients with obstructive sleep apnea

hypopnea: a meta-analysis of randomized controlled trials. Lung 2007;185:67–72.

63. Bazzano LA, Khan Z, Reynolds K, et al. Effect of nocturnal nasal continuous positive airway pressure on blood pressure in obstructive sleep apnea. Hypertension 2007;50:417–23.

64. Campos-Rodriguez F, Perez-Ronchel J, Grilo-Reina A, et al. Long-term effect of continuous positive airway pressure on BP in patients with hypertension and sleep apnea. Chest 2007;132:1847–52.

65. Becker HF, Jerrentrup A, Ploch T, et al. Effect of nasal continuous positive airway pressure treatment on blood pressure in patients with obstructive sleep apnea. Circulation 2003;107:68–73.

66. Hui DS, To KW, Ko FW, et al. Nasal CPAP reduces systemic blood pressure in patients with obstructive sleep apnoea and mild sleepiness. Thorax 2006;61:1083–90.

67. Robinson GV, Smith DM, Langford BA, et al. Continuous positive airway pressure does not reduce blood pressure in nonsleepy hypertensive OSA patients. Eur Respir J 2006;27:1229–35.

68. Kohler M, Pepperell JC, Casadei B, et al. CPAP and measures of cardiovascular risk in males with OSAS. Eur Respir J 2008;32:1488–96.

69. Kohler M, Stoewhas AC, Ayers L, et al. Effects of continuous positive airway pressure therapy withdrawal in patients with obstructive sleep apnea: a randomized controlled trial. Am J Respir Crit Care Med 2011;184:1192–9.

70. Drager LF, Pedrosa RP, Diniz PM, et al. The effects of continuous positive airway pressure on prehypertension and masked hypertension in men with severe obstructive sleep apnea. Hypertension 2011;57:549–55.

71. Barnes M, McEvoy RD, Banks S, et al. Efficacy of positive airway pressure and oral appliance in mild to moderate obstructive sleep apnea. Am J Respir Crit Care Med 2004;170:656–64.

72. Lam B, Sam K, Lam JC, et al. The efficacy of oral appliances in the treatment of severe obstructive sleep apnea. Sleep Breath 2011;15:195–201.

73. Zhang LQ, Zheng X, Wang JL, et al. Effects of oral appliance treatment upon blood pressure in mild to moderate obstructive sleep apnea-hypopnea syndrome. Zhonghua Yi Xue Za Zhi 2009;89:1807–10 [in Chinese].

74. Yoshida K. Effect on blood pressure of oral appliance therapy for sleep apnea syndrome. Int J Prosthodont 2006;19:61–6.

75. Otsuka R, Ribeiro de Almeida F, Lowe AA, et al. The effect of oral appliance therapy on blood pressure in patients with obstructive sleep apnea. Sleep Breath 2006;10:29–36.

76. Gotsopoulos H, Kelly JJ, Cistulli PA. Oral appliance therapy reduces blood pressure in obstructive sleep apnea: a randomized, controlled trial. Sleep 2004;27:934–41.

77. Andren A, Sjoquist M, Tegelberg A. Effects on blood pressure after treatment of obstructive sleep apnoea with a mandibular advancement appliance—a three-year follow-up. J Oral Rehabil 2009;36:719–25.

78. Collins R, Peto R, MacMahon S, et al. Blood pressure, stroke, and coronary heart disease. Part 2, short-term reductions in blood pressure: overview of randomised drug trials in their epidemiological context. Lancet 1990;335:827–38.

79. Harsch IA, Schahin SP, Radespiel-Troger M, et al. Continuous positive airway pressure treatment rapidly improves insulin sensitivity in patients with obstructive sleep apnea syndrome. Am J Respir Crit Care Med 2004;169:156–62.

80. Babu AR, Herdegen J, Fogelfeld L, et al. Type 2 diabetes, glycemic control, and continuous positive airway pressure in obstructive sleep apnea. Arch Intern Med 2005;165:447–52.

81. Shpirer I, Rapoport MJ, Stav D, et al. Normal and elevated HbA1C levels correlate with severity of hypoxemia in patients with obstructive sleep apnea and decrease following CPAP treatment. Sleep Breath 2012;16:461–6.

82. Dorkova Z, Petrasova D, Molcanyiova A, et al. Effects of continuous positive airway pressure on cardiovascular risk profile in patients with severe obstructive sleep apnea and metabolic syndrome. Chest 2008;134:686–92.

83. Oktay B, Akbal E, Firat H, et al. CPAP treatment in the coexistence of obstructive sleep apnea syndrome and metabolic syndrome, results of one year follow up. Acta Clin Belg 2009;64:329–34.

84. Mota PC, Drummond M, Winck JC, et al. APAP impact on metabolic syndrome in obstructive sleep apnea patients. Sleep Breath 2011;15:665–72.

85. Weinstock TG, Wang X, Rueschman M, et al. A controlled trial of CPAP therapy on metabolic control in individuals with impaired glucose tolerance and sleep apnea. Sleep 2012;35:617–625B.

86. Lam JC, Lam B, Yao TJ, et al. A randomised controlled trial of nasal continuous positive airway pressure on insulin sensitivity in obstructive sleep apnoea. Eur Respir J 2010;35:138–45.

87. Hecht L, Mohler R, Meyer G. Effects of CPAP-respiration on markers of glucose metabolism in patients with obstructive sleep apnoea syndrome: a systematic review and meta-analysis. Ger Med Sci 2011;9:Doc20.

88. Iftikhar IH, Blankfield RP. Effect of continuous positive airway pressure on hemoglobin A(1c) in patients with obstructive sleep apnea: a systematic review and meta-analysis. Lung 2012;190: 605–11.

89. Sarkhosh K, Switzer NJ, El-Hadi M, et al. The impact of bariatric surgery on obstructive sleep apnea: a systematic review. Obes Surg 2013;23: 414–23.

90. Buchwald H, Estok R, Fahrbach K, et al. Weight and type 2 diabetes after bariatric surgery: systematic review and meta-analysis. Am J Med 2009; 122:248–56.e5.

91. Schauer PR, Kashyap SR, Wolski K, et al. Bariatric surgery versus intensive medical therapy in obese patients with diabetes. N Engl J Med 2012;366: 1567–76.

92. Dixon JB, Schachter LM, O'Brien PE, et al. Surgical vs conventional therapy for weight loss treatment of obstructive sleep apnea: a randomized controlled trial. JAMA 2012;308:1142–9.

Effects of Obstructive Sleep Apnea Therapy on Cardiovascular Disease

Neomi Shah, MD, MPH[a], Jorge R. Kizer, MD, MSc[b],
H. Klar Yaggi, MD, MPH[c],*

KEYWORDS

- Obstructive sleep apnea • Subclinical atherosclerosis • Coronary heart disease
- Cardiac arrhythmias • Stroke

KEY POINTS

- Sleep apnea occurs when the upper airway collapses during sleep resulting in a cycle of hypoxemia, increased respiratory effort, frequent arousals, and increased sympathetic activity.
- OSA has been associated with numerous cardiovascular conditions.
- The impact of treatment of OSA on cardiovascular outcomes has been investigated.

OVERVIEW OF OBSTRUCTIVE SLEEP APNEA AND ASSOCIATED CARDIOVASCULAR OUTCOMES

Obstructive sleep apnea (OSA) is exceedingly prevalent in the United States. It occurs when the upper airway collapses during sleep resulting in a cycle of hypoxemia, increased respiratory effort, frequent arousals, and increased sympathetic activity. OSA syndrome (OSAS) is clinically defined as an apnea-hypopnea index (AHI) greater than or equal to five per hour in the presence of daytime sleepiness. However, sleep medicine has not determined precise definitions for this terminology and often OSA and OSAS are used interchangeably. It is estimated that among the western population, 24% of men and 9% of women have OSA (AHI ≥5).[1]

OSA has been associated with numerous cardiovascular conditions including hypertension,[2] coronary heart disease,[3,4] cardiac arrhythmias,[5] heart failure,[6,7] stroke,[8] and sudden death.[9] Although the specific mechanisms that explain these individual associations have not been fully delineated plausible factors that contribute to an overall increased vascular risk in the setting of underlying OSA have been investigated. They include (but are not limited to) sympathetic activation,[10] metabolic dysregulation,[11–14] endothelial dysfunction,[15,16] oxidative stress,[17] and autonomic dysfunction.[18]

The impact of treatment of OSA on cardiovascular outcomes has also been investigated, albeit not as extensively as the association studies mentioned previously (**Table 1**). Moreover, most OSA treatment investigations are predominantly observational in nature. A limited number of randomized trials exist because of ethical concerns pertaining to withholding treatment of OSA for prolonged periods of time (over 3–6 months).

[a] Pulmonary Sleep Lab, Department of Medicine, Montefiore Medical Center, Albert Einstein College of Medicine, 111 East 210th Street, Klau-3 Pulmonary Sleep Lab, Bronx, NY 10467, USA; [b] Department of Medicine, Department of Epidemiology and Population Health, Montefiore Medical Center, Albert Einstein College of Medicine, Block Room 114, 1300 Morris Park Avenue, Bronx, NY 10461, USA; [c] Program in Sleep Medicine, Section of Pulmonary, Critical Care, and Sleep Medicine, VA Clinical Epidemiology Research Center, Yale University School of Medicine, PO Box 208057, 300 Cedar Street, New Haven, CT 06520, USA
* Corresponding author.
E-mail address: henry.yaggi@yale.edu

Sleep Med Clin 8 (2013) 453–461
http://dx.doi.org/10.1016/j.jsmc.2013.07.015
1556-407X/13/$ – see front matter © 2013 Elsevier Inc. All rights reserved.

Table 1
Summary of key studies on impact of OSA treatment on CVD

CVD of Interest	Type of Study	Sample Size	Duration of Treatment	Impact of Treatment of OSA
Subclinical atherosclerosis[22]	Randomized controlled study	N = 24 (males only)	4 mo of CPAP	Significant decrease in carotid intima-media thickness in treatment group
Subclinical atherosclerosis[23]	Randomized, double-blind, placebo-controlled trial	N = 86 (cross-over design with 1 mo wash-out period)	3 mo of CPAP	Significant decrease in carotid intima-media thickness posttreatment
Subclinical atherosclerosis[24]	Nonrandomized study	N = 50	12 mo CPAP	Significant long-term beneficial impact of CPAP therapy on carotid intima-media thickness
Arrhythmias[29]	Nonrandomized study	N = 316	1 night of CPAP	Significant reduction in occurrence of paroxysmal atrial fibrillation, sinus bradycardia, and sinus pause
Arrhythmias[30]	Randomized controlled trial	N = 83 (males only)	1 mo	No significant change in the frequency of any cardiac arrhythmias
Arrhythmias[31]	Nonrandomized study	N = 29 (patients with heart failure with both obstructive and central sleep apnea)	1 night of CPAP	Significant reduction in nocturnal premature ventricular contractions and couplets
Arrhythmias[32]	Nonrandomized study	N = 23	14 mo CPAP	Significant decrease in sinus pauses and bradycardia No significant difference in supraventricular arrhythmias
Coronary artery disease and stroke[35]	Nonrandomized study	N = 1347 (men only)	10 y follow-up	Significantly fewer number of nonfatal and fatal coronary and cerebrovascular events in treated patients with OSA compared with untreated patients with severe OSA

Abbreviations: CPAP, continuous positive airway pressure; CVD, cardiovascular disease.

SUBCLINICAL ATHEROSCLEROSIS

Atherosclerosis, a chronic disorder characterized by lipid accumulation and inflammation in the vascular wall, has been proposed as a mechanistic link between OSA and cardiovascular disease. Atherosclerosis is usually asymptomatic for many years before its manifestation in the form of a cardiovascular event, such as myocardial infarction. This presence of clinically inapparent atherosclerosis (ie, subclinical atherosclerosis) can be measured using several noninvasive and invasive techniques including B-mode ultrasound, computed tomography, magnetic resonance imaging, and catheter-based angiography. Several noninvasive measures of subclinical atherosclerosis have been identified and include carotid intima-media thickness[19] and arterial stiffness,[20] with the latter determined using pulse wave velocity or other techniques.[21] This section reviews the studies that have examined the influence of continuous positive airway pressure (CPAP) treatment on the previously noted measures of subclinical atherosclerosis.

Drager and colleagues[22] designed a randomized controlled study to test the hypothesis, "treatment of OSA with CPAP therapy significantly improves validated markers of early signs of atherosclerosis, namely carotid intima-media thickness (primary outcome), arterial stiffness, and carotid diameter (secondary outcomes)". In this study they excluded individuals with any comorbidity including hypertension, diabetes, heart failure, coronary artery disease (CAD), stroke, smoking, and chronic use of medications. All patients underwent a routine attended, in-laboratory polysomnogram. They defined apnea as complete cessation of airflow for at least 10 seconds, associated with oxygen desaturation of 3% and hypopnea as a 50% reduction in airflow for at least 10 seconds associated with oxygen desaturation of 3%. The investigators only included those patients with severe OSA (AHI >30 events per hour) who were naive to treatment. A total of 400 patients with severe OSA were screened, of whom 24 males (age, 46 ± 6) met the rigorous inclusion criteria. The patients were randomized to receive no treatment (control, N = 12) or CPAP (N = 12) for 4 months. The CPAP intensity was determined by overnight CPAP titration studies and CPAP compliance was objectively measured throughout the course of the trial. The main outcome variables for the study were measured using a high-resolution echo-tracking system (for carotid intima-media thickness) and a noninvasive automatic device (for carotid-femoral pulse-wave velocity). The baseline characteristics were similar in the two groups with no significant difference in the mean age, body mass index (BMI), waist/hip ratio, day and night systolic and diastolic blood pressure, daytime sleepiness, and baseline levels of carotid intima-media thickness and carotid-femoral pulse-wave velocity. The mean AHI was 62 ± 22 in the control group and 56 ± 22 in the CPAP group ($P = .52$). The results of this study revealed a significant decrease in

carotid intima-media thickness (707 ± 105 vs 645 ± 95 μm; $P = .04$) and pulse-wave velocity (10.4 ± 1.0 vs 9.3 ± 0.9 m/s; $P<.001$) in patients with severe OSA who were treated with CPAP (4 months) versus those with severe OSA who received no CPAP treatment. No significant changes occurred in BMI, glucose, cholesterol, and blood pressure. The authors concluded that treatment of OSA with CPAP improved markers of subclinical atherosclerosis in middle-aged overweight men with severe OSA who were free of underlying risk factors including hypertension and smoking. This study supports the notion that OSA is an independent risk factor for atherosclerosis.

Sharma and colleagues[23] demonstrated similar findings in a randomized, double-blind, placebo-controlled trial to assess the impact of treatment of OSA with CPAP on metabolic syndrome and its constituents. As part of this trial, patients with OSA underwent 3 months of therapeutic CPAP with subsequent 3 months of sham-CPAP (interspersed with a 1-month washout period). They measured various components of metabolic syndrome, as well as carotid intima-media thickness. In this trial, they found that patients with OSA who were adherent with CPAP therapy (average use of 5 hours per night) had significantly reduced carotid intima-media thickness compared with those who were less adherent (carotid intima-media thickness 0.034 vs 0.014 mm; $P<.05$).

In contrast to the aforementioned studies, which assessed the short-term impact of CPAP on subclinical atherosclerosis, Hui and colleagues recently reported the long-term impact of CPAP treatment on carotid intima-media thickness.[24] They conducted a cohort study of 50 newly diagnosed patients with OSA (ages 20–80) who received CPAP (N = 28) or conservative treatment (N = 22, at patient's discretion) and were followed prospectively for 12 months. Carotid intima-media thickness was assessed with B-mode ultrasound of the far wall of the distal 10 mm of the common carotid arteries bilaterally at baseline, 6 months, and 12 months. In this study the authors defined OSA using an attended overnight sleep study showing AHI greater than or equal to five per hour of sleep plus excessive daytime sleepiness or the presence of choking or gasping during sleep and recurrent awakenings. At baseline there was no significant difference in the two groups for the following variables: age; BMI; daytime sleepiness; AHI; oxygen saturation (minimum); and existing comorbidities. Additionally, CPAP usage was similar in the two groups at 6 months and 12 months of follow-up. Carotid artery intima-media thicknesses at baseline, 6 months, and 12 months were 758 (30), 721 (20), and 705 (20) μm for the CPAP group versus 760 (30), 770 (30), and 778 (30) μm, respectively, for the group that received conservative treatment ($P = .002$). The authors concluded that CPAP therapy has long-term beneficial impact on the carotid artery intima-media thickness, but as noted, these findings were observational.

A recent study by Buchner and colleagues[25] has also demonstrated a beneficial role of CPAP therapy in patients with OSA on subclinical atherosclerosis. They conducted a nonrandomized 6-month study to determine the impact of CPAP therapy on arterial stiffness as measured by carotid-radial pulse wave velocity. Among patients with OSA who were effectively treated with CPAP, the pulse wave velocity decreased from 9.6 ± 1.5 at baseline to 8.7 ± 1.4 at follow-up ($P<.05$). Patients who were not treated effectively with CPAP had no improvement in arterial wall stiffness measurement. The study does not, however, report on the characteristics of the two groups (effective and noneffective users of CPAP) and it does not provide information on lifestyle and compliance with cardiovascular medications that can confound the relationship between CPAP and the outcome of interest.

In summary, there is accumulating evidence to support a beneficial impact of short- and long-term CPAP therapy on subclinical atherosclerosis in patients with OSA, although caution is warranted because the evidence comes from small studies, and much of it is non-randomized. It is important to acknowledge that most of the studies noted here emphasized the importance of "effective" CPAP therapy (ie, nightly CPAP use of at least 4 hours and up to 6 hours) to significantly improve markers of subclinical atherosclerosis.

ARRHYTHMIAS

OSA has been shown to be associated with cardiac arrhythmias.[5,26–28] This was documented in a cross-sectional study by Mehra and colleagues[5] using data from the Sleep Heart Health Study. In this study (N = 566), OSA was independently associated with atrial fibrillation (odds ratio [OR], 4.02; 95% confidence interval [CI], 1.03–15.74); nonsustained ventricular tachycardia (OR, 3.40; 95% CI, 1.03–11.20); and complex ventricular ectopy (OR, 1.74; 95% CI, 1.11–2.74).

Several studies have examined the effect of CPAP therapy on cardiac arrhythmias. Some of these studies have evaluated short-term impact (diagnostic night vs titration night), whereas others have evaluated a longer-term impact of CPAP therapy on cardiac arrhythmias.

A Japanese study[29] of 1394 participants (N= 108 men; all underwent overnight polysomnography for the diagnosis of OSA) evaluated the short-term impact of CPAP therapy on various cardiac arrhythmias. The investigators found a significant association between OSA status and the presence of cardiac arrhythmias, such as paroxysmal atrial fibrillation, premature ventricular complexes, sinus bradycardia, and sinus pauses. A total of 1047 of the study participants had an AHI of greater than or equal to 20 per hour. Of these, 316 participants accepted CPAP treatment and underwent a CPAP titration study (roughly 3–4 weeks after the diagnostic test). On the second night of effective CPAP therapy in patients with OSA, a significant reduction in the occurrence of paroxysmal atrial fibrillation ($P<.001$), premature ventricular complexes ($P = .016$), sinus bradycardia ($P = .001$), and sinus pauses ($P = .004$) was found.[29]

Contrary to the previously mentioned study, Craig and colleagues[30] found no beneficial role of CPAP therapy on cardiac arrhythmias in patients with OSA. They conducted a randomized controlled trial (N = 83 males; moderate to severe OSA) to investigate the impact of therapeutic CPAP therapy versus subtherapeutic CPAP (<1 cm H_2O) on the presence of pauses, bradycardias, and supraventricular and ventricular arrhythmias. Before initiation of the trial and 1 month post effective use of CPAP therapy, all participants underwent three-channel 24-hour electrocardiograms. The two groups were well matched for age, BMI, OSA severity, and cardiovascular history. The trial revealed that there was no significant change in the frequencies of any of the cardiac arrhythmias noted previously (day or night time) after 1 month of CPAP therapy.

Javaheri[31] has also investigated the role of CPAP therapy on cardiac arrhythmias, specifically studying patients with congestive heart failure with a mixture of obstructive and central sleep apnea. A total of 29 patients with heart failure with consecutive polysomnogram studies were recruited and patients with an AHI of 15 or more per hour of sleep (N = 21 central sleep apnea; N = 8 OSA) were identified. These patients were subjected to a second night of CPAP titration study. In patients whose sleep apnea was effectively treated by CPAP, there was a significant reduction in hourly episodes of nocturnal premature ventricular contractions (66 ± 117 vs 18 ± 20; $P = .055$) and couplets (3.2 ± 6 vs 0.2 ± 0.21; $P = .031$).

Another study[32] evaluated the long-term impact of CPAP therapy on arrhythmias in 23 patients (N = 16 men; mean age, 50 ± 11 years) with moderate to severe OSA. Using an insertable loop recorder capable of 16-month cardiac -arrhythmia monitoring, this group of investigators assessed the presence of cardiac pauses (>3 seconds) and bradycardic episodes (<40 bpm) during a 2-month period before and for 14 months after CPAP therapy. Holter recording (48 hours) was also done in this study before and after CPAP treatment. The investigators found the diagnostic capability of the Holter recording to be insufficient compared with the insertable loop recorder. After 8 weeks of CPAP therapy, the median number of bradycardia events dropped significantly (5.5 to 0.5; $P = .028$). Similarly, the number of pauses decreased 8 weeks post-CPAP treatment. The authors also commented, "Supra-ventricular arrhythmias were present to a lesser extent and did not seem to be affected significantly by CPAP treatment."

The previously cited studies and others[33,34] suggest a beneficial role of CPAP therapy on cardiac arrhythmias. The randomized controlled trial findings from Craig and colleagues[30] did not show any significant difference in the prevalence of cardiac arrhythmias before and after CPAP therapy among patients with OSA. Although this study[30] had numerous strengths, some of the limitations that could account for lack of benefit from CPAP therapy on cardiac arrhythmias included one-time 24-hour cardiac monitoring versus continuous monitoring, which seems to have better capability to detect arrhythmias as demonstrated by Simantirakis and colleagues;[32] and that the study was limited to a short-term follow-up (1 month), such that longer follow-up might have demonstrated benefit, as suggested by others.[32] Further investigations are needed to assess the impact of CPAP on cardiac arrhythmias among patients with OSA. These investigations should include women, use continuous cardiac monitoring, and have follow-up over an extended time period.

CORONARY HEART DISEASE

OSA has been shown to be an independent risk factor for coronary heart disease events.[3,4,7] The impact of treatment of OSA with CPAP on long-term cardiovascular outcomes has been investigated in numerous studies. These studies have been largely observational in nature.

A landmark study pertinent to this area was from Marin and colleagues.[35] In their study, the investigators recruited 1387 men from a sleep clinic–based sample and an additional 264 healthy men (age- and BMI- matched with an untreated severe OSA subgroup) from a population-based sample. All patients underwent in-laboratory attended polysomnogram. Patients with an AHI greater than 30 per hour and those with an AHI between 5 and 30 plus daytime sleepiness or cardiac failure were offered CPAP therapy. The rest of the patients were offered conservative advice including weight loss, avoidance of alcohol, smoking, and sedatives, and appropriate sleep hygiene. All patients were followed forward in time (10 years) with yearly clinic appointments for the major end point of fatal or nonfatal cardiovascular events (including acute coronary syndromes, myocardial infarction, and stroke).

Objective CPAP compliance was ascertained at each visit. Of the 1347 patients, 377 had simple snoring; 403 had mild-moderate OSA (untreated); 235 had severe OSA (untreated); and 372 had treated OSA with CPAP. The results from this study are detailed in **Table 2**. Patients with untreated severe OSA were found to have an increased risk of fatal and nonfatal cardiovascular events (after adjusting for confounding variables listed in **Table 2**). Patients with no sleep apnea (snorers), untreated mild-moderate OSA, and treated OSA with CPAP had no significant increase in the risk of either fatal or nonfatal cardiac events. The authors of this study did not provide specific ORs for component outcomes (ie, coronary or cerebrovascular event specific). Therefore, it is not possible to determine the impact of CPAP therapy on coronary heart disease–specific events (fatal or nonfatal).[35] Furthermore, the observational nature of this study leaves it open to unmeasured

Table 2		
Adjusted OR for nonfatal and fatal cardiovascular events		
	Adjusted OR[a] (CI, *P* Value)	
Diagnostic Group	**Nonfatal Cardiovascular Events**	**Fatal Cardiovascular Events**
Snoring	1.32 (0.64–3.01, 0.38)	1.03 (0.31–1.84, 0.88)
Mild-moderate OSA	1.57 (0.62–3.16, 0.22)	1.15 (0.34–2.69, 0.71)
Severe OSA	3.17 (1.12–7.52, 0.001)	2.87 (1.17–7.51, 0.025)
CPAP	1.42 (0.52–3.40, 0.29)	1.05 (0.39–2.21, 0.74)

[a] Variable in the fully adjusted mode includes age; diagnostic group; presence of cardiovascular disease; hypertension; diabetes; lipid disorders; smoking status; alcohol use; systolic and diastolic blood pressure; blood glucose; total cholesterol; triglycerides; and current use of antihypertensive, lipid-lowering, and antidiabetic drugs.

or residual confounding. Despite these limitations, this study was the first of its kind to demonstrate a significant impact of CPAP therapy on cardiovascular outcomes over a long-term period.

Another study by Milleron and colleagues[36] investigated the long-term effect of treating OSA on cardiovascular events in patients with underlying CAD. They found that OSA treatment significantly reduced the number of cardiovascular events (acute coronary syndrome, need for coronary revascularization, hospitalization for heart failure, or cardiovascular death), which occurred in 24% in the treated group versus 58% in the untreated group ($P<.01$) over a period of 86.5 ± 39 months. At baseline, the two groups were similar in risk factors for cardiovascular disease and in corresponding, non-OSA specific therapies. Most patients in the intervention group (N = 25) were treated with CPAP (N = 21), with a small fraction treated with upper airway surgery (N = 4). Similarly, others have shown that treatment of OSA is associated with improved cardiovascular outcomes in the setting of acute or chronic CAD. A recent cohort study[37] of 192 patients with acute myocardial infarction and 96 matched control subjects without CAD (ratio 2:1) revealed that treated patients with OSA (AHI $\geq$5 per hour) had a lower risk of recurrent myocardial infarction (adjusted hazard ratio, 0.16; 0.03–0.76, 0.021) and revascularization (adjusted hazard ratio, 0.15; 0.03–0.79, 0.025) compared with untreated patients with OSA.

Despite such data suggesting a beneficial role of treatment of OSA on cardiovascular outcomes (either in the setting of CAD[36] or outside of the setting of acute coronary syndromes[35]), there is as yet no evidence from large-scale randomized studies regarding this question. In the last few years, however, several randomized clinical trials have been launched to assess the impact of OSA treatment on the risk of cardiovascular disease. One such trial, currently underway in Europe, is the Randomized Intervention with CPAP in CAD and OSA (RICCADSA) Study[38] (N = 400 patients). It will assess the impact of CPAP on a composite end point of new coronary revascularization, myocardial infarction, stroke, and cardiovascular mortality among those with both CAD and OSA. Similarly, in the United States, a multicenter study called the Heart Biomarker Evaluation in Apnea Treatment was recently completed (August 2012). This study randomized patients with OSA and CAD or CAD risk factors to CPAP, nocturnal oxygen, and healthy lifestyle instruction. The major goal of this trial is to determine whether CPAP or oxygen alter cardiac biomarkers including (but not limited to) measures of systemic inflammation and oxidative stress, cardiac rhythm, impulse generation, and myocardial ischemia or stress. Finally, another clinical trial, Continuous Positive Airway Pressure Treatment of Obstructive Sleep Apnea to Prevent Cardiovascular Disease[39] (SAVE), is underway and will be the largest clinical trial to date in the sleep apnea field (anticipated completion September 2015). "The overall aim of SAVE is to determine if CPAP can reduce the risk of heart attack, stroke or heart failure for people with OSA." This trial plans to recruit 5000 participants and will be multicenter, involving various countries including China, India, Australia, and New Zealand. Similar to the RICCADSA trial, it will evaluate the impact of OSA treatment with CPAP on incidence of serious cardiovascular events among those with established cardiovascular disease.

Clinical trials such as these are essential to assessing the impact of CPAP therapy on important clinical outcomes, specifically those pertaining to the cardiovascular system. However, ethical and regulatory topics continue to be a major focus of concern for investigators in the field of sleep medicine. A recent article by Brown and colleagues[40] reviews important information (including follow-up duration) on ethical issues pertaining to the design and conduct of clinical trials in OSA.

STROKE

The incidence of stroke approaches 800,000 cases per year, and this disorder ranks as the fourth leading cause of death, in the United States.[41] Established risk factors for cerebrovascular disease include atrial fibrillation, age older than 65 years, arterial hypertension, heart disease, asymptomatic carotid stenosis, history of transient ischemic attack (TIA), alcohol abuse, smoking, diabetes mellitus, and hypercholesterolemia.[41] These factors account only partially for the variability in stroke incidence, however, so far efforts aimed at stroke prevention require identification of additional modifiable risk factors. One such factor that has emerged in recent years is the presence of sleep-related breathing disorders (SRBDs), which comprise OSA, snoring, upper airway resistance syndrome, and central sleep apnea (including Cheyne-Stokes breathing).[42,43] SDBDs are highly prevalent in the general population, affecting 2% to 4% of adults.[1] Much higher rates are consistently observed in the population of patients who have suffered a stroke or TIA, however, with estimates ranging from 44% to 72% across series.[42–45] Data accumulated from prospective observational studies implicate SRBDs in the

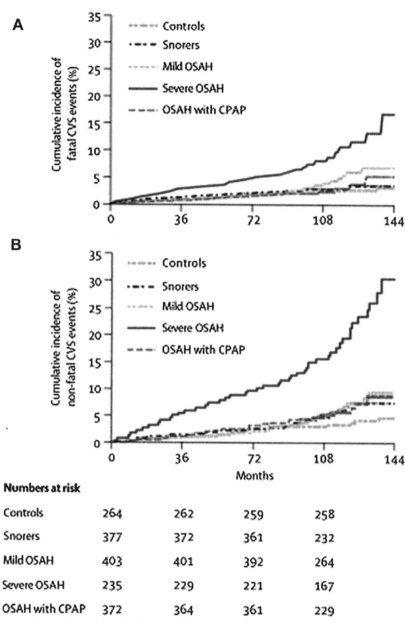

Numbers at risk				
Controls	264	262	259	258
Snorers	377	372	361	232
Mild OSAH	403	401	392	264
Severe OSAH	235	229	221	167
OSAH with CPAP	372	364	361	229

Fig. 1. Data from a large observational cohort study that compared rates of fatal and nonfatal cardiovascular events (including percutaneous or surgical coronary revascularization, myocardial infarction, stroke) in patients with OSA versus simple snorers or healthy participants. The presence of severe OSA (AHI >30) was associated with a significantly increased risk of fatal (A) and nonfatal (B) cardiovascular events. cardiovascular system; OSA. (*From* Marin JM, Carrizo SJ, Vicente E, et al. Long-term cardiovascular outcomes in men with obstructive sleep apnea-hypopnea with or without treatment with continuous positive airway pressure: an observational study. Lancet 2005;365:1046–53; with permission.)

pathogenesis of ischemic stroke.[42,43,45,46] Therefore, SRBDs offer an important target for future studies aimed at improving stroke outcomes.

The mainstay for treatment of SRBDs is positive airway pressure, with the particular type of therapy determined by the specific SRBD. Existing data have been mixed regarding whether CPAP use can improve outcomes in patients with stroke. Most studies to date have been limited by small sample sizes, methodologic flaws, and nonrandomized design. There are not yet data from randomized controlled trials supporting a benefit of CPAP for either primary or secondary stroke prevention.

One large observational study[35] followed more than 1000 individuals who were either diagnosed with OSA; simple snorers (AHI <5); or healthy adults. CPAP therapy was recommended to all patients with OSA and either AHI greater than 30 or AHI 5 to 30 with symptoms of excessive daytime sleepiness or coexistent heart failure. Over the course of 10 years, patients with untreated severe OSA (AHI >30) had a significantly higher incidence of fatal and nonfatal cardiovascular events than did healthy subjects (**Fig. 1**). By contrast, similar outcomes were seen in patients with OSA treated with CPAP and healthy participants. These data support a possible benefit of CPAP for improving cardiovascular and cerebrovascular outcomes in patients with severe OSA. Because this was not a randomized trial, however, it is possible that the poorer outcomes seen in the patients with severe OSA who refused CPAP may reflect confounding risk factors, such as poor adherence to other medical therapies and the presence of unaccounted comorbidities.

In summary, current knowledge remains limited regarding whether CPAP therapy can modify the natural history of stroke. At present there are no established guidelines recommending screening for SRBDs in patients with stroke or TIA. Because approximately 15% of strokes are preceded by a TIA, patients with TIA or minor stroke may represent particularly important candidates for CPAP as a means of prevention of subsequent cerebro vascular events. We await the results of several ongoing trials[47–49] examining the impact of CPAP therapy on clinical outcomes in patients with underlying cerebrovascular disease and SRBDs.

REFERENCES

1. Young T, Palta M, Dempsey J, et al. The occurrence of sleep-disordered breathing among middle-aged adults. N Engl J Med 1993;328:1230–5.
2. Peppard P, Young T, Palta M, et al. Prospective study of the association between sleep-disordered breathing and hypertension. N Engl J Med 2000; 342:1378–84.
3. Peker Y, Kraiczi H, Hedner J, et al. An independent association between obstructive sleep apnoea and coronary artery disease. Eur Respir J 1999;14(1): 179–84.
4. Shah NA, Yaggi HK, Concato J, et al. Obstructive sleep apnea as a risk factor for coronary events or cardiovascular death. Sleep Breath 2010;14(2): 131–6.
5. Mehra R, Benjamin EJ, Shahar E, et al. Association of nocturnal arrhythmias with sleep-disordered breathing: the sleep heart health study. Am J Respir Crit Care Med 2006;173(8):910–6.
6. Gottlieb DJ, Yenokyan G, Newman AB, et al. Prospective study of obstructive sleep apnea and incident coronary heart disease and heart failure: the sleep heart health study. Circulation 2010;122(4): 352–60.
7. Shahar E, Whitney C, Redline S, et al. Sleep-disordered breathing and cardiovascular disease: cross-sectional results of the Sleep Heart Health Study. Am J Respir Crit Care Med 2001;163:19–25.
8. Yaggi H, Brass L, Kernan W, et al. Obstructive sleep apnea as a risk factor for stroke. Stroke 2004;316:365.
9. Gami AS, Howard DE, Olson EJ, et al. Day-night pattern of sudden death in obstructive sleep apnea. N Engl J Med 2005;352(12):1206–14.
10. Wolk R, Shamsuzzaman AS, Somers VK. Obesity, sleep apnea, and hypertension. Hypertension 2003;42(6):1067–74.
11. Ip MS, Lam B, Ng MM, et al. Obstructive sleep apnea is independently associated with insulin resistance. Am J Respir Crit Care Med 2002;165(5):670–6.
12. Punjabi NM, Polotsky VY. Disorders of glucose metabolism in sleep apnea. J Appl Physiol 2005;99(5): 1998–2007.
13. Gottlieb DJ, Punjabi NM, Newman AB, et al. Association of sleep time with diabetes mellitus and impaired glucose tolerance. Arch Intern Med 2005; 165(8):863–7.
14. Van Cauter E, Holmback U, Knutson K, et al. Impact of sleep and sleep loss on neuroendocrine and metabolic function. Horm Res 2007;67(Suppl 1):2–9.
15. Nieto FJ, Herrington DM, Redline S, et al. Sleep apnea and markers of vascular endothelial function in a large community sample of older adults. Am J Respir Crit Care Med 2004;169(3):354–60.
16. Faulx MD, Larkin EK, Hoit BD, et al. Sex influences endothelial function in sleep-disordered breathing. Sleep 2004;27(6):1113–20.
17. Lavie L. Obstructive sleep apnoea syndrome: an oxidative stress disorder. Sleep Med Rev 2003; 7(1):35–51.
18. Narkiewicz K, Somers VK. Cardiovascular variability characteristics in obstructive sleep apnea. Auton Neurosci 2001;90(1–2):89–94.
19. Lorenz MW, Markus HS, Bots ML, et al. Prediction of clinical cardiovascular events with carotid intima-media thickness: a systematic review and meta-analysis. Circulation 2007;115(4):459–67.
20. Herrington DM, Brown WV, Mosca L, et al. Relationship between arterial stiffness and subclinical aortic atherosclerosis. Circulation 2004;110(4):432–7.
21. Nagahama H, Soejima M, Uenomachi H, et al. Pulse wave velocity as an indicator of atherosclerosis in obstructive sleep apnea syndrome patients. Intern Med 2004;43(3):184–8.
22. Drager LF, Bortolotto LA, Figueiredo AC, et al. Effects of continuous positive airway pressure on

early signs of atherosclerosis in obstructive sleep apnea. Am J Respir Crit Care Med 2007;176(7): 706–12.

23. Sharma SK, Agrawal S, Damodaran D, et al. CPAP for the metabolic syndrome in patients with obstructive sleep apnea. N Engl J Med 2011; 365(24):2277–86.

24. Hui DS, Shang Q, Ko FW, et al. A prospective cohort study of the long-term effects of CPAP on carotid artery intima-media thickness in obstructive sleep apnea syndrome. Respir Res 2012;13:22.

25. Buchner NJ, Quack I, Stegbauer J, et al. Treatment of obstructive sleep apnea reduces arterial stiffness. Sleep Breath 2012;16(1):123–33.

26. Monahan K, Storfer-Isser A, Mehra R, et al. Triggering of nocturnal arrhythmias by sleep-disordered breathing events. J Am Coll Cardiol 2009;54(19):1797–804.

27. Mehra R, Stone KL, Varosy PD, et al. Nocturnal arrhythmias across a spectrum of obstructive and central sleep-disordered breathing in older men: outcomes of sleep disorders in older men (MrOS sleep) study. Arch Intern Med 2009;169(12):1147–55.

28. Kohler U, Bredenbroker D, Fus E, et al. Cardiac arrhythmias in sleep apnea. Increased cardiovascular risk caused by nocturnal arrhythmia? Fortschr Med 1998;116(16):28–31.

29. Abe H, Takahashi M, Yaegashi H, et al. Efficacy of continuous positive airway pressure on arrhythmias in obstructive sleep apnea patients. Heart Vessels 2010;25(1):63–9.

30. Craig S, Pepperell JC, Kohler M, et al. Continuous positive airway pressure treatment for obstructive sleep apnoea reduces resting heart rate but does not affect dysrhythmias: a randomised controlled trial. J Sleep Res 2009;18(3):329–36.

31. Javaheri S. Effects of continuous positive airway pressure on sleep apnea and ventricular irritability in patients with heart failure. Circulation 2000; 101(4):392–7.

32. Simantirakis EN, Schiza SI, Marketou ME, et al. Severe bradyarrhythmias in patients with sleep apnoea: the effect of continuous positive airway pressure treatment: a long-term evaluation using an insertable loop recorder. Eur Heart J 2004;25(12):1070–6.

33. Harbison J, O'Reilly P, McNicholas WT. Cardiac rhythm disturbances in the obstructive sleep apnea syndrome: effects of nasal continuous positive airway pressure therapy. Chest 2000;118(3): 591–5.

34. Kanagala R, Murali N, Friedman P, et al. Obstructive sleep apnea and the recurrence of atrial fibrillation. Circulation 2003;107:2589–94.

35. Marin JM, Carrizo SJ, Vicente E, et al. Long-term cardiovascular outcomes in men with obstructive sleep apnoea-hypopnoea with or without treatment with continuous positive airway pressure: an observational study. Lancet 2005;365(9464):1046–53.

36. Milleron O, Pilliere R, Foucher A, et al. Benefits of obstructive sleep apnoea treatment in coronary artery disease: a long-term follow-up study. Eur Heart J 2004;25(9):728–34.

37. Garcia-Rio F, Alonso-Fernandez A, Armada E, et al. CPAP effect on recurrent episodes in patients with sleep apnea and myocardial infarction. Int J Cardiol 2013. [Epub ahead of print].

38. Peker Y, Glantz H, Thunstrom E, et al. Rationale and design of the Randomized Intervention with CPAP in Coronary Artery Disease and Sleep Apnoea–RICCADSA trial. Scand Cardiovasc J 2009;43(1):24–31.

39. McEvoy RD, Anderson CS, Antic NA, et al. The sleep apnea cardiovascular endpoints (SAVE) trial: rationale and start-up phase. J Thorac Dis 2010;2(3): 138–43.

40. Brown DL, Anderson CS, Chervin RD, et al. Ethical issues in the conduct of clinical trials in obstructive sleep apnea. J Clin Sleep Med 2011;7(1):103–8.

41. Go AS, Mozaffarian D, Roger VL, et al. Executive summary: heart disease and stroke statistics–2013 update: a report from the American Heart Association. Circulation 2013;127(1):143–52.

42. Yaggi H, Mohsenin V. Obstructive sleep apnoea and stroke. Lancet Neurol 2004;3(6):333–42.

43. Redline S, Yenokyan G, Gottlieb DJ, et al. Obstructive sleep apnea-hypopnea and incident stroke: the sleep heart health study. Am J Respir Crit Care Med 2010;182(2):269–77.

44. Bassetti CL, Milanova M, Gugger M. Sleep-disordered breathing and acute ischemic stroke: diagnosis, risk factors, treatment, evolution, and long-term clinical outcome. Stroke 2006;37(4): 967–72.

45. Yaggi HK, Concato J, Kernan WN, et al. Obstructive sleep apnea as a risk factor for stroke and death. N Engl J Med 2005;353(19):2034–41.

46. Mohsenin V. Is sleep apnea a risk factor for stroke? A critical analysis. Minerva Med 2004; 95(4):291–305.

47. Bravata DM, Ferguson J, Miech EJ, et al. Diagnosis and treatment of sleep apnea in patients' homes: the rationale and methods of the "GoToSleep" randomized-controlled trial. J Clin Sleep Med 2012;8(1):27–35.

48. Brown DL, Chervin RD, Kalbfleisch JD, et al. Sleep apnea treatment after stroke (SATS) trial: is it feasible? J Stroke Cerebrovasc Dis 2011. [Epub ahead of print].

49. Bravata DM, Concato J, Fried T, et al. Continuous positive airway pressure: evaluation of a novel therapy for patients with acute ischemic stroke. Sleep 2011;34(9):1271–7.

Complex Sleep Apnea

Richard J. Castriotta, MD[a,b,]*, Ruckshanda Majid, MD[a,c]

KEYWORDS

- Complex sleep apnea • Central sleep apnea • Obstructive sleep apnea • Cheyne-Stokes respiration
- Adaptive servoventilation (ASV) • Continuous positive airway pressure (CPAP)
- Bilevel positive airway pressure (BPAP) • Periodic breathing

KEY POINTS

- Complex sleep apnea entails the combination of obstructive and central sleep apnea during the same polysomnographic study.
- Treatment-emergent central sleep apnea during administration of positive airway pressure for obstructive sleep apnea is the most common form of complex sleep apnea.
- Predisposing factors for complex sleep apnea are baseline hypocapnia and heart disease with a long circulation time and low cardiac output, or the concurrent use of opioids.
- In most cases of treatment-emergent complex sleep apnea without cardiovascular comorbidity or opioid use, the central component may resolve with use of continuous positive airway pressure sufficient to eliminate the obstructive component.
- Effective treatment of persistent complex sleep apnea can be achieved with the use of adaptive servoventilation.

INTRODUCTION

Complex sleep apnea (CompSA) may be defined as the presence of both obstructive and repetitive central sleep apnea (CSA) occurring in the same individual during the same night. This definition is in contradistinction to the more common mixed apnea, which consists of central and obstructive components during the same apneic event (**Fig. 1**). The latter can be considered part of the clinical entity of obstructive sleep apnea (OSA), and would be counted in the overall obstructive apnea hypopnea index (AHI). With CompSA, on the other hand, the obstructive and central apneic events are separate and should be reported separately in an obstructive apnea index (OAI) and a central apnea index. The term was originally used to describe a third category of sleep-disordered breathing with its own phenotype.

This description by Gilmartin and colleagues[1] referred to a sleep-disordered breathing pattern that contained both obstructive and repetitive, problematic, nonhypercapneic central events, common to 1 individual. Patients with this pattern of breathing were described to manifest obstructive events, periodic breathing, mixed apneas, obstructive events in rapid eye movement (REM) and supine position, central events in non-REM and lateral position, and time of night variation (obstructive earlier and central events in the latter part of the night). Thomas and colleagues[2] described a combination of OSA during REM sleep and periodic breathing during non-REM sleep with dominant cyclic alternating pattern (CAP) as complex sleep-disordered breathing, and Morgenthaler and colleagues[3] used the term CompSA syndrome to refer to OSA with CPAP-emergent CSA. Later reports have frequently

Disclosures: Neither of the authors has any conflicts of interest to disclose.

[a] Division of Pulmonary and Sleep Medicine, University of Texas Medical School at Houston, 6431 Fannin Street, MSB 1.274, Houston, TX 77030, USA; [b] Sleep Disorders Center, Memorial Hermann Hospital - Texas Medical Center, 6411 Fannin Street, Houston, TX 77030, USA; [c] Harris Health Sleep Disorders Center, Quentin Meese Community Hospital, 3601 North Mac Gregor Way, Houston, TX 77004, USA
* Corresponding author.
E-mail address: Richard.J.Castriotta@uth.tmc.edu

Sleep Med Clin 8 (2013) 463–475
http://dx.doi.org/10.1016/j.jsmc.2013.07.006

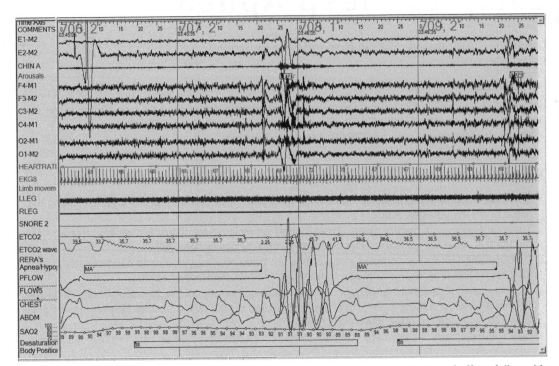

Fig. 1. Mixed apnea. Each apnea begins after deep breaths, leading to a total cessation of effort, followed by asynchronous abdominal and chest movements in an attempt to breathe against a closed airway. This condition may be scored as part of the obstructive AHI and is not considered CompSA.

used the term CompSA synonymously with CPAP-emergent CSA, but that term may more properly be reserved for the subtype of CompSA, which occurs only in the presence of positive airway pressure (PAP). This refers to the development of CSA during the administration of continuous PAP (CPAP), bilevel PAP (BPAP), or autotitrating PAP (APAP) as treatment of OSA. We use the term CompSA in the original sense. In all cases, the underlying causes of the obstructive component remains the same as in other patients, but the central component is a distinguishing feature. For practical purposes, there are 2 principal types of CSA: (1) CSA with Cheyne-Stokes pattern or Cheyne-Stokes respiration (CSR) (**Fig. 2**) and (2) CSA without CSR (**Fig. 3**). The former is usually associated with cardiac or neurologic disease, and the latter can be seen in many situations, including opioid use (cluster or ataxic breathing) and PAP-interface problems. When there is CSR with cardiac disease and systolic dysfunction, there is usually prolonged circulation time (>20 seconds). CompSA incorporates the following:

1. Primary CompSA: obstructive and central events de novo
   a. Intrinsic enhanced hypercapnic chemosensitivity
   b. Sleep stage dependent (REM, non-REM)
   c. Sleep duration-dependent (congestive heart failure with lower P_{CO_2} during later part of night)
   d. CAP-dependent (dominant cyclic alternating pattern)
2. Secondary CompSA: CSA occurring after medical intervention
   a. Treatment-emergent: arising during administration of PAP (CPAP, BPAP, APAP) for OSA
      i. Cardiac disease (high loop gain, enhanced chemosensitivity)
      ii. Hypopnea dominant
      iii. Respiratory effort-related arousal (RERAs) dominant
      iv. Mask leak
   b. Opioid-associated: low loop gain
   c. Associated with non-PAP treatment of OSA
      i. Tracheostomy
      ii. Maxillomandibular advancement surgery
      iii. Mandibular-advancing oral appliance

PATHOPHYSIOLOGY
Treatment-emergent CompSA

The pathophysiology of CompSA involves the development of both OSA and CSA with different mechanisms. Thus, there must be the usual

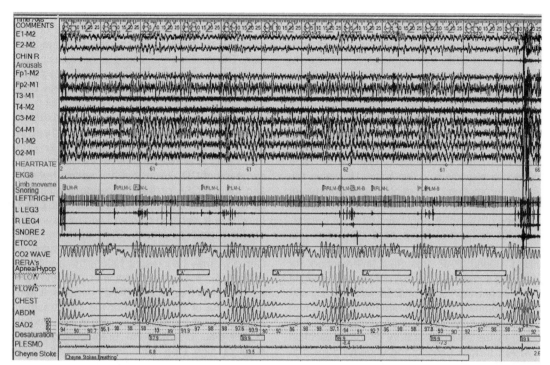

Fig. 2. CSA with CSR and long circulation time. There is a crescendo-decrescendo pattern, and the time between the end of the apnea (resumption of breathing) and the oxygen saturation nadir is more than 20 seconds. This finding suggests systolic cardiac dysfunction.

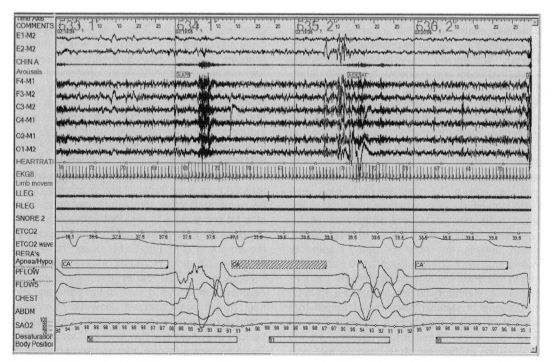

Fig. 3. CSA without Cheyne-Stokes pattern. This is an example of ataxic breathing, which can be seen with opioid use and in multiple other conditions. The circulation time is less than 20 seconds.

anatomic and physiologic predisposing features required for common OSA, plus the additional instability of the control of breathing, which produces CSA or CSR. The former are well known: anything that increases upper airway resistance plus the normal physiology of sleep, especially REM sleep, with its reduction in neuronal output of the muscles keeping the upper airways open, sometimes with the additional contributions of supine positioning. This subject is more fully discussed in the article by Ghamande and colleagues elsewhere in this issue. However, the factors promoting the central component of CompSA bear more discussion here. The various subtypes of CompSA may have different mechanisms for the central component. We begin with the most frequently seen type of CompSA: that arising during PAP treatment intervention for OSA. This subset of CompSA entails the presence of significant OSA without CSA at baseline, and the development of CSA during the application of PAP during either a titration study (CPAP or BPAP) in the sleep laboratory or the application of APAP. In these cases, the underlying mechanism is similar, and consists of a perturbation of the stability of the ventilatory control system. Under normal, waking conditions, there are 2 elements of the respiratory control system: behavioral and metabolic. During REM sleep, the behavioral system is dominant, with impaired ventilatory response to hypercapnia, especially during phasic REM sleep.[4] However, translation of sensory-stimulated central drive into muscle activity is compromised by the hyperpolarization of motor neurons.[5] This finding may explain the propensity of both hypercapnia and obstructive apnea during REM sleep. During non-REM sleep, in contrast, the metabolic control of breathing is dominant, with minimal to absent behavioral control. The system is dependent mostly on CO_2, pH, O_2 (central and peripheral chemoreceptors), and the vagus nerve (regarding lung mechanics).[6] For this reason, in adults, significant central apnea is more frequently and sometimes exclusively seen during non-REM sleep, whereas obstructive apnea is more frequently, and sometimes exclusively, seen in REM sleep.[7] Also, for this reason, central apneas (or more properly respiratory pauses) may occur during sleep/wake transitions, even in those without significant disease. The stability of the respiratory control system depends on the balance of stimulant/depressant forces that promote or inhibit breathing and the rapidity of those responses. These forces depend on the amplification of the ventilatory changes that produce CO_2 changes (plant gain) and the strength of the chemoreflexive ventilatory responsiveness

to changes in CO_2 (controller gain). The stability of the system depends on the product of plant gain and controller gain, and this is termed loop gain. Those with a high loop gain have an unstable ventilatory control system, with oscillatory behavior resulting from small changes. Those with cardiac disease may have a high loop gain with enhanced chemosensitivity exacerbated by baseline hypocapnia at sleep onset. In these patients, the application of CPAP, BPAP, or APAP may result in increased alveolar ventilation with a decrease of CO_2 lower than the apneic threshold and induce CSA or the crescendo-decrescendo pattern of CSR. Patients on opioid medications may have a low loop gain and central apnea with ataxic breathing pattern. Both occur predominantly during non-REM sleep. In both cases, the CompSA may be present before the application of PAP, but in some patients with OSA, the application of PAP, especially BPAP, may result in the emergence of CSA only after the PAP treatment has caused the lower CO_2. In those with underlying cardiac disease, the predisposing factors entail a high loop gain and enhanced carotid body chemosensitivity to CO_2, because baseline hypocapnia alone may not result in CSA.[8] Within this group of treatment-emergent CompSA, there may also be some patients with OSA without significant heart disease for whom the PAP treatment itself may have provoked central apneas as a response to increasing pressures used to more completely eliminate all traces of sleep-disordered breathing. This finding may be especially important with BPAP, in which there is pressure support with increased tidal volumes and minute ventilation ($\dot{V}_E$) with consequent reduction in CO_2.[9,10] It is theoretically possible that misinterpreted signals with some models of APAP may result in inappropriately high pressures and induced or worsening CSA, but it is also clear that attended in-laboratory titrations of CPAP or BPAP for OSA may result in the same phenomenon. This finding is because most sleep laboratories do not have the ability to clearly distinguish between obstructive and central hyopneas. There may be some clues to the obstructive nature of a hypopnea (eg, asynchronous abdominal and chest movement during non-REM sleep, termination with loud snorting, increased intercostal electromyogram), in most cases the hypopneas are deemed obstructive in view of the company they keep (obstructive apneas). However, there are some extremely obese patients who have a paucity of apneas and few apneas[11] for guidance. The other possible cause for overtitration may be the attempt to eradicate RERAs, as indicated by flattening of the nasal pressure signal without oxygen desaturation. It is possible that many of these arousals during CPAP titration may not be caused by increased upper airway resistance, but may be related to other mechanisms, including discomfort with the PAP delivery interface. It is possible to bring about the appearance of CSA during PAP titration with a large mask leak or mouth breathing with high pressures. The resultant decrease in CO_2 from washout may decrease the CO_2 lower than the apneic threshold. But overtitration or high PAP cannot be implicated as the dominant mechanism for treatment-emergent CompSA. The resolution of OSA may result in the development of CSA after treatment with tracheostomy,[12] maxillomandibular advancement surgery,[13] and mandibular-advancing oral appliances.[14,15] The pathophysiology of these cases is uncertain. The prevalence of CompSA in those without opioid use or heart failure is low.[16] Most, but not all, patients with treatment-emergent CompSA show resolution with continued PAP treatment.[17] One final pathophysiologic possibility remains to be discussed and provides a potential argument for the need to effectively treat the CSA component of CompSA. In patients with systolic heart failure and CSA, there is a high failure rate of resolution with CPAP.[18,19] In those patients whose CSA resolves on CPAP, there is an improved survival, but in those with persisting CSA on CPAP, mortality is increased.[20] According to the Javaheri hypothesis, in some patients with heart disease, PAP may increase intrathoracic pressures enough to decrease venous return to the right ventricle, shift the interventricular septum to the left, decrease stroke volume and cardiac output, and hence, worsen the chances of longer-term survival. This situation would, of course, result in a heightened loop gain, longer circulation time, and the development or persistence of the central component in those with CompSA. This may be the most compelling argument for more aggressive management of CompSA, at least in those with chronic heart failure (CHF).

Primary CompSA

Some patients with idiopathic CSA have enhanced hypoxic and hypercapnic chemosensitivity (controller gain).[21] Because there are differences among individuals with regard to hypercapnic and hypoxic chemosensitivity,[22] those who present with primary CompSA, before attempted treatment with PAP, may be patients with OSA who also have a high loop gain because of an intrinsically enhanced hypoxic or hypercapnic chemosensitivity. Among these cases of primary CompSA (not

brought about by treatment with PAP or opioid medication), some may represent the combination of OSA in REM sleep with CSA in non-REM sleep because of the different ventilatory control mechanisms in play with the different sleep states, based on the differences in the normal physiology between the wake, REM sleep, and non-REM sleep states. In other cases, the CSA develops over the course of the night in some patients with CHF coincident with a progressive decrease in P_{CO_2} as a result of increased minute ventilation, increased circulation time, and increased periodic breathing cycle length.[23] Some patients with primary CompSA may have sleep instability with transient arousals characterized by a predominant CAP.[2,24] These patients may have increased sleep instability, variable arousal thresholds, and unstable ventilatory control leading to fluctuations in CO_2 and central apnea. Gilmartin and colleagues[1] have constructed an alternative model of unstable non-REM sleep characterized by unstable breathing, low-frequency narrow-band electroencephalographic-respiratory coupling, and CAP to characterize the phenotype of those with primary CompSA.

PREVALENCE

A wide range in the prevalence of CompSA has been reported, and some variance is caused by the variable definitions used. The high prevalence rates described by some with a lower burden of disease may be explained by several factors likely related to the type of PAP titration study and associated patient comorbidities. A few studies have shown a prevalence of 13% to 20%. In a retrospective review,[3] the prevalence of patients with CompSA was 15% (after excluding patients with CHF or a left ventricular ejection fraction [LVEF] $\leq$40%). Dernaika and colleagues[25] reported that 20% of their patients with split-night studies had CPAP-emergent CSA. In a third retrospective study of 99 patients with a primary diagnosis of OSA, Lehman and colleagues[26] reported a prevalence of 13%. In this study, a history of ischemic heart disease or heart failure was more frequent among patients with CPAP-emergent CSA than among those without a history of ischemic heart disease or heart failure. These patients had a higher frequency of cardiac and cerebrovascular complications, which was presumably the reason for their higher reported prevalence. Javaheri and colleagues[17] estimated a lower prevalence of CompSA at an average of 6.5% during a 1-year period. This study was the largest study to date (n = 1286), and 2 separate nights were used for diagnostic polysomnography (PSG) and CPAP titration. Another study[27] in a Japanese population (also looking at 2 separate study nights) reported a similar lower overall prevalence of CompSAs of 5% (n = 66) after retrospectively looking at 1312 patients with sleep apnea syndrome (AHI>20). Javaheri[28] postulated that the lower prevalence he observed compared with earlier reports may be a reflection of fewer arousals and transitions in sleep stages when less aggressively titrating CPAP. Single-night split studies may lead to more sleep disruption brought about by placement of the mask and rapidly escalating pressures, with consequently more fluctuation in P_{CO_2}, which could promote instability of breathing. Overtitration may have also increased the likelihood of oral leaks, which may appear as central apneas. Pressure toxicity has been described as worsening of central apneas after increases in PAP pressure after obstructive events have been treated with increased sleep fragmentation secondary to poor tolerance to higher CPAP pressures. Lung overinflation may also cause central apneas,[29] explained by the Hering-Breuer reflex. Increased ventilation through a newly patent airway could also lead to a decrease of the P_{CO_2} lower than the apnea threshold, culminating in a central apnea and an absent drive to breathe. This situation may explain the worsening of central apneas on BPAP in the spontaneous mode with an augmentation in minute ventilation. The prevalence of CompSA therefore may vary depending on CPAP titration strategies and subject referring base.

CLINICAL CHARACTERISTICS

Clinical heterogeneity of patients with CompSA branch from the host of pathophysiologic processes and their interactions. Several studies have looked at distinguishing patient characteristics that may help predict the development of central apneas while treating underlying sleep apnea. For example, nonhypercapneic central events are seen in patients with heart disease.[28,30] However, this same complexity may make it difficult to reliably identify patients who are at risk for developing central apneas on CPAP. Identifying patients earlier may allow prescription of alternative, more effective therapies for the complex syndrome. Comparing demographics of patients with OSA, CSA, and CompSA, male sex has been found to be more common in patients with CompSAs than in those with obstructive sleep apnea/hypopnea syndrome (OSAHS) or CSA in several studies.[3,26,31] In another similar review, Thomas and colleagues[38] also noted a male predominance in patients with CompSA. There may be a physiologic explanation for the male predominance. Men

have a higher awake hypercapneic ventilatory response than women[32,33] and have a higher ventilatory response to arousals from non-REM sleep. Men hence develop greater subsequent hypoventilation on resumption of sleep.[34] This ventilatory response combined with the observation that men develop CSA after smaller reduction in end tidal CO_2 than women may add to the higher male prevalence of CSA.[35,36] Men also tend to have lighter and more disturbed sleep, again resulting in more frequent central events, which often occur during disrupted and lighter stages of sleep. Morgenthaler and colleagues[3] found no difference in body mass index (BMI, calculated as weight in kilograms divided by the square of height in meters), Epworth Sleepiness Score (ESS), hypertension (HTN), snoring, ejection fraction (they did not evaluate patients with an EF <40%), atrial fibrillation, or right ventricular systolic pressure. Another review[37] also reported no difference in clinical findings (HTN, CHF, and atrial fibrillation) and no differences in mean age, initial ESS, and total diagnostic AHI. Patients with CompSA were almost described as an entity intermediate in the spectrum spanning from OSA to CSA. Patients with CompSA had a BMI intermediate between that of patients with OSA and CSA (although not statistically different from one another).[3] Although in the largest comparative study to date,[37] patients with CompSA were found to have lower BMIs than patients with OSA. The diagnostic AHI for CompSA was also intermediate in rank (CSA = 38.3 ± 36.2 vs CompSA = 32.3 ± 26.8 vs OSAHS = 20.6 ± 23.7 per hour, P = .005). In this study, there was also a trend toward longer apnea durations in patients with CompSAs compared with OSAHS, possibly reflecting a difference in respiratory chemoreflex gain. There seem to be more reports of a higher AHI in patients with CompSA.[3,26,27,38] Javaheri and colleagues[17] also found that patients who had CompSA had a higher AHI (57 ± 27 vs 39 ± 24, P = .001), OAI, central apnea index, and apnea index compared with patients who did not develop central apneas. Some studies[3,31] have reported a higher arousal index on the baseline study in patients with CompSAs, whereas other studies[17,39,40] did not show a difference. At diagnosis, they had more central and mixed apneas in addition to more periodic breathing on the baseline (18% vs 0.8, P<.001), which may also be an indicator of persistent CompSA.[30] Sleep architectural differences in patients with CompSA have also been shown to reflect increased disturbance. This disturbance includes decreased sleep efficiency, increased sleep stage 1%, sleep stages shift, wake time after sleep onset, and total arousals compared with control individuals.[25] One study[31] showed a trend toward a higher arousal index (51.4 vs 46.9 events/h, $P = .06$) and significantly more awakenings during the study (66 vs 56, $P = .028$). These patients also were reported to have more problems with wearing CPAP, specifically air hunger, dyspnea, and mask removal, although they have similar compliance. The presence of CompSA may be suggested if a patient diagnosed with OSA on CPAP has incomplete response to therapy, has a high AHI on the adherence data download available on the PAP machine,[41] persistent hypersomnia, or mask/interface complaints.[37] Nasal resistance was found to be significantly higher in the CompSA group than in the obstructive sleep apnea syndrome group.[42] It has been hypothesized that CPAP intolerance associated with an increased nasal resistance might precipitate an increase of arousals from sleep, thus facilitating CompSA. A cardiovascular comorbidity has also been seen in some reports to be more prevalent in CompSA. Lehman and colleagues[26] reported that a history of ischemic heart disease or heart failure was more frequent among patients with CPAP-emergent CSA than those without (38% vs 14%, $P = .03$). Cassel and colleagues[31] reported that their CompSA group were diagnosed with more HTN (76.7 vs 56.2%, $P = .028$) and coronary artery disease (40 vs 8.4%, $P<.001$). It is not clear if there is a link between CompSA and the development of cardiovascular disease, but the reverse is clearly probable. In cardiac failure, the increased central CO_2 ventilatory response lowers P_{CO_2} toward the apnea threshold at rest, narrowing the difference between ambient P_{CO_2} levels and the apnea threshold, thereby predisposing to CSA.[28,30,43] Moreover the activity of the faster-acting peripheral CO_2 ventilatory response then oscillates ventilation and is responsible for the periodicity and severity of CSA in patients with heart failure.[30] A long circulation also increases the loop gain.[28,43] Patients with CHF often have hypocapnia secondary to lung edema, which may cause hyperventilation and lead to a baseline P_{CO_2} being closer to the apneic threshold.

NATURAL HISTORY

Much of the debate surrounding the management of CompSA revolves around the question of whether the central apneas improve with time on CPAP or whether they persist. There are conflicting results in the literature as to whether CompSA is transient. In 1 retrospective review,[26] patients were evaluated with 2 sleep studies and those who were diagnosed with CompSA were followed up with a subsequent PSG. Thirteen patients

were identified, with a median follow-up of 195 (49–562) days. The residual AHI decreased from 26 (23–40) on the first PSG to 7 (3–21) on the follow-up PSG. There were 7 patients who reached an AHI less than 10 and were regarded as CPAP responders. The 6 nonresponders were found to be sleepier by ESS ($P = .03$) and trended toward a lower BMI ($P = .06$). Both groups showed similar adherence to CPAP. In contrast, Dernaika and colleagues,[25] in a cross-sectional study, evaluated a group who developed central apneas on PAP therapy (n = 14) and found significant improvement in the central apneas. Twelve of the 14 patients had a decrease in central apneas from 20 ± 14.2 to 2 ± 4.5 in a follow-up study 2 to 3 months later with a prevalence of CPAP-persistent CSA in only about 1.5%. The investigators concluded that the CSA events that emerged during CPAP titration were only transient and hypothesized that they may have emerged as a result of sleep fragmentation. Jahaveri and colleagues[17] also reported a continued prevalence of CompSA of only 1.5% (18 patients of 1286) after 8 weeks of CPAP therapy. This transient nature of the central apneas has not only been shown in patients with treatment of their OSA with CPAP but also after surgical tracheostomy. Guilleminault and colleagues[12] noted that patients with OSA who had undergone tracheostomy were found to initially have emergent central events, which decreased with time when looked at again with a repeat PSG. Coccagna and colleagues[44] found a similar finding toward resolution of central events with time. In this study, the central apneas improved 6 months after tracheostomy. A possible physiologic explanation for a high-resolution rate of CompSA after prolonged CPAP treatment may be normalization of the underdamped chemoreflex control system with increased CO_2 reserve and decreased controller gain under CPAP.[45] Javaheri[17] tried to identify risk factors for persistent central events. He found that patients with persistent CompSA had more severe OSA and a larger number of central apneas on the baseline study. A third potential risk factor was the use of opioids, which are known to cause central apneas. In The Canadian Continuous Positive Airway Pressure for Patients with Central Sleep Apnea and Heart Failure (CANPAP) trial,[20] there was no significant change in AHI (mostly central) between the 1-month and the 6-month follow-up. However, these were patients with known congestive heart failure, not CompSA. Cassel and colleagues[31] documented resolution of CompSA in some patients (the prevalence of CompSA decreased from 12.2% to 6.9% in 3 months), but he also reported de novo appearance of complex activity in a significant proportion of patients

(4.2%) with OSA treated with CPAP. This is the only study that longitudinally examined patients who had CompSA initially but also those who did not. Patients with and without follow-up CompSA showed no pronounced difference in CPAP adherence.

TREATMENT
PAP

CPAP

CPAP has been used for the treatment of CompSA, with several reviews investigating the clinical effectiveness of this modality to eliminate the OSA quickly and the central apneas over a longer period. A proposed mechanism by which CPAP therapy may modulate this condition is by steady improvement in chemoreceptor sensitivity,[46] decrease of the arousal threshold,[47] control of airway obstruction, and improvement of airway edema. This situation leads to apparent resolution of CompSA over a period of weeks to months of treatment, as is seen in some patients.[16,17,25,48] Dernaika and colleagues[25] reported that 12 of 14 patients (92%) with CPAP-emergent CSA showed complete or near-complete resolution of CSA events on the repeat PSG. Continued CSA events (although significantly decreased) were seen in a patient with diastolic dysfunction on baseline transesophageal echocardiography. However, several studies have shown CPAP to be ineffective in eliminating the residual central apneas with continued use of this treatment.[17,31,48] There have also been cases of the development of central apneas on CPAP that were not initially seen on the initial studies.[31] Pusalavidyasagar and colleagues[37] in their retrospective review of 133 patients with OSA and 34 with CompSA prescribed CPAP to 93.7% and 87.9% of the patients, respectively. No significant differences in CPAP pressure were reported. Mean time to first follow-up was shorter in the CompSA group (46.2 ± 47.3 vs 53.8 ± 36.8 days; P = .022). The adherence to CPAP and improvement in Epworth scores were similar between the 2 groups. However, interface problems were significantly more common in the CompSA group, especially air hunger, dyspnea (0.8 vs 8.8%), and difficulties with the mask with mask removal (2.6 vs 17.7%, P<.05 for both). Pusalavidyasagar and colleagues[37] reported that patients with CompSA treated with CPAP reported more difficulty with the mask interface than patients with OSA. These difficulties include feelings of suffocation and air hunger in addition to mask leakage. These patients also are less adherent to CPAP therapy than those in whom the CompSA

resolves.[17] The adherence data download on the CPAP devices, which also is equipped to look for persistent respiratory events, may allow for better follow-up of patients with CompSA in order to document the resolution of all sleep-disordered breathing, allowing the option of CPAP as initial treatment before moving onto other more sophisticated PAP devices. Whether continued CPAP therapy leads to resolution of the emergent central events in most patients with continued treatment is of therapeutic significance. The answer to this question would determine whether patients with CompSA need to be treated with a different device, versus a more conservative approach with an observation period on CPAP. Additional categorization of the subsets of CompSA may be needed, which would in turn help to determine optimal treatment strategies for the individual patient groups. It is not possible to reliably predict in whom the central apneas improve or resolve.

BPAP and APAP

Standard BPAP should be avoided in CompSA when possible, because of the possibility of augmented tidal volumes and minute ventilation with resultant hypocapnia and central apnea or periodic breathing.[9,10] BPAP in spontaneous timed mode is an option to treat CSA in the American Academy of Sleep Medicine Practice Parameters[49] only after CPAP, adaptive servoventilation (ASV), and oxygen have failed. There is a paucity of data concerning APAP with CompSA, and a great deal of variability among the various models available. There are theoretic reasons to avoid APAP in CompSA, especially with primary CompSA in those with cardiovascular disease, but much of this may be specific to individual models and the algorithms used to detect flow limitation, obstructive and central events. APAP is not recommended for the treatment of CompSA.

ASV

ASV is a new mode of PAP treatment that was developed to address the problems entailed in the management of CSA, CSR, and CompSA. It is an attempt to allow, via algorithms, the computer-controlled management of breathing with variable ventilation, pressure support, and PAP. It is effective in the management of CSA and CompSA that remain unresolved with CPAP, BPAP, or APAP. It has its developmental roots in the first attempts to provide a means of APAP for OSA[50] and later an attempt at computer-controlled ventilators for invasive mechanical ventilation in the intensive care environment.[51] The first ASV model (ResMed AutoSet CS, ResMed Ltd, North Ryde NSW, Australia) was used in 2001 for the successful treatment of CSR in patients with CHF.[52] This model has evolved into the current VPAP Adapt SV (ResMed Ltd, North Ryde NSW, Australia), which is volume triggered (using $\dot{V}_E$). The Respironics BiPAP AutoSV (Phillips Respironics, Murrysville, Pennsylvaia, USA) was then introduced in 2006 as a flow-triggered (peak inspiratory flow) device, also with successful treatment of CSR in CHF.[53] This model has evolved into the BiPAP AutoSV Advanced with the addition of an autotitrating expiratory PAP (EPAP) algorithm aimed at CompSA. The last model to be introduced was the Weinmann SOMNOvent CR (Weinmann Geräte für Medizin GmbH & Co., Hamburg, Germany), which was successfully used for CompSA in 2009.[54] This model is volume and flow driven with auto-EPAP and auto-IPAP algorithms. Both of the other models (VPAP Adapt SV and BiPAP Auto SV) have been shown to be effective in CompSA, even when not associated with CHF.[14] The VPAP Adapt SV has been used successfully in the treatment of CompSA associated with opioid use,[55,56] but only when the end-expiratory pressure (EEP) is adjusted during the titration. It was not successful when using a fixed EEP and rate.[57] ASV works in CompSA by providing enough EPAP/EEP to resolve OSA, then addressing CSA or CSR by automatically adjusting pressure support breath by breath, monitoring $\dot{V}_E$ (Resmed) or peak flow (Respironics) or both (Weinmann) to stabilize the breathing pattern and maintain a moving-target ventilation set at 90% of the recent average $\dot{V}_E$. This strategy stabilizes breathing, reducing any respiratory alkalosis with an increase in P_{CO_2}. The ASV is designed to provide ventilation that is anticyclic to the patient's own respiratory drive periodicity. In the hyperventilatory phase, it gives minimal support (not enough to worsen hypocapnia), whereas in the hypoventilatory or apneic phase, it increases ventilation. This pattern dampens the oscillations of the patient's own respiratory drive, which would otherwise result in CSA or CSR. ASV has been designated as an option for the treatment of primary CSA and as standard treatment of CSA related to CHF in the current Practice Parameters of the American Academy of Sleep Medicine.[49] The most recent meta-analysis of the use of ASV in sleep-disordered breathing with heart failure[58] showed that ASV was better than CPAP, BPAP, O_2, sham ASV, and no treatment in reducing the severity of sleep-disordered breathing (reducing AHI), improving cardiac function (increasing LVEF), and increasing exercise capacity (6-minute walk distance). There was no statistically significant difference in the change in hypercapnic ventilatory drive ($\dot{V}_E/\dot{V}_{CO_2}$ slope) between the ASV and other modalities. Patients with heart failure and CSR have shown better long-term adherence to ASV compared with CPAP,[59] but these did not have CompSA.

Non-PAP Management

Pharmacotherapy

Avoidance of drugs that induce complex disease such as opiates, including methadone and baclofen, is of importance. There has been no proven role for any medications in the treatment of CompSA. Theophylline and acetazolamide may help with periodic breathing; however, the lack of consistent effectiveness and the significant side effect profile limit the use of these drugs, even as adjunct therapy.[60] There is only 1 report of a patient with opioid-associated CompSAs with successful control of their CompSA with CPAP and azetazolamide.[61] An alternative strategy for minimizing the central component of CompSA theoretically could include medications that increase the percentage of stable non-REM sleep. These medications include drugs that modulate γ-aminobutyric acid transmission, the 5-HT$_{2C}$ receptor (eg, mirtazapine), and sodium oxybate.[1] However, these drugs have not yet been investigated. Studies have also shown that hypnotics and sedatives such as triazolam, clonazepam, and zolpidem[62-64] have improved central apneas in central apnea syndromes by possibly improving sleep continuity and avoiding fluctuations in CO_2. No studies have been performed in the CompSA population. However, these medications may be useful as an adjunct to CPAP therapy and may be an area of future investigation.

Dead space

During sleep, ventilation decreases and there is a subsequent decrease in arterial carbon dioxide. Hyperventilation during sleep may cause a decrease lower than the apneic threshold, and in those with increased sensitivity, this can cause cycles of central apneas. Minimizing hypocapnea by minimizing the PAP pressure may lessen the contribution of CO_2 dyscontrol to the development of CompSA. Inhalation of 1% to 4% CO_2 has been seen to improve central apneas, particularly in CSR in patients with CHF.[65-67] The use of a nonvented mask and enhancing expiratory rebreathing space could produce controlled increases of CO_2 concentrations in the inhaled air.[65] Gilmartin and colleagues[1] suggest nonvented masks, which would enhance rebreathing of CO_2 and increase dead space as an initial option. Increase in dead space alone has been shown to improve CSA and heart failure. However, it may be impractical to add 500 to 600 mL to inspiratory volume alone.

However, adding 100 to 150 mL to PAP may have a synergistic benefit to patients. Experimental new devices allow flow-dependent, precisely controlled increases in CO_2 in the inspired air, which would help in stabilizing respiratory instability.[38] Thomas and colleagues[38] introduced CO_2 via a PAP gas modulator in 6 patients with residual mixed apneas on PAP, resulting in the elimination of sleep-disordered breathing. The challenge of attaining medical grade CO_2 and possible side effects limit its practical use.

Oxygen

Oxygen supplementation reduces responsiveness of peripheral chemoreceptors, hence stabilizing ventilatory drive and reducing loop gain.[68–70] Allam and colleagues[71] reported that the addition of oxygen to CPAP in patients with CompSA led to an improvement in respiratory events. The use of oxygen in patients who are not hypoxemic may be difficult to justify. However, it may be of use in patients who require oxygen and in addition have CompSA.

CLINICAL IMPLICATIONS

There is an ongoing debate focused around the best and most appropriate initial treatment of CompSA. This treatment should entail the understanding of the pathophysiology present in a given patient and individualizing therapy according to the type of CompSA (primary vs treatment-emergent) and comorbidities. This treatment should also take into account the relative severity of the various components of CompSA. Thus, someone with severe OSA and mild CPAP-emergent CSA may be expected to do well on CPAP, whereas someone with primary CompSA and CHF who has mild OSA but severe CSR might not be expected to do so well, and would have more risks with standard CPAP. This situation might result in limiting the higher cost of newer PAP devices versus conventional CPAP, with the potential of resolving central apneas with continued use[17,25,48] and reserving the more sophisticated devices for the more resistant central apneas in higher-risk patients. However, poor initial experience to CPAP has been reported to predict poor subsequent treatment to CPAP in addition to alternative PAP therapies.[72,73] Patients with heart failure and CSA have shown better long-term adherence to ASV compared with CPAP.[59] Several studies suggest superiority of ASV over CPAP and BPAP in eliminating central events, the respiratory arousals, and residual events.[59,74–77] Therefore, recognizing those who may respond better to CPAP,

distinguishing individuals who are more unlikely to resolve their central apneas, and possibly moving to ASV if there is an early concern for CPAP intolerance is of importance. ASV works well for CompSA and is well-tolerated. We know that most treatment-emergent CompSA resolves over time, with elimination of OSA by CPAP. "There are currently no clear clinical or PSG predictors of this resolution."[78] Those with cardiac dysfunction are particularly vulnerable to adverse effects of persisting CSA and CSR. Perhaps this situation represents the patient population who may most benefit from early use of ASV, particularly when presenting as primary CompSA rather than treatment-emergent CompSA.

REFERENCES

1. Gilmartin GS, Daly RW, Thomas RJ. Recognition and management of complex sleep-disordered breathing. Curr Opin Pulm Med 2005;11:485–93.
2. Thomas RJ, Terzano MG, Parrino L, et al. Obstructive sleep disordered breathing with a dominant cyclic alternating pattern–a recognizable polysomnographic variant with practical clinical implications. Sleep 2004;27:229–34.
3. Morgenthaler TI, Kagramanov V, Hanak V, et al. Complex sleep apnea syndrome: is it a unique clinical syndrome? Sleep 2006;29(9):1203–9.
4. Phillipson EA. Regulation of breathing during sleep. Am Rev Respir Dis 1977;115(Suppl): 217–24.
5. Glenn LL, Foutz AS, Dement EC. Membrane potential of spinal motoneurons during natural sleep in cats. Sleep 1978;1:199–204.
6. Fink BR. Influence of cerebral activity of wakefulness on regulation of breathing. J Appl Physiol 1961;16:15–20.
7. Lugaresi E, Cocogna G, Mantovani M, et al. Pathophysiological, clinical and nosographic considerations regarding hypersomnia with periodic breathing. Bull Eur Physiopathol Respir 1972;8: 1249–56.
8. Javaheri S, Almoosa KF, Saleh K, et al. Hypocapnia is not a predictor of central sleep apnea in patients with cirrhosis. Am J Respir Crit Care Med 2005; 171:908–11.
9. Meza S, Mendez M, Ostrowski M, et al. Susceptibility to periodic breathing with assisted ventilation during sleep in normal subjects. J Appl Physiol 1998;85:1929–40.
10. Johnson KG, Johnson DC. Bilevel positive airway pressure worsens central apneas during sleep. Chest 2005;128:2141–50.
11. Mathew R, Castriotta RJ. Preponderance of hypopneas over apneas in morbid obesity. Chest 2011;140:942A.

12. Guilleminault C, Commiskey J. Progressive improvement in apnea index and ventilatory response to CO_2 after tracheostomy in obstructive sleep apnea syndrome. Am Rev Respir Dis 1982; 126:14–20.

13. Corcoran S, Mysliwwiec V, Niven AS, et al. Development of central sleep apnea after maxillofacial surgery for obstructive sleep apnea. J Clin Sleep Med 2009;5:151–3.

14. Gindre L, Gagnadoux F, Meslier N, et al. Central apnea developing during treatment with mandibular advancement device. Rev Mal Respir 2006; 23:477–80 [in French].

15. Kuzniar TJ, Kovacevic-Ristanovic R, Freedom T. Complex sleep apnea unmasked by the use of a mandibular advancement device. Sleep Breath 2011;15(2):249–52.

16. Westhoff M, Arzt M, Literst P. Prevalence and treatment of central sleep apnoea emerging after initiation of continuous positive airway pressure in patients with obstructive sleep apnoea without evidence of heart failure. Sleep Breath 2012;16: 71–8.

17. Javaheri S, Smith J, Chung E. The prevalence and natural history of complex sleep apnea. J Clin Sleep Med 2009;5(3):205–11.

18. Javaheri S. Effects of continuous positive airway pressure on sleep apnea and ventricular irritability in patients with heart failure. Circulation 2000;101: 292–7.

19. Arzt M, Floras J, Logan A, et al. Suppression of central sleep apnea by continuous positive airway pressure and transplant-free survival. Circulation 2007;31:73–80.

20. Bradley DB, Logan AG, Kimoff RJ, et al. Continuous positive airway pressure for central sleep apnea and heart failure. N Engl J Med 2005;353: 2025–33.

21. Xie A, Rutherford R, Rankin F, et al. Hypocapnia and increased ventilatory responsiveness in patients with idiopathic sleep apnea. Am J Respir Crit Care Med 1995;152:1950–5.

22. Khoo MC. Determinants of ventilatory instability and variability. Respir Physiol 2000;122:167–82.

23. Tkacova R, Niroumand M, Loenzi-Filho G, et al. Overnight shift from obstructive to central apneas in patients with heart failure. Circulation 2001;103: 238–43.

24. Terzano MG, Parrino L, Boselli M, et al. The cyclic alternating pattern (CAP) as a physiological mechanism of EEG synchronization during NREM sleep. J Sleep Res 1994; 3(Suppl 1):251.

25. Dernaika T, Tawk M, Nazir S, et al. The significance and outcome of continuous positive airway pressure-related central sleep apnea during split-night sleep studies. Chest 2007;132:81–8.

26. Lehman S, Anic N, Thompson C, et al. Central sleep apnea on commencement of continuous positive airway pressure in patient with primary diagnosis of obstructive sleep apnea-hyperpnoea. J Clin Sleep Med 2007;3:462–6.

27. Endo Y, Suzuki M, Inoue Y, et al. Prevalence of complex sleep apnea among Japanese patients with sleep apnea syndrome. Tohoku J Exp Med 2008;215(4):349–54.

28. Javaheri S. A mechanism of central sleep apnea in patients with heart failure. N Engl J Med 1999;341: 949–54.

29. Hamilton RD, Winning AJ, Horner RL, et al. The effect of lung inflation on breathing in man during wakefulness and sleep. Respir Physiol 1988; 73(2):145–54.

30. Solin P, Roebuck T, Johns DP, et al. Peripheral and central ventilatory responses in central sleep apnea with and without congestive heart failure. Am J Respir Crit Care Med 2000;162:2194–200.

31. Cassel W, Canisius S, Becker HF, et al. A prospective polysomnographic study on the evolution of complex sleep apnoea. Eur Respir J 2011; 38(2):329–37.

32. Aiken ML, Franklin JL, Pierson DJ, et al. Influence of body size and gender on control of ventilation. J Appl Physiol 1986;60:1894–9.

33. White DP, Douglas NJ, Pickett CK, et al. Sexual influence on the control of breathing. J Appl Physiol 1983;54:874–9.

34. Jordan AS, Eckert DJ, Catcheside PG, et al. Ventilatory response to brief arousal from non-rapid eye movement sleep is greater in men than in women. Am J Respir Crit Care Med 2003;168:1512–9.

35. Xie A, Wong B, Phillipson EA, et al. Interaction of hyperventilation and arousal in the pathogenesis of idiopathic central sleep apnea. Am J Respir Crit Care Med 1994;150:489–95.

36. Zou XS, Shahabuddin S, Zahn BR, et al. Effect of gender on the development of hypocapnic apnea/hypopnea during NREM sleep. J Appl Physiol 2000;89:192–9.

37. Pusalavidyasagar SS, Olsen EJ, Gay PC, et al. Treatment of complex sleep apnea syndrome; a retrospective comparative review. Sleep Med 2006;7:474–9.

38. Thomas RJ, Daly RW, Weiss JW. Low concentration carbon dioxide is an effective adjunct to positive airway pressure in the treatment of refractory mixed obstructive and central sleep-disordered breathing. Sleep 2005;28:69–77.

39. Yaegashi H, Fujimoto K, Abe H, et al. Characteristics of Japanese patients with complex sleep apnea syndrome: a retrospective comparison with obstructive sleep apnea syndrome. Intern Med 2009;48(6):427–32.

40. Pusalavidyasagar S, Kuzniar TJ, Olson EJ, et al. Periodic limb movements in complex sleep apnea syndrome. Open Sleep J 2009;2:43–7.

41. Mulgrew AT, Lawati NA, Ayas NT, et al. Residual sleep apnea on polysomnography after 3 months of CPAP therapy: clinical implications, predictors and patterns. Sleep Med 2010;11:119–25.

42. Nakazaki C, Noda A, Yasuda Y, et al. Continuous positive airway pressure intolerance associated with elevated complex sleep apnea syndrome. Sleep Breath 2012;16:747–52.

43. Wilcox I, McNamara SG, Dodd MJ, et al. Ventilatory control in patients with sleep apnea and left ventricular dysfunction: comparison of obstructive and central sleep apnea. Eur Respir J 1998;11:7–13.

44. Coccagna G, Mantovani M, Brignani F, et al. Tracheostomy in hypersomnia with periodic breathing. Bull Physiopathol Respir (Nancy) 1972;8:1217–27.

45. Salloum A, Rowley JA, Mateika JH, et al. Increased propensity for central apnea in patients with obstructive sleep apnea: effect of nasal continuous positive airway pressure. Am J Respir Crit Care Med 2010;181:189–93.

46. Spicuzza L, Bernardi L, Balsamo R, et al. Effect of treatment with nasal continuous positive airway pressure on ventilatory response to hypoxia and hypercapnia in patients with sleep apnea syndrome. Chest 2006;130(3):774–9.

47. Loewen A, Ostrowski M, Laprairie J, et al. Determinants of ventilatory instability in obstructive sleep apnea: inherent or acquired. Sleep 2009;32(10):1355–65.

48. Kuzniar TJ, Pusalavidyasagar S, Gay PC, et al. Natural course of complex sleep apnea–a retrospective study. Sleep Breath 2008;12:135–9.

49. Aurora RN, Chowdhuri S, Ramar K, et al. The treatment of central sleep apnea syndromes in adults: practice parameters with an evidence-based literature review and meta-analysis. Sleep 2012;35:17–40.

50. Burk JR, Lucas EA, Axe JR, et al. Auto-CPAP in the treatment of obstructive sleep apnea: a new approach. In: Chase MH, Krueger J, O'Connor C, editors. Sleep Research. Los Angeles, CA: Brain Information Service/Brain Research Institute, University of California; 1992. p. 182.

51. Laubscher TP, Heinrichs W, Weiler N, et al. An adaptive lung ventilation controller. IEEE Trans Biomed Eng 1994;41:51–9.

52. Teschler H, Dohring J, Wang YM, et al. Adaptive pressure support servo-ventilation: a novel treatment for Cheyne-Stokes respiration in heart failure. Am J Respir Crit Care Med 2001;164:614–9.

53. Kasai T, Narui K, Dohi T, et al. First experience of using new adaptive servo-ventilation device for Cheyne-Stokes respiration with central sleep apnea among Japanese patients with congestive heart failure. Report of 4 clinical cases. Circ J 2006;70:1148–54.

54. Randerath WJ, Galetke W, Kenter M, et al. Combined adaptive servo-ventilation and automatic positive airway pressure (anticyclic modulated ventilation) in co-existing obstructive and central sleep apnea syndrome and periodic breathing. Sleep Med 2009;10:898–903.

55. Javaheri S, Malik A, Smith J, et al. Adaptive servo-ventilation: a novel treatment for sleep apnea associated with use of opioids. J Clin Sleep Med 2008;4:305–10.

56. Ramar K, Rmar P, Morgenthaler TI. Adaptive servo-ventilation in patients with central or complex sleep apnea related to chronic opioid use and congestive heart failure. J Clin Sleep Med 2012;8:569–76.

57. Farney RJ, Walker JM, Boyle KM, et al. Adaptive servoventilation (ASV) in patients with sleep-disordered breathing associated with chronic opioid medications for non-malignant pain. J Clin Sleep Med 2008;4:311–9.

58. Sharma B, Bakker JP, McSharry DG, et al. Adaptive servoventilation for the treatment of sleep-disordered breathing in heart failure. A systematic review and met-analysis. Chest 2012;142:1211–21.

59. Philippe C, Stoïca-Herman M, Drouot X, et al. Compliance with and effectiveness of adaptive servoventilation versus continuous positive airway pressure in the treatment of Cheyne-Stokes respiration in heart failure over a six month period. Heart 2006;92:337–42.

60. Orth MM, Grootoonk S, Duchna HW, et al. Short term effects of oral theophylline in addition to PAP in mild to moderate OSAS. Respir Med 2005;99:471–6.

61. Glidewell RN, Orr WC, Imes N. Acetazolamide as an adjunct to CPAP treatment: a case of complex sleep apnea in a patient on long-acting opioid therapy. J Clin Sleep Med 2009;5:63–4.

62. Quadri S, Drake C, Hudgel DW. Improvement of idiopathic central sleep apnea with zolpidem. J Clin Sleep Med 2009;5(2):122–9.

63. Grimaldi D, Provini F, Vetrugno R, et al. Idiopathic central sleep apnoea syndrome treated with zolpidem. Neurol Sci 2008;29(5):355–7.

64. Guilleminault C, Crowe C, Quera-Salva MA, et al. Periodic leg movement, sleep fragmentation and central sleep apnoea in two cases: reduction with clonazepam. Eur Respir J 1988;1:762–5.

65. Szollosi I, Jones M, Morrell MJ, et al. Effect of CO_2 inhalation on central sleep apnea and arousals from sleep. Respiration 2004;71:493–8.

66. Lorenzi-Filho G, Rankin F, Bies I, et al. Effects of inhaled carbon dioxide and oxygen on Cheyne-Stokes respiration in patients with heart failure.

Am J Respir Crit Care Med 1999;159(5 pt 1): 1490–8.

67. Steens RD, Millar TW, Su X, et al. Effect of inhaled 3% CO_2 on Cheyne-Stokes respiration in congestive heart failure. Sleep 1994;17:61–8.

68. Mohan R, Duffin J. The effect of hypoxia on the ventilator response to carbon dioxide in man. Respir Physiol 1997;108(2):101–15.

69. Duffin J, Mohan RM, Vasiliou P, et al. A model of the chemoreflex control of breathing in humans: model parameters measurement. Respir Physiol 2000; 120:13–26.

70. Wellman A, Malhotra A, Jordan AS, et al. Effect of oxygen in obstructive sleep apnea: role of loop gain. Respir Physiol Neurobiol 2008;162:144–51.

71. Allam JS, Olson EJ, Gay PC, et al. Efficacy of adaptive servoventilation in treatment of complex and central sleep apnea syndromes. Chest 2007; 132(6):1839–46.

72. Budhiraja R, Parthasarathy S, Drake CL, et al. Early CPAP use identifies subsequent adherence to CPAP therapy. Sleep 2007;30:320–4.

73. Ballard RD, Gay PC, Strollo PJ. Interventions to improve compliance in sleep apnea patients previously non-compliant with continuous positive airway pressure. J Clin Sleep Med 2007;3:706–12.

74. Pepperell JC, Maskell NA, Jones DR, et al. A randomized controlled trial of adaptive ventilation for Cheyne-Stokes breathing in heart failure. Am J Respir Crit Care Med 2003;168:1109–14.

75. Brown LK. Filling in the gaps: the role of noninvasive adaptive servoventilation for heart failure-related central sleep apnea. Chest 2008;134:4–7.

76. Arzt M, Wensel R, Montalvan S, et al. Effects of dynamic bilevel positive airway pressure support on central sleep apnea in men with heart failure. Chest 2008;134:61–6.

77. Morgenthaler TI, Gay PC, Gordon N, et al. Adaptive servoventilation versus noninvasive positive pressure ventilation for central, mixed, and complex sleep apnea syndromes. Sleep 2007;30: 468–75.

78. Kuzniar TJ, Morganthaler TI. Treatment of complex sleep apnea syndrome. Chest 2012;142:1049–57.

Mask Interfaces

Leslie D. Wilke, DO*, Shekhar Ghamande, MD, FCCP, FAASM

KEYWORDS

- Mask interfaces • Nasal masks • Nasal pillows • Obstructive sleep apnea • Pediatriac sleep apnea
- Complication • Compliance

KEY POINTS

- Mask interfaces have evolved to promote better compliance with positive airway therapy machines. Patient preference and tolerance determines initial choice.
- Nasal masks or nasal pillows are generally preferred. Close follow-ups are necessary to change or adjust masks.
- Mouth breathers, patients with nasal irritation, or patients with higher positive airway pressures may need orofacial masks. A pressure adjustment may be necessary during the switch.
- Children may need custom-made masks for proper fit and compliance.
- Dermatologic and ocular side effects may contribute to noncompliance.

INTRODUCTION

Successful use of continuous (CPAP) and bilevel (BiPAP) positive airway pressure therapy requires an adequate and comfortable mask interface. It has been noted that the type of mask interface prescribed may have a significant impact on influencing acceptance and adherence to CPAP therapy.[1,2] Poorly fitting interfaces can permit air leak. The optimum interface remains unclear because of the limited number of studies available.[3] The pros and cons of different mask interfaces are reviewed.

NASAL MASK

The nasal interface was first described in 1981 and used in long-term therapy by 1985.[2] The nasal mask seals around the bridge of the nose superiorly, above the superior lips inferiorly, and just lateral to the medial cheeks bilaterally (**Fig. 1**). Typically, the smallest mask size that encompasses the nose without pinching the nares is used.[2] Positive airway pressure delivered nasal masks has been confirmed by many studies to act as a pneumatic

splint to prevent collapse of the pharyngeal airway and has been shown to be effective in both obstructive and mixed apneas.[2] The nasal mask is frequently the first choice offered to patients.[2] Patients can expectorate and can speak and it allows more physiologic breathing as well as natural humidification.[2]

Compared with full face masks, CPAP therapy with nasal masks revealed that the nasal masks provided a higher compliance rate, were rated to be significantly more comfortable, and led to improved overall symptoms and Epworth Sleepiness Scale scores.[4] Subsequently, in a small study, 16 patients who were on nasal mask were randomized to nasal mask or full face mask for 2 separate nights. Both interfaces were found to be equally effective in maintaining nocturnal gas exchange and preventing sleep-disordered breathing. However, the nasal mask provided fewer air leaks. Also, there was a subjective increase in comfort on the nasal mask as found by the visual analog score.[5]

The most common adverse effect of the nasal mask is nasal congestion from the vasodilation and mucus production, which can be mitigated by using heated humidification, and treatment of

Department of Medicine, Division of Pulmonary, Critical Care, and Sleep Medicine, Scott & White Memorial Hospital, Texas A&M Health & Science Center, 2401 South 31st Street, Temple, TX 76508, USA
* Corresponding author.
E-mail address: LWILKE@swmail.sw.org

Sleep Med Clin 8 (2013) 477–481
http://dx.doi.org/10.1016/j.jsmc.2013.07.004
1556-407X/13/$ – see front matter © 2013 Elsevier Inc. All rights reserved.

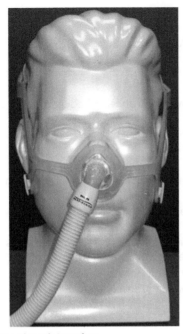

Fig. 1. Nasal mask interface.

allergic rhinitis. Mouth leaks occur in subjects with a tendency to sleep with open mouths but this could be alleviated by using a chin strap.[2] Irritant contact dermatitis has been described to occur even several years later.[6]

FULL FACE MASK/ORONASAL MASK

A full face mask seals across the forehead, around the temples and the chin, encompassing the eyes, nose, and mouth (**Fig. 2**A). Oronasal masks, which are more commonly used, seal around the bridge of the nose to the chin, encompassing the nose and mouth (see **Fig. 2**B). A full face or oronasal mask may be indicated when mouth leaks are significant and prevents adequate ventilator support. Adequate ventilator support is particularly relevant for predominant nocturnal mouth breathers. For simplicity, both of these masks are used synonymously. Sanders and colleagues[7] reviewed 30 patients with oronasal mask use after failure from nasal mask and concluded that the oronasal mask can be an effective alternative for OSA patients. In the first randomized controlled trial, Teo and colleagues[8] studied 24 patients who underwent 2 consecutive CPAP titration studies and were randomized to a nasal mask with chin strap or oronasal mask. The patients completed a visual analog scale after each study. There was no difference in sleep quality; however, there was a higher leak noted in the oronasal mask. Patients also rated the nasal masks higher in satisfaction because they were better fitting and more comfortable. The apnea-hypopnea index (AHI) was higher while using an oronasal mask even though the CPAP pressures were similar.

Simultaneous application of pressure via an oronasal mask in the nose and mouth may lead to posterior displacement of upper airway structures, resulting in reduced airway opening. The tongue may fall back due to airway pressure while using an oronasal mask in some patients, potentially leading to failure of CPAP therapy.[9]

A large study compared nasal mask, nasal pillows, and an oronasal mask in a randomized trial during CPAP titration. The final AHI did not differ

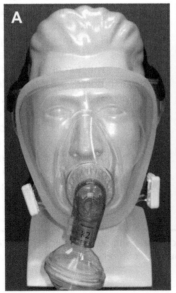
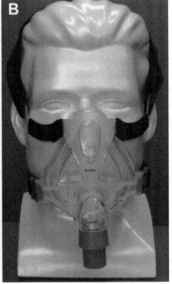

Fig. 2. Total facemask (*A*); oronasal facemask (*B*).

between the 3 groups. Oronasal mask use led to higher mask leakage compared with nasal pillows but not nasal mask. Importantly, considerably higher pressures were needed when oronasal mask was used.[10] In these patients, CPAP pressure requirements were higher on an average by 2.8 cm H_2O in the moderate OSA patients and by 6 cm H_2O in the severe OSA patients. There was no difference in pressures needed when either a nasal mask or nasal pillows were used, similar to the results of the Ryan study.[11]

These findings may imply inadequacy of pressures while switching over from a nasal mask or pillows to an oronasal mask without a change in CPAP pressure.

Adverse effects of full face/oronasal masks include increased dead space in which noninvasive ventilator settings may need to be adjusted.[2] Claustrophobia and facial skin necrosis may occur.[2] Patients may have swallowing difficulties and a potential aspiration risk, especially with underlying esophageal reflux or vomiting.[2] A full face mask may be too uncomfortable for long-term use secondary to airway and mucous membrane dryness, even despite heated humidification.[1]

ORAL MASK

Oral masks, such as the Oracle Mask, are butterfly-shaped interfaces that rest in the oral vestibule between the lips and the teeth (**Fig. 3**). This type of device ensures that the desired airway pressure is delivered with minimal leakage.[12] In a small study of 7 patients, the oral mask was found to have pressure-flow relationships with positive airway pressure comparable to the nasal interface.[13] Beecroft and colleagues[12] compared the oral mask to nasal and oronasal interface devices in patients with a new diagnosis of OSA with a 6-month follow-up. There was no significant difference in the proportion of nonadherence between the groups. Patients appreciated the lack of headgear and reported higher satisfaction with the oral Mask. However, a common complaint included choking or gagging. They concluded that the oral mask is efficacious for long-term CPAP therapy and may be more acceptable than oronasal masks for patients who do not tolerate nasal CPAP therapy.

Adverse effects of the oral mask include dental pain, orthodontic problems, nasal leaks, initial hypersalivation, and aerophagia.[2]

NASAL PILLOWS

Nasal pillows, or prongs, can be useful when there is skin breakdown on the nasal bridge, when the nasal mask is considered too obtrusive, or in patients with limited arm movement (**Fig. 4**).[2] Nasal pillows are usually reserved for patients who do not tolerate nasal masks. The use of headgear may enhance patient comfort.[1] In 2003, Massie and colleagues compared nasal pillows to nasal masks in 39 patients in a 6-week randomized, crossover study. This study showed a significant increase in percentage of days used in the nasal pillows group compared with the nasal mask group. There was no difference in the Epworth Sleepiness Scale and the Functional Outcomes of Sleep Questionnaire between the 2 groups. They noted that the nasal pillows may not be

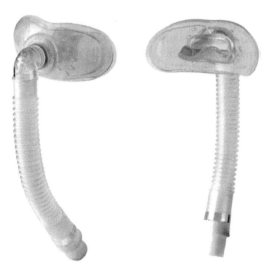

Fig. 3. Oracle CPAP mask. (*Courtesy of* Fisher & Paykel Healthcare, Auckland, New Zealand; with permission.)

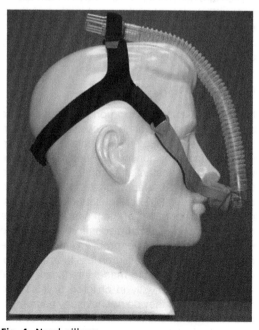

Fig. 4. Nasal pillows.

appropriate for patients with higher CPAP pressures as there were concerns of the mask seal and the possibility of inadequate pressure delivery. They concluded that nasal pillows are well-tolerated as patients have reported less discomfort with their use, and is an effective interface for patients with OSA at a CPAP pressure of ≤14 cm H_2O.[1]

More recently in 2011, Ryan and colleagues studied 21 patients in an 8-week crossover design with randomization to nasal pillows or nasal mask. The nasal pillows had less reported pressure on the face and a significant improvement in the Social Functioning and Change of Health Score, but there was not a significant improvement in compliance. The nasal mask had less reported complaints of cold face/nose, and at the end of the trial, 12 patients stated they preferred the nasal mask over the nasal pillows. With these results, they concluded that patients should be evaluated on an individual basis for usage of nasal pillows.[9]

COMBINATION DEVICES

In some patients, high pressures prevent adequate fitting of the mask, leading to CPAP intolerance. At the same time a mandibular advancement device (MAD) may be inadequate to control the sleep-disordered breathing. In such circumstances, using an MAD with the CPAP or BiPAP via nasal masks may be helpful. In a pilot study of 10 patients combining MAD with CPAP therapy using a nasal mask, there was a decrease in the amount of pressure needed for CPAP; the AHI normalized, and patients tolerated the combination of the 2 treatment modalities.[14] Further studies are warranted to determine the combination therapy concept in selected cases.

PEDIATRIC POPULATION

In children, finding an appropriate mask may be challenging and the range of choices is smaller. In a study reporting on a large cohort of children needing long-term noninvasive positive pressure ventilation (a substantial number had OSA on CPAP or BiPAP) the appropriate interface could be determined in 80% of patients during the first night of study but 21% of them needed a change mostly because of facial discomfort. Leaks were not reported to be a major problem in the absence of facial deformities.[15] Children less than 2 years of age may need custom-made interfaces. Facial masks are used mostly in children 5 years and older especially if they do not have any neuromuscular disease or craniofacial anomalies that may impair their ability to pull off the mask. It is important to remember that 60% of facial development occurs by 4 years of age and can be potentially altered by positive pressure. Midface hypoplasia has been described with prolonged use of nasal CPAP.[16] Facial alterations such as maxillary retrusion can occur with use of a nasal mask and need to be watched for during follow-up.[15] Nasal prongs may be more appropriate in this setting.

Interestingly, long-term nasal CPAP use has been associated with maxillary and dental changes in an adult Japanese cohort followed by cephalometric radiographs. In 46 patients (only 5 women) with an average age of 56 years followed over 35 months, a significant retrusion of the anterior maxilla, a decrease in maxillary-mandibular discrepancy, a setback of the supramentale and chin positions, a retroclination of maxillary incisors, and a decrease of convexity occurred[17] but did not lead to any significant facial morphology changes or malocclusions.

GENERAL CONSIDERATIONS

When prescribing any of the available interfaces for OSA, it is always preferable to follow the manufacturer's suggestion for proper sizing, avoid over tightening, and check skin regularly for signs of pressure ulcers, which may occur if the mask is too tight.[2] If an ulcer does develop, it is recommended to use mask or skin barriers or switch to an alternate type of interface.[2] Edentulous patients may find an inadequate seal, thus necessitating dentures to be worn at night.[2]

Claustrophobia is a common complaint as well as a predecessor for reluctance to a trial of CPAP treatment. Use of nasal mask has decreased the incidence of patient-reported claustrophobia.[12] Nasal pillows have been reserved for use in patients who do not tolerate a full face mask.[1,11] Patients may benefit from counseling before and during treatment of CPAP to help decrease perceived claustrophobia. A trial of using the CPAP machine with the mask may be done during the evening time while awake to see if this would help the patient be more comfortable with it at night.

Other factors than the type of interface may also contribute to a patient's noncompliance of CPAP. For example, most contemporary masks and nasal pillows have silicone rubber and may lead to contact allergic dermatitis. Mask straps may contain neoprene made of dialkylthioureas and can cause a scalp allergic dermatitis.[18]

Ocular complications of CPAP occur in 10% to 30% of patients using noninvasive mask ventilation. These complications can occur because of air blowing into the eyes around the superior portion of nasal or oronasal masks, compression of venous drainage from eyes because of mask pressure, and from retrograde lacrimal flow of air and mucus into the eye.[19,20] Bacterial conjunctivitis, corneal abrasions and ulcers, dry eyes, and increased ocular pressure have been described. Retrograde lacrimal flow may be more prevalent in patients with neuromuscular disease.[20] Nocturnal lubricants or artificial tears may provide relief from dry eyes in the morning. Nasal pillows or lowering of pressure may be necessary in other cases.

SUMMARY

It is important to match the interface to individual patients and follow them closely to assess their clinical response to CPAP therapy.[1] Full face or oronasal mask may not be recommended as first-line interface because of the compliance rates as described above. However, they should be considered if a nasal mask is not tolerated secondary to nasal congestion, dryness, or persistent mouth leaks despite use of a chin strap. Nasal pillows and, in selected cases, oral masks may be useful alternatives for patients who do not tolerate conventional nasal masks.[18] Studies of higher power and longer duration are necessary for further determination of superior interface for different patient groups.

REFERENCES

1. Massie CM, Hart RW. Clinical outcomes related to interface type in patients with obstructive sleep apnea/hypopnea syndrome who are using continuous positive airway pressure. Chest 2003;123:1112–8.
2. Kryger MH, Buchanan P, Grunstein R. Principles and practice of sleep medicine. 5th edition. St Louis (MO): WB Saunders; 2010. p. 1233–49, 1318–1330.
3. Chai CL, Pathinathan A, Smith BJ. Continuous positive airway pressure delivery interfaces for obstructive sleep apnoea. Cochrane Database Syst Rev 2011;(4):CD005308.
4. Mortimore IL, Whittle AT, Douglas NJ. Comparison of nose and face mask CPAP therapy for sleep apnoea. Thorax 1998;53:290–2.
5. Willson GN, Piper AJ, Norman M, et al. Nasal versus full face mask for noninvasive ventilation in chronic respiratory failure. Eur Respir J 2004;23:605–9.
6. Egesi A, Davis MD. Irritant contact dermatitis due to the use of a continuous positive airway pressure nasal mask: 2 case reports and review of the literature. Cutis 2012;90(3):125–8.
7. Sanders MH, Kern NB, Stiller RA, et al. CPAP therapy via oronasal mask for obstructive sleep apnea. Chest 1994;106:774–9.
8. Teo M, Amis T, Lee S, et al. Equivalence of nasal and oronasal masks during initial CPAP titration for obstructive sleep apnea syndrome. Sleep 2011;34: 951–5.
9. Schorr F, Genta PR, Gregório MG, et al. Continuous positive airway pressure delivered by oronasal mask may not be effective for obstructive sleep apnoea. Eur Respir J 2012;40(2):503–5.
10. Ebben MR, Oyegbile T, Pollak CP. The efficacy of three different mask styles on a PAP titration night. Sleep Med 2012;13(6):645–9.
11. Ryan S, Garvey JF, Swan V, et al. Nasal pillows as an alternative interface in patients with obstructive sleep apnoea syndrome initiating continuous positive airway pressure therapy. J Sleep Res 2011;20: 367–73.
12. Beecroft J, Zanon S, Lukic D, et al. Oral continuous positive airway pressure for sleep apnea. Chest 2003;124:2200–8.
13. Smith PL, O'Donnell CP, Allan L, et al. A physiologic comparison of nasal and oral positive airway pressure. Chest 2003;123:689–94.
14. El-Solh AA, Moitheennazima B, Akinnusi ME, et al. Combined oral appliance and positive airway pressure therapy for obstructive sleep apnea: a pilot study. Sleep Breath 2011;15:203–8.
15. Ramirez A, Delord V, Khirani S, et al. Interfaces for long-term non-invasive positive pressure ventilation in children. Intensive Care Med 2012;38: 655–62.
16. Li KK, Riley RW, Guilleminault C. An unreported risk in the use of home nasal continuous positive airway pressure and home nasal ventilation in children: mid-face hypoplasia. Chest 2000;117:916–8.
17. Tsuda H, Almeida FR, Tsuda T, et al. Craniofacial changes after 2 years of nasal continuous positive airway pressure use in patients with obstructive sleep apnea. Chest 2010;138:870–4.
18. Parthasarathy S. Mask interface and CPAP adherence. J Clin Sleep Med 2008;4:511–2.
19. Waller EA, Bendel RE, Kaplan J. Sleep disorders and the eye. Mayo Clin Proc 2008;83:1251–61.
20. Zandieh S, Katz ES. Retrograde lacrimal duct airflow during nasal positive pressure ventilation. J Clin Sleep Med 2010;6(6):603–4.

Therapies for Children with Obstructive Sleep Apnea

Christopher Cielo, DO[a], Lee J. Brooks, MD[b],*

KEYWORDS

- Children • Obstructive sleep apnea • Adenotonsillectomy • Positive airway pressure
- Polysomnography

KEY POINTS

- The mainstays of therapy for obstructive sleep apnea in children are adenotonsillectomy and positive airway pressure.
- Nonsurgical therapies, including anti-inflammatory medications, dental devices, and weight loss, may be useful in specific circumstances.
- Airway surgery has been shown to be effective in children with craniofacial abnormalities, but not in the general pediatric population.
- Children with Down syndrome, craniofacial abnormalities, obesity, or Prader-Willi syndrome are at increased risk for obstructive sleep apnea syndrome and may require more frequent polysomnography and specific therapies.

DIAGNOSIS OF OBSTRUCTIVE SLEEP APNEA SYNDROME IN CHILDREN

Obstructive sleep apnea syndrome (OSAS) in children is a "disorder of breathing during sleep characterized by prolonged partial upper airway obstruction and/or intermittent complete obstruction (obstructive apnea) that disrupts normal ventilation during sleep and normal sleep patterns."[1] Symptoms vary by age in children with OSAS, and may include neurobehavioral problems in younger children, daytime sleepiness or headaches in older children, and habitual snoring with or without observed apnea at any age. The sequelae of untreated OSAS in children includes excessive daytime sleepiness,[2] neurocognitive impairment and behavioral problems,[3,4] blood pressure dysregulation,[5] diastolic hypertension, and less commonly pulmonary hypertension and failure to thrive.[6] Risk factors for OSAS in children include adenotonsillar hypertrophy,[7] neuromuscular disorders,[8] craniofacial abnormalities,[9] and obesity.[10]

History and physical examination alone are unreliable for predicting the presence and severity of OSAS in children.[11,12] The gold standard for evaluating sleep apnea in the pediatric population is overnight, attended, in-laboratory polysomnography. Children who snore on a regular basis and for whom parents report observed apnea, sleep enuresis, sleeping while sitting or with the neck in a hyperextended position, cyanosis, headaches on awakening, daytime sleepiness, attention-deficit/hyperactivity disorder, or learning problems should be referred to a sleep specialist or for polysomnography. Children who habitually snore and have physical findings including underweight or overweight, tonsillar hypertrophy, adenoidal facies, micrognathia or retrognathia, high-arched palate, failure to

Disclosure: Dr Brooks has stock holdings in various publicly-traded, health-related companies. None are relevant to the topic of this article.

[a] Division of Pulmonary Medicine, The Children's Hospital of Philadelphia, Colket Building, 11th Floor, 3501 Civic Center Boulevard, Philadelphia, PA 19104, USA; [b] Division of Pulmonary Medicine, Sleep Center, The Children's Hospital of Philadelphia, University of Pennsylvania, 9 Northwest 50 Main Building, 34th and Civic Center Boulevard, Philadelphia, PA 19104, USA

* Corresponding author.

E-mail address: brooksl@email.chop.edu

Sleep Med Clin 8 (2013) 483–493

http://dx.doi.org/10.1016/j.jsmc.2013.07.010

thrive, or hypertension should also be referred for polysomnography.[13] Evidence-based guidelines defining OSAS severity in children do not exist, and the polysomnogram must be interpreted in the clinical context of each individual case. The decision to treat OSAS in children involves consideration of both the severity of clinical signs and symptoms and the polysomnographic findings. Many therapies, both surgical (**Table 1**) and nonsurgical (**Table 2**), are available for select groups of children.

SPECIFIC THERAPIES
Adenotonsillectomy

Tonsillectomy is a surgical procedure in which the peritonsillar space between the tonsil capsule and muscular wall is dissected, completely removing the tonsil. When performed in conjunction with surgical removal of the adenoids, this procedure is referred to as *adenotonsillectomy*. If a child has OSAS and has adenotonsillar hypertrophy, adenotonsillectomy is usually recommended as the first-line treatment.[13]

In most children, adenotonsillectomy is effective in treating OSAS and improving quality of life. Relative contraindications include very small tonsils/adenoids, morbid obesity with small tonsils/adenoids, bleeding disorders refractory to

treatment, and medical instability. The rate of complete resolution of OSAS after adenotonsillectomy depends on many factors. Retrospective studies have found that adenotonsillectomy is highly effective in reducing the apnea-hypopnea index (AHI) and 25% to 71% of children have a postoperative AHI of less than 1 event per hour.[14–16] Older age, obesity, and higher preoperative AHI are negative predictors of successful resolution of OSAS after adenotonsillectomy.[11,14,16]

Treatment of obstructive sleep apnea (OSA) is cost-effective. Adenotonsillectomy has been associated with a reduction in health care costs by one-third, a 39% reduction in emergency department visits, and 60% fewer hospital admissions.[17] The efficacy of treating OSAS with adenotonsillectomy has not been compared with tonsillectomy or adenoidectomy alone, but in children without enlarged tonsils, particularly those younger than 1 year, adenoidectomy is often performed without tonsillectomy.

Adenotonsillectomy is a relatively safe procedure, and as many as 93% of patients have no intraoperative or postoperative problems.[18] The most common complications include pain and poor oral intake, with more severe complications including hemorrhage, dehydration, infection, respiratory complications, and atlantoaxial subluxation. The rate of major complications, including

Table 1
Surgical therapies for OSAS in children

Therapy	Population	Benefits	Risks/Challenges
Adenotonsillectomy	Children with enlarged tonsils and/or adenoids	Highly effective Well-tolerated in most children	Common adverse effects include pain, decreased oral tolerance, rare hemorrhaging, respiratory complications
Partial tonsillectomy	Children with enlarged tonsils with or without adenoids	Shorter recovery time and fewer postoperative complications than adenotonsillectomy	Efficacy in treating OSAS less-established Effect of tonsillar regrowth on OSAS unknown
Tracheostomy	Children with severe OSAS and no other therapeutic option	Highly effective	Requires increased level of support at home Increased risk of significant complications
Bariatric surgery	Select obese teenagers for whom other therapies have failed	Small studies show high short-term success rate in select populations	Significant complications No long-term efficacy data Success varies by center/ type of surgery
Craniofacial surgery (mandibular distraction osteogenesis, lip-tongue adhesion)	Children with micrognathia, craniosynostosis, other craniofacial conditions	Highly effective in select population	Minimal long-term follow-up data Success varies by center/ type of surgery Significant complications

Table 2
Nonsurgical therapies for OSAS in children

Therapy	Population	Benefits	Risks/Challenges
Positive airway pressure (PAP)	Any child	Strong evidence for efficacy, even if OSAS severe	Some will have trouble tolerating Few mask options for some children
Nasal steroids & leukotriene receptor antagonists	Children with mild-to-moderate OSAS	Minimally invasive	Overall weak evidence Length of therapy needed is unknown Unclear which children will benefit
Rapid maxillary expansion	Children with narrow maxilla or constricted maxillary arch, nonobese, without adenotonsillar enlargement	Therapy is short-term, minimally invasive	Few studies showing efficacy Unclear which children will benefit most
Oral appliances	Unclear	In some children, may be better tolerated than PAP	Dry mouth and dental discomfort seen Few studies showing efficacy Can be expensive
Weight loss	Older, obese children	Noninvasive, good for overall health Can be performed in conjunction with PAP	Difficult No evidence for sustained resolution of OSAS
Supplemental oxygen	Unclear Possibly infants or those with no other therapeutic options	May prevent hypoxemia	Does not treat airway obstruction May cause hypercapnia

hemorrhage and dehydration, ranges from 0.7% to 3.1% depending on the surgical technique used.[19] A study of 475 consecutive adenotonsillectomies found that 11.2% of children had some respiratory complication postoperatively, most commonly multiple episodes of desaturation requiring an oropharyngeal or nasopharyngeal airway. Risk factors for complications included young age, obesity, and high preoperative AHI.[20] Both the American Academy of Otolaryngology-Head and Neck Surgery and the American Academy of Pediatrics recommend that children at increased risk for respiratory complications be observed overnight in a facility with experience in caring for children with airway problems.[13,21] Children considered high risk include those younger than 3 years and those with severe OSA, cardiac complications of OSAS, failure to thrive, obesity, craniofacial abnormalities, neuromuscular disorders, or current respiratory infections.

Although most otolaryngologists rely on clinical judgment to determine which patients require adenotonsillectomy, and only 10% of children undergoing adenotonsillectomy have a polysomnography before surgery,[22] several studies have shown that history and physical examination alone are unreliable in predicting the presence and severity of OSAS in children.[11,12,23] The American Academy of Otolaryngology-Head and Neck Surgery suggests that polysomnography should be performed before adenotonsillectomy in children with obesity, Down syndrome, craniofacial abnormalities, neuromuscular disorders, sickle cell disease, or mucopolysaccharidoses. Additionally, clinicians should advocate for polysomnography before adenotonsillectomy when the benefit of surgery is unclear or when tonsil size on examination seems small in relation to the symptoms of sleep-disordered breathing.[21]

Understanding the severity of OSAS before adenotonsillectomy is useful for several reasons. First, it allows anesthesia personnel and the surgeon to better evaluate risk for perioperative complications. Second, it permits clinicians to plan for postoperative management, which may include hospital admission or observation in an intensive care unit. Finally, it helps determine which patients should be reevaluated for residual OSAS after surgery.

Partial Tonsillectomy

In an attempt to decrease postoperative complications related to adenotonsillectomy and reduce recovery time, significant interest has been shown in developing less-invasive surgical techniques. A variety of partial tonsillectomy procedures exist, including powered intracapsular tonsillectomy and radiofrequency tonsillectomy. Powered intracapsular tonsillectomy uses a microdebrider and spares the tonsillar capsule. A variety of radiofrequency techniques use heat to perform a similar function.

Limited data are available comparing polysomnography outcomes using these newer techniques. For intracapsular tonsillectomy, one study of 14 children with moderate OSA found that 93% had an AHI of less than 1 event per hour at 4 to 8 weeks postoperatively.[24] A small retrospective study with several limitations comparing intracapsular tonsillectomy with total tonsillectomy found no differences in the rate of residual AHI of greater than 5 events per hour.[25] For radiofrequency tonsillectomy, one group reported similar rates of snoring at follow-up compared with total tonsillectomy, but no follow-up polysomnography was performed.[26] Randomized studies comparing partial tonsillectomy surgeries with traditional adenotonsillectomy, including follow-up polysomnography, are needed to evaluate efficacy of these newer techniques as treatments for OSAS.

Advantages to partial tonsillectomy include shorter recovery times and fewer complications than traditional adenotonsillectomy. Children are able to return to normal activity earlier, are less likely to require pain medication postoperatively, are able to return to full diet sooner, or have had less postoperative bleeding than those who undergo traditional adentonsillectomy.[27–30]

Unlike traditional tonsillectomy, however, partial tonsillectomy is associated with a risk of tonsillar regrowth. Studies of children who underwent partial tonsillectomy have shown tonsillar regrowth rates between 7.2% and 16.6%, but have varied in the follow-up duration and type of procedure.[31,32] The implications of this regrowth on sleep-disordered breathing are unknown.

Positive Airway Pressure

If OSAS persists after adenotonsillectomy or if adenotonsillectomy is not performed, positive airway pressure (PAP) is often the next line of therapy.[13]

Therapy with PAP involves air that is pressurized by an electronic device and delivered during sleep via a nasal mask, acting as a pneumatic stent of the airway. PAP can be delivered as continuous positive airway pressure (CPAP) or as bilevel pressure (BPAP). PAP is effective in eliminating OSAS in children, even those younger than 2 years of age, but adherence can be challenging even with close follow-up, and parental report of PAP use can be unreliable.[33–35] PAP is titrated in the sleep laboratory to determine the pressures required to normalize breathing. Limited evidence is available to guide clinicians in titrating PAP in young children.[36]

Autotitration of PAP is not recommended for children, because the lower pressures they generate may be insufficient to properly trigger the machine. Unlike adults, children may not need PAP for life.[37] Periodic retitration may be required to assess the continuing need and efficacy of PAP, particularly if significant growth or weight gain or loss has occurred, surgical procedures have been performed, or in the presence of other factors that may affect upper airway anatomy or physiology.

The challenges in treating children with OSAS using PAP include finding the appropriate equipment and achieving tolerance of that equipment. Some evidence shows that behavioral therapy can improve adherence to PAP in children who are willing to participate in this type of therapy.[38,39] The availability of appropriate equipment for children with OSAS has also been a challenge, particularly in younger patients. Machines that generate pressure for CPAP and BPAP are designed for adults, and algorithms used in these machines to adequately ventilate young children requiring more advanced settings have not been well studied. Smaller children may not be able to adequately trigger a BPAP machine because of smaller pressures and tidal volumes. Furthermore, few nasal masks are available that fit the faces of children with OSAS, particularly those younger than 2 years and those with craniofacial abnormalities.

Although most children who are able to effectively use PAP do so without side effects, the technique has several potential complications. Children may experience skin erythema or breakdown from poorly fitting masks or those applied too tightly. Global facial flattening and midface hypoplasia has also been observed.[40] Nasal symptoms, including congestion or dry nose, are relatively common and can often be treated by adjusting the machine's humidification. Epistaxis is seen occasionally. Other potential complications include headache, irritation of the eyes from air leak, and aerophagia.

Pharmacologic Therapies

Nasal steroids

Enlarged tonsils and adenoids consist of hypertrophied lymphoid tissue, and topical steroids may be capable of reducing this inflammation. In the presence of residual lymphoid tissue from adenoidal regrowth after adenotonsillectomy or when adenotonsillectomy cannot performed, intranasal steroids have been considered to treat OSA. One small study of children younger than 10 years found that those randomized to nasal fluticasone propionate had an AHI that decreased from 10.7 $\pm$ 2.6 to 5.8 $\pm$ 2.2 in the treatment group, but increased in the control group.[41] A slightly larger similar study of intranasal budesonide also demonstrated short-term polysomnographic improvement but not overall resolution of OSAS after steroid administration.[42] Side effects include nasal irritation and epistaxis, and a potential risk exists for adrenal and growth suppression if used long-term. The long-term efficacy of nasal steroids for OSAS and the length of therapy required remain unknown.

Leukotriene receptor antagonists

Leukotrienes regulate inflammation in the respiratory system, and mediators of this pathway, such as human cysteinyl leukotriene receptor 1, have been shown to be overexpressed in tonsillar tissue of children with OSAS. Leukotriene receptor antagonists such as montelukast have been proposed to treat OSAS through their anti-inflammatory action on this pathway. Two small trials (by the same group) of montelukast in children with mild OSAS showed modest improvement in AHI after 12 to 16 weeks of therapy without significant side effects.[43,44] Larger studies are needed to know whether these findings can be generalized to children with more severe OSAS or those who are not surgical candidates.

Combination therapy with montelukast and intranasal steroids has also been studied. In a study of children who had residual mild OSAS after adenotonsillectomy, 22 patients who received daily montelukast and intranasal budesonide had reductions in AHI and improvement in several other sleep parameters.[45]

Other Nonsurgical Therapies

Rapid maxillary expansion

Rapid maxillary expansion (RME) involves placing a dental appliance in the child's mouth, which is worn during sleep. The device is connected to the posterior teeth and provides lateral pressure on the maxillary surface of the mouth. This reopens the midpalatal suture to increase the transverse diameter of the hard palate over a period of several months. Over 2 to 3 weeks, the device is expanded through daily turning of screws, followed by a fixed retention phase, in which the device remains in place for an additional 6 to 13 months.

RME has been proposed to treat OSAS in specific pediatric populations, including those with constricted maxillary arches. In a study of 31 nonobese children with upper jaw constriction but without adenotonsillar hypertrophy who had a mean AHI of 12 events per hour, maxillary expansion for 10 to 20 days resulted in resolution of OSAS, with all subjects having an AHI of less than 1 event per hour at follow-up.[46] A smaller study of school-aged children with dental malocclusion showed more modest improvements in more mild OSAS at a 24-month follow-up.[47] RME has also been considered as a second-line therapy when OSAS persists after adenotonsillectomy. One study of 31 prepubertal children with OSA who had both tonsillar enlargement and a narrow maxilla were sequentially treated with either adenotonsillectomy or RME, and then the other intervention. Although 30 patients had persistent OSAS after one intervention, all but 2 had complete resolution of OSAS after both interventions, regardless of the order of intervention.[48] Larger, more inclusive studies are needed to better define which pediatric populations will benefit from RME and whether the benefit is sustainable.

Oral appliances

Oral appliances are another dental option available for the treatment of OSAS. These devices, worn during sleep, advance the mandible or tongue, increasing the size of the upper airway. A Cochrane review found that in adults, oral appliances can cause a decrease in AHI, but are not curative in those with more severe OSAS.[49] A single small study of children with mostly mild-to-moderate OSAS showed general improvement in AHI and daytime symptoms but not resolution of OSAS after 6 months of orthodontic therapy.[50] Reported side effects of oral appliances include dental discomfort and dry mouth.

Positional therapy

Among adults, 50% with mild and 19% with moderate OSAS can normalize their sleep-disordered breathing through sleeping in a nonsupine position. Devices are available that have been successful in treating adults with positional obstructive apnea through preventing them from rolling on their backs during sleep.[51] Less evidence is available in children that positional OSAS exists, with some studies actually showing more apnea in the lateral than supine position, and others not finding any correlation between sleep position and OSAS.[52,53] No studies have evaluated the role of positional therapy in treating pediatric OSAS.

Weight loss

Weight loss has been shown to be effective in improving OSAS in adults, but not curing it.[54] In a study of 49 obese children aged 10 to 18 with OSAS, weight loss was associated with resolution of OSAS in 71%.[55] A previous study by the same group also found that weight loss improved OSAS in obese teens.[56] However, sustained weight loss is difficult without continued intervention. The limited data available suggest that weight loss could be considered adjunctive therapy for older children and teenagers with OSAS, especially considering that adenotonsillectomy is less likely to be successful in this group. CPAP could be used simultaneously until OSAS is shown to have resolved. If significant weight gain occurs, patients should be reevaluated for OSAS.

Supplemental oxygen

Although it does not reduce airway obstruction, supplemental oxygen has been used to normalize oxyhemoglobin saturation during sleep in children with OSAS. In one small study of young children with OSAS caused by adenotonsillar hypertrophy, supplemental oxygen was effective in increasing mean oxyhemoglobin saturation, reducing scorable obstructive apneas, and increasing rapid eye movement (REM) sleep, but did not worsen alveolar ventilation.[57] Another small study of children around the same age found no change in the number of obstructive events, but 2 children had significant elevation in end-tidal carbon dioxide with the addition of supplemental oxygen.[58] With the paucity of data available, supplemental oxygen should be used with caution in treating OSAS because of concerns for hypercapnia, and its inability to actually treat upper airway obstruction. Especially in young children who are normoxemic except for brief intermittent obstructive events, prolonged supplemental oxygen exposure can be associated with toxicity, and the titration of oxygen can be problematic.

Other Surgical Therapies

Uvulopalatopharyngoplasty

Although uvulopalatopharyngoplasty is commonly performed in adults with OSAS, no studies in children evaluating its efficacy include polysomnograms. Case series of children who have undergone uvulopalatopharyngoplasty for OSAS are limited to patients with neurologic impairment,

and use parental report of symptoms as a metric of successful resolution of OSAS.[59,60]

Tracheostomy

Tracheostomy is a highly effective means of treating upper airway obstruction.[61] Through simply bypassing the site of obstruction with an artificial airway in the trachea, this therapy is virtually 100% effective in eliminating OSAS. Tracheostomy allows patients to receive PAP without the need for a mask. However, the burden of a tracheostomy in children is great, requiring increased care and having increased risk for complications, including tracheitis and death. Because of the invasive nature of this procedure and alternative therapies such as PAP, tracheostomy is usually reserved for children with refractory OSAS and no available alternative.

Bariatric surgery

A variety of surgeries exist to restrict stomach size or impair micronutrient absorption to aid in weight loss. Weight loss surgery can be effective in treating OSAS in children, with success rates of 77% to 100% in resolving OSAS, depending on AHI criteria used.[62] Limitations in these studies include minimal polysomnographic follow-up and lack of long-term polysomnographic follow-up. The Roux-en-Y gastric bypass, which can be performed laparoscopically, creates a small gastric pouch and bypasses the duodenum and proximal jejunum. Laparoscopic adjustable gastric band surgery places a restrictive band around the proximal stomach, but has not been approved for use in children in the United States. Bariatric surgery can be effective in sustained weight loss, but complications can be serious, including wound infection, stricture, dehydration, micronutrient deficiency, peripheral neuropathy, beriberi, and death.[63]

SPECIAL POPULATIONS
Infants

Infants are particularly susceptible to OSAS because of the laryngeal chemoreflex and a REM-predominant sleep state distribution. Diagnosis and treatment of OSAS in infants are challenging for several reasons. First, no well-established normative polysomnographic respiratory data exist for infants, making the diagnosis of OSAS somewhat problematic. With regard to management, adenotonsillectomy has been shown to be less effective in resolving OSAS in young children. One study of 73 children younger than 24 months undergoing adenotonsillectomy for OSAS found that 66% had moderate to severe residual OSAS postoperatively.[64] Younger children and infants are also more likely to have respiratory complications postoperatively, and should be observed in-hospital after adenotonsillectomy. CPAP can be used to effectively treat OSAS in infants, although the lack of appropriately sized interfaces and head-gear available for conventional CPAP units can make this particularly challenging. Some centers choose to initiate CPAP in a hospital setting to facilitate acceptance of a mask, whereas others may be able to do this at home with appropriate parental and medical support.

Children with Craniofacial Abnormalities

Children with craniofacial abnormalities, such as Pierre Robin sequence, craniosynostosis, and conditions causing midface hypoplasia, are at increased risk for OSA because of isolated or multiple sites of upper airway narrowing.[65] Even nonsyndromic isolated cleft palate significantly increases the risk of OSAS in young children.[66] In children with micrognathia, OSAS can be seen beginning in infancy because of tongue-based airway obstruction. Conservative therapies include prone positioning, nasopharyngeal tube placement, and CPAP, but all can be difficult for parents to initiate and may be ineffective in eliminating OSAS. Surgical therapies include lip-tongue adhesion, in which the mucosa and muscles of the lip and tongue are surgically fixed, and mandibular distraction osteogenesis (MDO), which involves osteotomies of the mandibular rami and the placement of a distraction apparatus that is extended gradually over several weeks. Case series of these procedures suggest that MDO may be more successful at resolving OSAS,[67] but this surgery carries the risk of several complications, including nerve damage and infection. For children with midface hypoplasia caused by craniosynostosis, gradual frontofacial distraction or single-stage midface advancement are available surgical therapies, but data regarding improvement in OSAS are limited and variable.[68] Adenotonsillectomy should be considered in older children with craniofacial abnormalities and OSAS, although some populations have a high risk for residual OSAS. Tracheostomy should be considered in patients in whom surgical correction is not possible, who have multiple sites of obstruction, and/or for whom CPAP trials have failed.

Obese Children

As in adults, obesity is an independent risk factor for OSAS in children, and the combination of OSAS and obesity can exacerbate the risks associated with both disorders.[69] Although not as common as in adults with severe obesity, the prevalence of OSAS in adolescents with body mass index greater than 40 kg/m^2 has been shown to be approximately 50%, with boys at greater risk than girls.[62] A weight loss plan may be used in conjunction with medical or surgical therapy directed at OSAS. Adenotonsillectomy should still be considered first-line therapy in obese children with enlarged tonsils or adenoids, particularly in younger children. If significant weight loss or gain is seen, repeat polysomnogram or PAP titration should be performed to reevaluate the need for CPAP and the appropriate pressure required.

Down Syndrome

Children with Down syndrome are at increased risk for OSAS because of midface hypoplasia, reduced upper airway volume, glossoptosis, decreased upper airway tone, and increased rates of obesity compared with children without Down syndrome. Similar to what has been published in studies of otherwise healthy children with adenotonsillar hypertrophy, children with Down syndrome usually have improvement of OSAS after adenotonsillectomy, but only between 27% and 54% have complete resolution according to polysomnography.[70–72] Children with Down syndrome are also at higher risk for complications after adenotonsillectomy, and postoperative in-hospital monitoring and follow-up polysomnography should be strongly considered.[73,74] In children with Down syndrome who are unable to undergo adenotonsillectomy or who have persistent OSAS postoperatively, CPAP treatment should be considered, although adherence can be challenging.[75] Other surgical procedures that have been reported in children with Down syndrome include MDO, midface advancement, genioglossus advancement, tongue reduction surgery, or tracheostomy.

Prader-Willi Syndrome

In Prader-Willi syndrome (PWS), a period of failure to thrive and hypotonia is seen during infancy, followed by hyperphagia, obesity, and short stature in older children. Although growth hormones can be an effective and important part of therapy for these children, patients with PWS should be monitored carefully, particularly those who are sick with respiratory illnesses. Respiratory disorders are a leading cause of death in infants with PWS, and case reports exist of infants who have died from respiratory illnesses soon after starting growth hormone.[76] Studies evaluating the effect of growth hormone on sleep-disordered breathing in children with PWS show mixed results, depending on the age of children studied and the length of time patients are followed.[77,78] One small case series of children with PWS with OSAS who underwent adenotonsillectomy showed that most of those with mild OSAS had normalization of AHI postoperatively, but a few patients with more severe OSAS had no improvement or worsening after surgery.[79] This finding suggests that children with PWS and OSAS who have adenotonsillar enlargement may be good candidates for adenotonsillectomy, but that they should have a repeat polysomnography postoperatively to reevaluate for residual OSAS.

SUMMARY

The mainstays of therapy for OSA in children are adenotonsillectomy and PAP. Nonsurgical therapies, including anti-inflammatory medications, dental devices, and weight loss, may be useful in specific circumstances. Airway surgery has been shown to be effective in children with craniofacial abnormalities, but not in the general pediatric population. Children with Down syndrome, craniofacial abnormalities, obesity, or PWS are at increased risk for OSAS and may require more frequent polysomnography and specific therapies.

REFERENCES

1. Standards and indications for cardiopulmonary sleep studies in children. American Thoracic Society. Am J Respir Crit Care Med 1996;153(2):866–78.
2. Chervin RD, Weatherly RA, Ruzicka DL, et al. Subjective sleepiness and polysomnographic correlates in children scheduled for adenotonsillectomy vs other surgical care. Sleep 2006;29(4):495–503.
3. Gozal D, Crabtree VM, Sans Capdevila O, et al. C-reactive protein, obstructive sleep apnea, and cognitive dysfunction in school-aged children. Am J Respir Crit Care Med 2007;176(2):188–93.
4. Kheirandish L, Gozal D. Neurocognitive dysfunction in children with sleep disorders. Dev Sci 2006;9(4):388–99.
5. Amin RS, Carroll JL, Jeffries JL, et al. Twenty-four-hour ambulatory blood pressure in children with sleep-disordered breathing. Am J Respir Crit Care Med 2004;169(8):950–6.
6. Bonuck K, Parikh S, Bassila M. Growth failure and sleep disordered breathing: a review of the literature. Int J Pediatr Otorhinolaryngol 2006;70(5):769–78.
7. Li AM, Wong E, Kew J, et al. Use of tonsil size in the evaluation of obstructive sleep apnoea. Arch Dis Child 2002;87(2):156–9.
8. Pinard JM, Azabou E, Essid N, et al. Sleep-disordered breathing in children with congenital muscular dystrophies. Eur J Paediatr Neurol 2012;16(6):619–24.
9. Marcus CL, Smith RJ, Mankarious LA, et al. Developmental aspects of the upper airway: report from an NHLBI Workshop, March 5-6, 2009. Proc Am Thorac Soc 2009;6(6):513–20.
10. Narang I, Mathew JL. Childhood obesity and obstructive sleep apnea. J Nutr Metab 2012;2012:134202.
11. Suen JS, Arnold JE, Brooks LJ. Adenotonsillectomy for treatment of obstructive sleep apnea in children. Arch Otolaryngol Head Neck Surg 1995;121(5):525–30.
12. Brietzke SE, Katz ES, Roberson DW. Can history and physical examination reliably diagnose pediatric obstructive sleep apnea/hypopnea syndrome? A systematic review of the literature. Otolaryngol Head Neck Surg 2004;131(6):827–32.
13. Marcus CL, Brooks LJ, Draper KA, et al. Clinical practice guideline: diagnosis and management of childhood obstructive sleep apnea syndrome. Pediatrics 2012;130(3):1–9.
14. Bhattacharjee R, Kheirandish-Gozal L, Spruyt K, et al. Adenotonsillectomy outcomes in treatment of obstructive sleep apnea in children: a multicenter retrospective study. Am J Respir Crit Care Med 2010;182(5):676–83.
15. Tauman R, Gulliver TE, Krishna J, et al. Persistence of obstructive sleep apnea syndrome in children after adenotonsillectomy. J Pediatr 2006;149(6):803–8.
16. Mitchell RB. Adenotonsillectomy for obstructive sleep apnea in children: outcome evaluated by pre- and postoperative polysomnography. Laryngoscope 2007;117(10):1844–54.
17. Tarasiuk A, Simon T, Tal A, et al. Adenotonsillectomy in children with obstructive sleep apnea syndrome reduces health care utilization. Pediatrics 2004;113(2):351–6.
18. Spencer DJ, Jones JE. Complications of adenotonsillectomy in patients younger than 3 years. Arch Otolaryngol Head Neck Surg 2012;138(4):335–9.
19. Gallagher TQ, Wilcox L, McGuire E, et al. Analyzing factors associated with major complications after adenotonsillectomy in 4776 patients: comparing three tonsillectomy techniques. Otolaryngol Head Neck Surg 2010;142(6):886–92.
20. Ye J, Liu H, Zhang G, et al. Postoperative respiratory complications of adenotonsillectomy for obstructive sleep apnea syndrome in older children: prevalence, risk factors, and impact on clinical outcome. J Otolaryngol Head Neck Surg 2009;38(1):49–58.
21. Roland PS, Rosenfeld RM, Brooks LJ, et al. Clinical practice guideline: polysomnography for sleep-disordered breathing prior to tonsillectomy in children. Otolaryngol Head Neck Surg 2011;145(Suppl 1):S1–15.

22. Mitchell RB, Pereira KD, Friedman NR. Sleep-disordered breathing in children: survey of current practice. Laryngoscope 2006;116(6):956–8.

23. Carroll JL, McColley SA, Marcus CL, et al. Inability of clinical history to distinguish primary snoring from obstructive sleep apnea syndrome in children. Chest 1995;108(3):610–8.

24. Tunkel DE, Hotchkiss KS, Carson KA, et al. Efficacy of powered intracapsular tonsillectomy and adenoidectomy. Laryngoscope 2008;118(7): 1295–302.

25. Mangiardi J, Graw-Panzer KD, Weedon J, et al. Polysomnography outcomes for partial intracapsular versus total tonsillectomy. Int J Pediatr Otorhinolaryngol 2010;74(12):1361–6.

26. Ericsson E, Ledin T, Hultcrantz E. Long-term improvement of quality of life as a result of tonsillotomy (with radiofrequency technique) and tonsillectomy in youths. Laryngoscope 2007;117(7): 1272–9.

27. Derkay CS, Darrow DH, Welch C, et al. Post-tonsillectomy morbidity and quality of life in pediatric patients with obstructive tonsils and adenoid: microdebrider vs electrocautery. Otolaryngol Head Neck Surg 2006;134(1):114–20.

28. Koltai PJ, Solares CA, Koempel JA, et al. Intracapsular tonsillar reduction (partial tonsillectomy): reviving a historical procedure for obstructive sleep disordered breathing in children. Otolaryngol Head Neck Surg 2003;129(5):532–8.

29. Sobol SE, Wetmore RF, Marsh RR, et al. Postoperative recovery after microdebrider intracapsular or monopolar electrocautery tonsillectomy: a prospective, randomized, single-blinded study. Arch Otolaryngol Head Neck Surg 2006;132(3):270–4.

30. Chaidas KS, Kaditis AG, Papadakis CE, et al. Tonsilloplasty versus tonsillectomy in children with sleep-disordered breathing: short- and long-term outcomes. Laryngoscope 2013;123(5):1294–9.

31. Celenk F, Bayazit YA, Yilmaz M, et al. Tonsillar regrowth following partial tonsillectomy with radiofrequency. Int J Pediatr Otorhinolaryngol 2008;72(1): 19–22.

32. Zagolski O. Why do palatine tonsils grow back after partial tonsillectomy in children? Eur Arch Otorhinolaryngol 2010;267(10):1613–7.

33. Marcus CL, Rosen G, Ward SL, et al. Adherence to and effectiveness of positive airway pressure therapy in children with obstructive sleep apnea. Pediatrics 2006;117(3):e442–51.

34. Uong EC, Epperson M, Bathon SA, et al. Adherence to nasal positive airway pressure therapy among school-aged children and adolescents with obstructive sleep apnea syndrome. Pediatrics 2007;120(5):e1203–11.

35. Downey R 3rd, Perkin RM, MacQuarrie J. Nasal continuous positive airway pressure use in children

with obstructive sleep apnea younger than 2 years of age. Chest 2000;117(6):1608–12.

36. Kushida CA, Chediak A, Berry RB, et al. Clinical guidelines for the manual titration of positive airway pressure in patients with obstructive sleep apnea. J Clin Sleep Med 2008;4(2):157–71.

37. Marcus CL, Ward SL, Mallory GB, et al. Use of nasal continuous positive airway pressure as treatment of childhood obstructive sleep-apnea. J Pediatr 1995;127(1):88–94.

38. Koontz KL, Slifer KJ, Cataldo MD, et al. Improving pediatric compliance with positive airway pressure therapy: the impact of behavioral intervention. Sleep 2003;26(8):1010–5.

39. Rains JC. Treatment of obstructive sleep apnea in pediatric patients. Behavioral intervention for compliance with nasal continuous positive airway pressure. Clin Pediatr (Phila) 1995;34(10):535–41.

40. Fauroux B, Lavis JF, Nicot F, et al. Facial side effects during noninvasive positive pressure ventilation in children. Intensive Care Med 2005;31(7): 965–9.

41. Brouillette RT, Manoukian JJ, Ducharme FM, et al. Efficacy of fluticasone nasal spray for pediatric obstructive sleep apnea. J Pediatr 2001;138(6): 838–44.

42. Kheirandish-Gozal L, Gozal D. Intranasal budesonide treatment for children with mild obstructive sleep apnea syndrome. Pediatrics 2008;122(1): e149–55.

43. Goldbart AD, Goldman JL, Veling MC, et al. Leukotriene modifier therapy for mild sleep-disordered breathing in children. Am J Respir Crit Care Med 2005;172(3):364–70.

44. Goldbart AD, Greenberg-Dotan S, Tal A. Montelukast for children with obstructive sleep apnea: a double-blind, placebo-controlled study. Pediatrics 2012;130(3):e575–80.

45. Kheirandish L, Goldbart AD, Gozal D. Intranasal steroids and oral leukotriene modifier therapy in residual sleep-disordered breathing after tonsillectomy and adenoidectomy in children. Pediatrics 2006;117(1):e61–6.

46. Pirelli P, Saponara M, Guilleminault C. Rapid maxillary expansion in children with obstructive sleep apnea syndrome. Sleep 2004;27(4):761–6.

47. Villa MP, Rizzoli A, Miano S, et al. Efficacy of rapid maxillary expansion in children with obstructive sleep apnea syndrome: 36 months of follow-up. Sleep Breath 2011;15(2):179–84.

48. Guilleminault C, Monteyrol PJ, Huynh NT, et al. Adeno-tonsillectomy and rapid maxillary distraction in pre-pubertal children, a pilot study. Sleep Breath 2011;15(2):173–7.

49. Lim J, Lasserson TJ, Fleetham J, et al. Oral appliances for obstructive sleep apnoea. Cochrane Database Syst Rev 2006;(1):CD004435.

50. Villa MP, Bernkopf E, Pagani J, et al. Randomized controlled study of an oral jaw-positioning appliance for the treatment of obstructive sleep apnea in children with malocclusion. Am J Respir Crit Care Med 2002;165(1):123–7.

51. Permut I, Diaz-Abad M, Chatila W, et al. Comparison of positional therapy to CPAP in patients with positional obstructive sleep apnea. J Clin Sleep Med 2010;6(3):238–43.

52. Fernandes do Prado LB, Li X, Thompson R, et al. Body position and obstructive sleep apnea in children. Sleep 2002;25(1):66–71.

53. Dayyat E, Maarafeya MM, Capdevila OS, et al. Nocturnal body position in sleeping children with and without obstructive sleep apnea. Pediatr Pulmonol 2007;42(4):374–9.

54. Greenburg DL, Lettieri CJ, Eliasson AH. Effects of surgical weight loss on measures of obstructive sleep apnea: a meta-analysis. Am J Med 2009; 122(6):535–42.

55. Van Hoorenbeeck K, Franckx H, Debode P, et al. Weight loss and sleep-disordered breathing in childhood obesity: effects on inflammation and uric acid. Obesity (Silver Spring) 2012;20(1):172–7.

56. Verhulst SL, Franckx H, Van Gaal L, et al. The effect of weight loss on sleep-disordered breathing in obese teenagers. Obesity (Silver Spring) 2009; 17(6):1178–83.

57. Aljadeff G, Gozal D, Bailey-Wahl SL, et al. Effects of overnight supplemental oxygen in obstructive sleep apnea in children. Am J Respir Crit Care Med 1996;153(1):51–5.

58. Marcus CL, Carroll JL, Bamford O, et al. Supplemental oxygen during sleep in children with sleep-disordered breathing. Am J Respir Crit Care Med 1995;152(4 Pt 1):1297–301.

59. Kosko JR, Derkay CS. Uvulopalatopharyngoplasty: treatment of obstructive sleep apnea in neurologically impaired pediatric patients. Int J Pediatr Otorhinolaryngol 1995;32(3):241–6.

60. Kerschner JE, Lynch JB, Kleiner H, et al. Uvulopalatopharyngoplasty with tonsillectomy and adenoidectomy as a treatment for obstructive sleep apnea in neurologically impaired children. Int J Pediatr Otorhinolaryngol 2002;62(3):229–35.

61. Guilleminault C, Simmons FB, Motta J, et al. Obstructive sleep apnea syndrome and tracheostomy. Long-term follow-up experience. Arch Intern Med 1981;141(8):985–8.

62. Kalra M, Inge T. Effect of bariatric surgery on obstructive sleep apnoea in adolescents. Paediatr Respir Rev 2006;7(4):260–7.

63. Lawson ML, Kirk S, Mitchell T, et al. One-year outcomes of Roux-en-Y gastric bypass for morbidly obese adolescents: a multicenter study from the Pediatric Bariatric Study Group. J Pediatr Surg 2006;41(1):137–43 [discussion: 137–43].

64. Brigance JS, Miyamoto RC, Schilt P, et al. Surgical management of obstructive sleep apnea in infants and young toddlers. Otolaryngol Head Neck Surg 2009;140(6):912–6.

65. Alexiou S, Brooks L. Congenital disorders affecting sleep. Sleep Med Clin 2012;7:689–702.

66. Maclean JE, Fitzsimons D, Fitzgerald DA, et al. The spectrum of sleep-disordered breathing symptoms and respiratory events in infants with cleft lip and/or palate. Arch Dis Child 2012;97(12):1058–63.

67. Bookman LB, Melton KR, Pan BS, et al. Neonates with tongue-based airway obstruction: a systematic review. Otolaryngol Head Neck Surg 2012; 146(1):8–18.

68. Mathijssen I, Arnaud E, Marchac D, et al. Respiratory outcome of mid-face advancement with distraction: a comparison between Le Fort III and frontofacial monobloc. J Craniofac Surg 2006; 17(5):880–2.

69. Doherty LS, Kiely JL, Swan V, et al. Long-term effects of nasal continuous positive airway pressure therapy on cardiovascular outcomes in sleep apnea syndrome. Chest 2005;127(6):2076–84.

70. Shete MM, Stocks RM, Sebelik ME, et al. Effects of adeno-tonsillectomy on polysomnography patterns in Down syndrome children with obstructive sleep apnea: a comparative study with children without Down syndrome. Int J Pediatr Otorhinolaryngol 2010;74(3):241–4.

71. Merrell JA, Shott SR. OSAS in Down syndrome: T&A versus T&A plus lateral pharyngoplasty. Int J Pediatr Otorhinolaryngol 2007;71(8):1197–203.

72. Marcus CL, Keens TG, Bautista DB, et al. Obstructive sleep apnea in children with Down syndrome. Pediatrics 1991;88(1):132–9.

73. Goldstein NA, Armfield DR, Kingsley LA, et al. Postoperative complications after tonsillectomy and adenoidectomy in children with Down syndrome. Arch Otolaryngol Head Neck Surg 1998; 124(2):171–6.

74. Marcus CL, Brooks LJ, Draper KA, et al. Diagnosis and management of childhood obstructive sleep apnea syndrome. Pediatrics 2012;130(3): e714–55.

75. Brooks L, Bacevice A, Beebe A, et al. Relationship between neuropsychological function and success of treatment for OSA in children with Down syndrome. Am J Respir Crit Care Med 1997;155: A710.

76. Van Vliet G, Deal CL, Crock PA, et al. Sudden death in growth hormone-treated children with Prader-Willi syndrome. J Pediatr 2004;144(1):129–31.

77. Al-Saleh S, Al-Naimi A, Hamilton J, et al. Longitudinal evaluation of sleep-disordered breathing in children with Prader-Willi syndrome during 2 years of growth hormone therapy. J Pediatr 2013;162(2): 263–8.e261.

78. Miller J, Silverstein J, Shuster J, et al. Short-term effects of growth hormone on sleep abnormalities in Prader-Willi syndrome. J Clin Endocrinol Metab 2006;91(2):413–7.

79. Meyer SL, Splaingard M, Repaske DR, et al. Outcomes of adenotonsillectomy in patients with Prader-Willi syndrome. Arch Otolaryngol Head Neck Surg 2012;138(11):1047–51.

Surgical Treatment of Obstructive Sleep Apnea

Macario Camacho, MD[a],*, Richard L. Jacobson, DMD, MS[b],
Stephen A. Schendel, MD, DDS[c]

KEYWORDS

- Obstructive sleep apnea • Uvulopalatopharyngoplasty • Tonsillectomy • Hypopharyngeal surgery
- Genial tubercle advancement • Maxillomandibular advancement • Sleep surgery

KEY POINTS

- Obstructive sleep apnea is a common disorder that adversely affects one's health and if left untreated can lead to cardiovascular complications and a higher overall mortality rate.
- First-line treatment of obstructive sleep apnea should be medical management to include positive airway pressure devices, oral appliances, weight loss, and positional therapy.
- Surgical management includes soft tissue and skeletal surgeries, which are specifically targeted to the areas of airway obstruction.
- Maxillomandibular advancement is highly effective in treating sleep apnea of all severities.
- A multidisciplinary team is necessary and should include an experienced surgeon as well as a sleep-trained orthodontist to maximize short- and long-term success.

INTRODUCTION

Obstructive sleep apnea (OSA) is a common sleep disorder and is associated with an increased incidence of myocardial infarctions, cardiac arrhythmias, hypertension, and stroke.[1] Classically, treatment consists of medical management usually with continuous positive airway pressure (CPAP) and surgery in selected patients. Individuals with OSA will seek medical treatment for complaints of snoring and/or excessive daytime hypersomnolence. Typically these patients will undergo overnight polysomnography to diagnose the extent of their sleep-disordered breathing. Sleep-disordered breathing is a spectrum of respiratory patterns, which includes primary snoring, upper airway resistance syndrome, and OSA (**Fig. 1**).

OSA is caused by a combination of factors of which the position of the jaws, body mass index (BMI), and lymphoid tissue seem to be the most important.

The first effective treatment described for OSA in adults was a tracheostomy.[2] Because of the significant morbidity associated with tracheostomies, alternative treatments were investigated. Sullivan and colleagues[3] described CPAP as highly effective therapy for OSA in 1981. Since then, medical management with CPAP as treatment of OSA is considered to be first-line therapy. For those patients with mild to moderate OSA who cannot tolerate CPAP, an oral appliance may serve as an effective alternative or adjunct for travel.[4] Oral appliances should be custom-made and function by decreasing the upper airway's collapsibility

Disclaimer: The views herein are the private views of the authors and do not reflect the official views of the Department of the Army or the Department of Defense.
Disclosures: None.
a Sleep Division, Department of Otolaryngology-Head and Neck Surgery, Stanford University, 801 Welch Road, Stanford, CA 94305, USA; b Department of Orthodontics, School of Dentistry, University of California, 10833 Le Conte Avenue, CHS - Box 951668, Los Angeles, CA 90095-1668, USA; c Department of Plastic Surgery, Stanford University School of Medicine, 770 Welch Road, Stanford, CA 94304, USA
* Corresponding author.
E-mail address: drcamachoent@yahoo.com

Sleep Med Clin 8 (2013) 495–503
http://dx.doi.org/10.1016/j.jsmc.2013.07.012
1556-407X/13/$ – see front matter Published by Elsevier Inc.

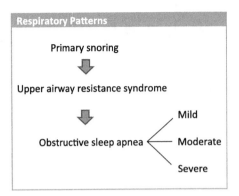

Fig. 1. Respiratory patterns in sleep-disordered breathing.

and enlarging the airway during sleep.[5] Greater compliance with oral appliances is seen when compared with CPAP, which results in improved therapeutic effectiveness.[6] Additional medical management includes weight loss and positional therapy. Unfortunately, many patients will fail medical management. It is estimated that more than 50% of patients do not effectively use or tolerate CPAP.[7] Surgical treatment of OSA is generally reserved for those patients who have failed medical interventions.

The anatomic areas treated surgically for OSA include the nose, nasal cavity, nasopharynx, soft palate, hard palate, oral cavity, oropharynx, hypopharynx, craniofacial, and neck locations (**Table 1**).

Because each patient is unique in their anatomy and pathophysiology, there is great variability in the treatment options. Surgical treatment of OSA is divided based on the location of the obstruction

and can start as high as the nose and extend down to the neck (see **Table 1**). Surgical success is contingent on properly identifying the site of obstruction and effectively treating it. Several modalities are used to identify the levels of obstruction and include physical exam, flexible fiberoptic laryngoscopy, Mueller maneuver, drug-induced sleep endoscopy, endoscopy under sedation, pressure recordings during sleep, lateral cephalograms, three-dimensional (3D) cone-beam computed tomography (CT) scan imaging and dynamic sleep magnetic resonance imaging.[8–12] There is currently no single modality that is used exclusively by all sleep surgeons, rather it is more often accepted to use multiple modalities to determine which procedure is best for the patient.

Categorizing the severity of sleep-disordered breathing is key to management and in achieving successful outcomes. Sher and colleagues[13] performed a literature review and classified surgical success as a decrease in respiratory disturbance index greater than or equal to 50% and a total of less than 20 events/h or a decrease in apnea index greater than or equal to 50% and a total of less than 10 events/h. This definition of success and cure is currently one of the most frequently used definitions in the literature.

NOSE, NASAL CAVITY, AND NASOPHARYNX

Nasal obstruction is a common complaint in patients who have OSA. Nasal obstruction can lead to oral breathing, which is associated with increased airway resistance. One study used polysomnography to demonstrate that healthy

Table 1
Surgical treatments for OSA

Location	Types of Surgeries
Nose	Rhinoplasty
Nasal cavity	Turbinoplasty, septoplasty, polypectomy
Nasopharynx	Adenoidectomy
Soft palate	Uvulopalatopharyngoplasty, laser assisted uvulopalatoplasty, cautery-assisted palatal stiffening operation, pillar implants, injection snoreplasty
Hard palate	Rapid maxillary expansion, transpalatal pharyngoplasty
Oropharynx	Tonsillectomy, tongue suspension, radiofrequency ablation of the tongue, midline glossectomy, lingual tonsillectomy, transoral robotic glossectomy
Hypopharynx	Genial tubercle advancement, hyoid suspension
Epiglottis	Epiglottopexy, epiglottoplasty
Larynx	Supraglottoplasty, arytenoidopexy
Craniofacial	Maxillomandibular advancement
Neck	Tracheostomy

non-OSA patients without nasal obstruction can develop partial or total obstructive respiratory events if their noses are experimentally obstructed.[14] Nasal procedures are commonly performed for functional improvement in daytime breathing and to improve CPAP compliance. However, nasal surgeries are not very successful in treating OSA, as demonstrated by a review performed by Verse and Pirsig[15] that demonstrated a pooled nasal surgical success rate of 17.5%. There is no study in which adenoidectomy alone has been evaluated as treatment of OSA.[16] Despite the low success rate in treating OSA, the improvement in nasal breathing may significantly improve patients' quality of life, sleep, and CPAP compliance.

SOFT PALATE

Initially described for snoring, the uvulopalatopharyngoplasty (UPPP) was eventually used as treatment of OSA.[17] There are modifications of the UPPP that have been developed to treat OSA. Unfortunately, there are variable success rates and in an improperly selected patient, the success rate may approach 0%.[18] In a patient with significant tonsillar hypertrophy (size 3, 4), a Friedman palate position of 1 or 2, and a BMI less than 40, the success rate approaches 80%.[18] One of the most commonly accepted modifications is the technique described by Dr Powell and colleagues,[19] which uses a reversible flap, is conservative and reduces the risk of postoperative velopharyngeal insufficiency. **Figs. 2** and **3** demonstrate the typical appearance of the oral cavity and oropharynx pre- and post-UPPP. Pillar implants, radiofrequency ablation of the soft palate, and injection snoreplasty are more commonly used in the treatment of snoring or upper airway resistance syndrome and are less likely to be used to treat OSA.

HARD PALATE

Rapid maxillary expansion (RME) is a procedure that is used to correct maxillary deficiency in the transverse dimension.[20] It is essential for the operating surgeon to work closely with an experienced orthodontist, as their expertise and knowledge in treating sleep apnea patients is critical for perioperative management. RME has a surgical success rate of 90% and cure rate of 70% when used in adults with transverse maxillary deficiency.[21] Transverse maxillary deficiency can be assessed using a cone-beam CT anterior-posterior cephalometric image. Severe constriction of the maxilla relative to the mandible results in a cross-bite,

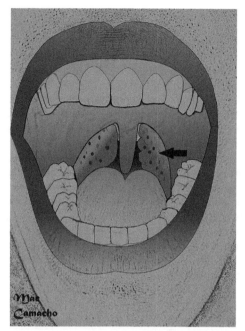

Fig. 2. Presurgical anatomy. Note the elongated uvula and partially obstructing tonsillar tissue (*right arrow*), both of which obstruct the airway.

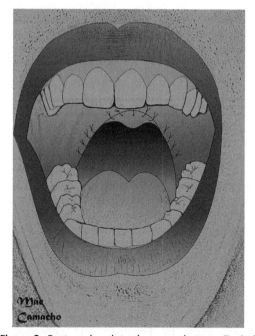

Fig. **3.** Post-uvulopalatopharyngoplasty. Typical appearance after the mucosa over the anterior aspect of the uvula and inferior soft palate is removed, with preservation of the underlying muscle. The flap is then reflected superiorly and is sutured into position.

where the maxillary teeth occlude edge to edge with, or inside the mandibular teeth. This type of malocclusion is abnormal and usually dysfunctional. In the pooled data for 88 children, the apnea-hypopnea index (AHI) decreased from 10.9 ± 4.7events/h to 0.8 ± 1.3 events/h.[21]

Transpalatal advancement pharyngoplasty (TAP) was first described for use in patients who were not good candidates for UPPP by Woodson and Toohill.[22] With this technique a segment of the hard palate and redundant mucosa is removed and advanced forward. In a case series of comparable preoperative AHI in patients classified as Friedman Stage 3, there is an improvement in AHI compared with UPPP alone, 17.1 ± 30.1 events/h versus 28.5 ± 25.6 events/h respectively, with a P<.02.[23] However, the mean post-operative AHI in the TAP patients was still consistent with moderate OSA.

OROPHARYNX
Tonsillectomy

In children, and in young, thin adults with no other anatomic abnormality other than significantly hypertrophied tonsils, a tonsillectomy may be first-line management.[24,25] Children typically undergo an adenoidectomy simultaneously with a tonsillectomy. A meta-analysis determined the pooled success rate to be 82.9%.[26] Adenotonsillectomy is more likely to fail in children who have craniofacial abnormalities, down syndrome, significant lingual tonsillar hypertrophy, collapse at the level of the soft palate, and who are obese or have occult laryngomalacia.[26–28]

Tongue Surgeries

During deep sleep, tongue muscles relax and may be displaced posteriorly and occlude the oropharynx. Several tongue modification procedures have been developed to attempt to either reduce the volume of the tongue or to prevent posterior displacement of the tongue. These procedures include tongue suspension devices, radiofrequency ablation of the tongue (RFBOT), midline glossectomy, submucosal minimally invasive lingual excision (SMILE), lingual tonsillectomy, and transoral robotic glossectomy (TORS). These procedures are performed in conjunction with other surgeries, so it is difficult to determine their effectiveness of performing them in isolation. A recent study by Friedman and colleagues[29] compared patients who underwent a z-plasty with TORS, z-plasty with RFBOT, and z-plasty with SMILE. The study demonstrated no major bleeding or airway complications. The combination of the z-plasty with these techniques yielded a surgical cure of 66.7% for the TORS group, 20.8% for the RFBOT, and 45.5% for SMILE.[29]

HYPOPHARYNX

Genial tubercle advancement (GTA) with hyoid suspension was first described by Dr Riley and colleagues[30] in 1984. Initially described as a mandibular horizontal sliding osteotomy, the GTA procedure has undergone several modifications over the years, to the current osteotomy design, which creates a rectangular osteotomy that encompasses the genial tubercle and most or all of the genioglossus tendon that attaches to it (**Figs. 4** and **5**). The GTA rectangular osteotomy typically measures about 8 to 10 mm × 20 mm. The advancement of the segment places tension on the tongue and repositions this complex anteriorly, which restricts collapse of the tongue posteriorly during hypotonic states of sleep.[31] Initially, the GTA procedures were performed in combination with hyoid suspension; however, today they are more often performed simultaneously with either uvulopalatopharyngoplasty or maxillomandibular advancement surgeries. A systematic review of hypopharyngeal surgeries demonstrated a 35% to 62% success rate in treating OSA.[32] Hyoid suspension alone has a surgical success rate of 17%, and thus is not recommended as an isolated procedure, but

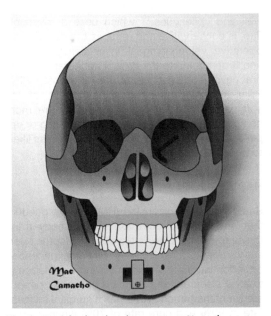

Fig. 4. Genial tubercle advancement. Note the rectangular osteotomy. The genioglossus muscle is attached to the genial tubercle, which is pulled anteriorly and rotated 30° to 90°. The cancellous bone and outer cortex are removed and the inner cortex is fixated to the lower mandibular border with a single screw.

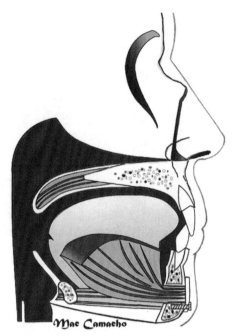

Fig. 5. Genial tubercle advancement. The genioglossus muscle is attached to the genial tubercle, which is pulled anteriorly; the outer cortex and cancellous bone are removed, leaving the inner cortex only, which is attached to the lower mandible with a single screw.

may improve outcomes if performed as part of a multilevel surgery.[33]

EPIGLOTTIS

In some patients with OSA, the epiglottis may collapse posteriorly during sleep. Negative pressure may build up in these patients and cause partial or complete obstruction. The 2 procedures used to correct the retrodisplacement include epiglottopexy (suspending the epiglottis to the tongue base with a suture) and epiglottoplasty (removing a portion of the superior part of the epiglottis). The procedures are rarely performed, but if performed, they are often done so as part of a multilevel surgery.[34] In children, epiglottoplasty is sometimes used as treatment of laryngomalacia.[35]

LARYNX

Laryngomalacia consists of the triad of an omega-shaped epiglottis, medially displaced arytenoids, and redundant aryepiglottic folds. Classic laryngomalacia presents with stridor and chronic cough. About 85% of patients with classic laryngomalacia can be managed medically with positional therapy and proton-pump inhibitors. A recent systematic review by Hartl and Chadha demonstrated that although there is a coexistence of laryngomalacia

and GERD, there is only limited evidence of causation.[36] Patients with chronic aspiration and failure to thrive are candidates for supraglottoplasty and/or arytenoidopexy. Koltai and colleagues have identified a variant of laryngomalacia (occult laryngomalacia) in post-adenotonsillectomy failures for OSA, which only manifests itself during sleep and can be diagnosed with drug-induced sleep endoscopy.[27] Supraglottoplasty has been noted to be highly effective for treating occult laryngomalacia, with a statistically significant reduction in AHI from 15.4 to 5.4 ($P<.001$).[37]

CRANIOFACIAL

Mandibular advancement was first described in 1979 by Kuo and colleagues,[38] as a successful treatment of OSA in 3 patients with mandibular deficiency. These patients had mandibular deficiency caused by trauma or congenital causes.[38] With the addition of the maxilla, the procedure becomes a maxillomandibular advancement (MMA). MMAs are performed with the creation of a LeForte 1 osteotomy to the maxilla and a bilateral split sagittal osteotomy to the mandible (**Figs. 6–9**). The airway is enlarged in the pharyngeal and hypopharyngeal regions by the expansion of the facial skeleton and the soft tissues attached to them. Specifically, the anterior movement of the maxillomandibular complex decreases collapsibility and increases the tension at the level of the velopharyngeal and suprahyoid musculature.[39]

Maxillomandibular advancement increases the anterior-posterior and lateral dimensions of the airway. Schendel and Hatcher described automated 3D airway analysis with cone-beam CT data, which allow for the calculation of airway

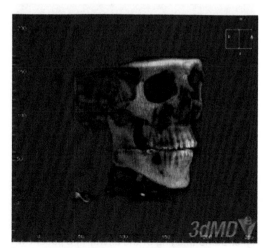

Fig. 6. 3dMD imaging reconstruction of the facial skeleton, premaxillomandibular advancement.

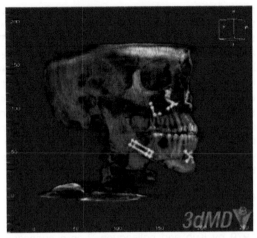

Fig. 7. 3dMD imaging reconstruction of the facial skeleton, post-maxillomandibular advancement. There is anterior and counterclockwise rotation of the advanced segments. Note the plates at the Le-Forte 1 osteotomies, bilateral split sagittal osteotomies, and inferior mandibular osteotomy site.

volume pre- and post-operatively.[12] The article describes the technique used and a patient who was analyzed with 3dMD. The imaging modality allows for calculation of the area for each level of the airway, and also can calculate the total volume of the upper airway.[12] **Figs. 8** and **9** demonstrate significant airway improvement in a patient with OSA who underwent a maxillomandibular advancement. A recent case series of 11 patients evaluating airway volume with 3DCT airway analysis demonstrated the average preoperative upper airway volume of 12.8 ± 5.1 mL and post-operative upper airway volume of 20.6 ± 8.7 mL, $P = .02$.[40]

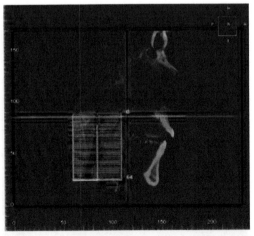

Fig. 8. 3dMD imaging of the airway in a patient with OSA, this is premaxillomandibular advancement. Note the retropalatal and retroglossal obstruction.

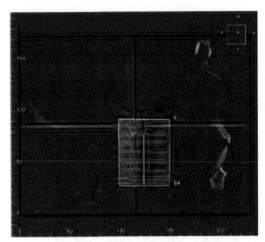

Fig. 9. 3dMD imaging of the airway, post-maxillomandibular advancement. Note the significant improvement of the entire upper airway, especially at the retropalatal and retroglossal levels.

Over the years, maxillomandibular advancement outcomes have demonstrated the procedure to be highly effective treatment for OSA. Riley and Powell developed the Stanford protocol, in which soft tissue surgeries were performed as part of phase 1 surgery, followed by a 6 month post-operative polysomnography and if there was residual OSA, then a maxillomandibular advancement would then be performed as phase 2 surgery.[41] If followed, the surgical success rate approaches 100%.[41] When assessing all the outcomes for MMAs as treatment of OSA, a recent systematic review demonstrated a pooled success rate of 86% and a cure rate of 43%.[21] A meta-analysis demonstrated that of the 627 adult patients in the study, the mean AHI improved from 63.9 ± 26.7 events/h to 9.5 ± 10.7 events/h with a $P<.001$.[42] Predictors of success and cure include an advancement greater than equal to 10 mm, lower BMI, and younger age.[42] Although upper airway surgery is not traditionally recommended for morbidly obese patients (BMI of >40 kg/m^2), one study by Li and colleagues[39] demonstrated that in patients with a BMI of 45 ± 5.4 kg/m^2 there was a surgical success in 17 out of 21 (81%) of the patients, with 2 out of the 4 treatment failures having had underlying obesity hypoventilation syndrome.

NECK

Tracheostomy is the only procedure that completely bypasses upper airway obstruction. Two types of tracheostomies are used: tubed (temporary, **Fig. 10**) and tubeless (permanent). Indications for tubed tracheostomies include

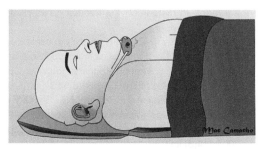

Fig. 10. Tracheostomy in an obese patient.

patients who have severe OSA with an AHI greater than 60 events/h; lowest oxygen saturations less than 70%; in patients who are undergoing other surgeries are performed such as UPPP, base of tongue reduction, MMA, and/or GTA.[39] If patients are undergoing a long-term tracheostomy as the primary surgical treatment of their OSA, a permanent, reversible tracheostomy is recommended as there are fewer complications.[43–45] Outcomes for tracheostomy as treatment of OSA demonstrate that the apnea index significantly decreases (88.4 ± 25.7 event/h to 0.5 ± 1.9 events/h, $P<.001$).[21] Even with a decrease in the apnea index, there is often an increase in central apneas (for about 3–6 months) and also an increase in hypopneas after surgery.[21] Because of the increase in hypopneas, the surgical success is 73%, which is lower than that for MMAs; however, tracheostomies are more often performed in morbidly obese patients, so it is difficult to compare the outcomes for the 2 surgeries. As in MMA failures,

morbidly obese patients may have obesity hypoventilation syndrome, which would require positive airway pressure via the tracheostomy during sleep to overcome the obstruction.[46]

SUMMARY

In summary, there are several possible surgeries that may be performed on patients with OSA (**Table 2** summarizes the maxillomandibular advancement, tracheostomy and uvulopalatophayrngoplasty results). However, the most effective surgeries in adults are maxillomandibular advancement surgeries and tracheostomies, with success rates of 86% and 73%, respectively. Tracheostomies have a higher rate of patient dissatisfaction than maxillomandibular advancement. Surgical success in children is currently 83% when adenotonsillectomy is performed. Improved surgical success is obtained with careful preoperative planning and assessment for areas of obstruction as demonstrated by surgical success of uvulopalatopharyngoplasty in 52% of patients with retropalatal obstruction only, compared with surgical success rate of only 5% in those with any component of retrolingual obstruction.[47] Sleep surgery failures should be evaluated with modalities that allow for assessment of the specific area of obstruction. A multidisciplinary team is necessary and should include an experienced surgeon as well as a sleep-trained orthodontist to maximize short- and long-term surgical success.

Table 2
Comparison of polysomnogram data for maxillomandibular advancement, tracheostomy, and uvulopalatopharyngoplasty based on recent systematic reviews or meta-analyses. Note: uvulopalatopharyngoplasty results demonstrate the clear indication for careful preoperative patient evaluation and surgical planning to reduce the likelihood of unsuccessful surgeries

Surgical Procedure (Reference)	Preprocedural Pooled PSG Data	Post-Procedural Pooled PSG Data	Pooled Success Rate	P-Value
Maxillomandibular advancement[42]	AHI 63.9 ± 26.7 events/h	AHI 9.5 ± 10.7 events/h	86%	<.001
Tracheostomy[21]	AHI during REM 63.8 ± 31.9 events/h	AHI during REM 26.2 ± 29.2 events/h	73%	<.001
	AHI during NREM 98.9 ± 36.0 events/h	AHI during NREM 21.6 ± 25.8 events/h		<.001
Uvulopalatopharyngoplasty[47]	RDI Type 1 57 events/h	RDI Type 1 38 events/h	Type 1 52%	N/A
	RDI Type 2 or 3 65 events/h	RDI Type 2 or 3 62 events/h	Type 2 or 3 5%	N/A

Abbreviations: AHI, apnea-hypopnea index; N/A, not available; NREM, non-rapid eye movement sleep; PSG, polysomnogram; RDI, respiratory disturbance index; REM, rapid eye movement sleep; Type 1, retropalatal obstruction only; Type 2, retropalatal and retrolingual obstruction; Type 3, retrolingual obstruction only.

REFERENCES

1. Shepard JW Jr. Hypertension, cardiac arrhythmias, myocardial infarction, and stroke in relation to obstructive sleep apnea. Clin Chest Med 1992; 13(3):437–58.

2. Valero A, Alroy G. Hypoventilation in Acquired Micrognathia. Arch Intern Med 1965;115:307–10.

3. Sullivan CE, Issa FG, Berthon-Jones M, et al. Reversal of obstructive sleep apnoea by continuous positive airway pressure applied through the nares. Lancet 1981;1(8225):862–5.

4. Kushida CA, Littner MR, Hirshkowitz M, et al. Practice parameters for the use of continuous and bilevel positive airway pressure devices to treat adult patients with sleep-related breathing disorders. Sleep 2006;29(3):375–80.

5. Jacobson RL, Schendel SA. Treating obstructive sleep apnea: the case for surgery. Am J Orthod Dentofacial Orthop 2012;142(4):435, 437, 439, 441–2.

6. Lowe AA. Treating obstructive sleep apnea: the case for oral appliances. Am J Orthod Dentofacial Orthop 2012;142(4):434, 436, 438, 440.

7. Weaver TE, Grunstein RR. Adherence to continuous positive airway pressure therapy: the challenge to effective treatment. Proc Am Thorac Soc 2008;5(2): 173–8.

8. Barrera JE, Chang RC, Popelka GR, et al. Reliability of airway obstruction analyses from Sleep MRI sequences. Otolaryngol Head Neck Surg 2010; 142(4):526–30.

9. Kezirian EJ, Hohenhorst W, de Vries N. Drug-induced sleep endoscopy: the VOTE classification. Eur Arch Otorhinolaryngol 2011;268(8):1233–6.

10. George JR, Chung S, Nielsen I, et al. Comparison of drug-induced sleep endoscopy and lateral cephalometry in obstructive sleep apnea. Laryngoscope 2012;122(11):2600–5.

11. Stuck BA, Maurer JT. Airway evaluation in obstructive sleep apnea. Sleep Med Rev 2008;12(6):411–36.

12. Schendel SA, Hatcher D. Automated 3-dimensional airway analysis from cone-beam computed tomography data. J Oral Maxillofac Surg 2010; 68(3):696–701.

13. Sher AE, Schechtman KB, Piccirillo JF. The efficacy of surgical modifications of the upper airway in adults with obstructive sleep apnea syndrome. Sleep 1996;19(2):156–77.

14. Olsen KD, Kern EB, Westbrook PR. Sleep and breathing disturbance secondary to nasal obstruction. Otolaryngol Head Neck Surg 1981;89(5):804–10.

15. Verse T, Pirsig W. Impact of impaired nasal breathing on sleep-disordered breathing. Sleep Breath 2003;7(2):63–76.

16. Caldwell P, Hensley R, Machaalani R, et al. How effective is adenoidectomy alone for treatment of obstructive sleep apnoea in a child who presents with adenoid hypertrophy? J Paediatr Child Health 2011;47(8):568–71.

17. Fujita S, Conway W, Zorick F, et al. Surgical correction of anatomic azbnormalities in obstructive sleep apnea syndrome: uvulopalatopharyngoplasty. Otolaryngol Head Neck Surg 1981;89(6):923–34.

18. Friedman M, Ibrahim H, Joseph NJ. Staging of obstructive sleep apnea/hypopnea syndrome: a guide to appropriate treatment. Laryngoscope 2004;114(3):454–9.

19. Powell N, Riley R, Guilleminault C, et al. A reversible uvulopalatal flap for snoring and sleep apnea syndrome. Sleep 1996;19(7):593–9.

20. Lagravere MO, Major PW, Flores-Mir C. Long-term skeletal changes with rapid maxillary expansion: a systematic review. Angle Orthod 2005;75(6):1046–52.

21. Holty JE, Guilleminault C. Surgical options for the treatment of obstructive sleep apnea. Med Clin North Am 2010;94(3):479–515.

22. Woodson BT, Toohill RJ. Transpalatal advancement pharyngoplasty for obstructive sleep apnea. Laryngoscope 1993;103(3):269–76.

23. Woodson BT, Robinson S, Lim HJ. Transpalatal advancement pharyngoplasty outcomes compared with uvulopalatopharygoplasty. Otolaryngol Head Neck Surg 2005;133(2):211–7.

24. Sussman D, Podoshin L, Alroy G. The Pickwickian syndrome with hypertrophy of tonsils: a re-appraisal. Laryngoscope 1975;85(3):565–9.

25. Stow NW, Sale PJ, Lee D, et al. Simultaneous tonsillectomy and nasal surgery in adult obstructive sleep apnea: a pilot study. Otolaryngol Head Neck Surg 2012;147(2):387–91.

26. Brietzke SE, Gallagher D. The effectiveness of tonsillectomy and adenoidectomy in the treatment of pediatric obstructive sleep apnea/hypopnea syndrome: a meta-analysis. Otolaryngol Head Neck Surg 2006;134(6):979–84.

27. Chan DK, Jan TA, Koltai PJ. Effect of obesity and medical comorbidities on outcomes after adjunct surgery for obstructive sleep apnea in cases of adenotonsillectomy failure. Arch Otolaryngol Head Neck Surg 2012;138(10):891–6.

28. Wiet GJ, Bower C, Seibert R, et al. Surgical correction of obstructive sleep apnea in the complicated pediatric patient documented by polysomnography. Int J Pediatr Otorhinolaryngol 1997;41(2):133–43.

29. Friedman M, Hamilton C, Samuelson CG, et al. Transoral robotic glossectomy for the treatment of obstructive sleep apnea-hypopnea syndrome. Otolaryngol Head Neck Surg 2012;146(5):854–62.

30. Riley R, Guilleminault C, Powell N, et al. Mandibular osteotomy and hyoid bone advancement for obstructive sleep apnea: a case report. Sleep 1984;7(1):79–82.

31. Li KK, Riley RW, Powell NB, et al. Obstructive sleep apnea surgery: genioglossus advancement

revisited. J Oral Maxillofac Surg 2001;59(10):1181–4 [discussion: 1185].

32. Kezirian EJ, Goldberg AN. Hypopharyngeal surgery in obstructive sleep apnea: an evidence-based medicine review. Arch Otolaryngol Head Neck Surg 2006;132(2):206–13.

33. Bowden MT, Kezirian EJ, Utley D, et al. Outcomes of hyoid suspension for the treatment of obstructive sleep apnea. Arch Otolaryngol Head Neck Surg 2005;131(5):440–5.

34. Vicini C, Frassineti S, La Pietra MG, et al. Tongue Base Reduction with Thyro-Hyoido-Pexy (TBRTHP) vs. Tongue Base Reduction with Hyo-Epiglottoplasty (TBRHE) in mild-severe OSAHS adult treatment. Preliminary findings from a prospective randomised trial. Acta otorhinolaryngol Ital 2010;30(3):144–8.

35. Marcus CL, Crockett DM, Ward SL. Evaluation of epiglottoplasty as treatment for severe laryngomalacia. J Pediatr 1990;117(5):706–10.

36. Hartl TT, Chadha NK. A systematic review of laryngomalacia and acid reflux. Otolaryngol Head Neck Surg 2012;147(4):619–26.

37. Chan DK, Truong MT, Koltai PJ. Supraglottoplasty for occult laryngomalacia to improve obstructive sleep apnea syndrome. Arch Otolaryngol Head Neck Surg 2012;138(1):50–4.

38. Kuo PC, West RA, Bloomquist DS, et al. The effect of mandibular osteotomy in three patients with hypersomnia sleep apnea. Oral Surg Oral Med Oral Pathol 1979;48(5):385–92.

39. Li KK, Powell NB, Riley RW, et al. Morbidly obese patients with severe obstructive sleep apnea: is airway reconstructive surgery a viable treatment option? Laryngoscope 2000;110(6):982–7.

40. Abramson Z, Susarla SM, Lawler M, et al. Three-dimensional computed tomographic airway analysis of patients with obstructive sleep apnea treated by maxillomandibular advancement. J Oral Maxillofac Surg 2011;69(3):677–86.

41. Riley RW, Powell NB, Guilleminault C. Obstructive sleep apnea syndrome: a surgical protocol for dynamic upper airway reconstruction. J Oral Maxillofac Surg 1993;51(7):742–7 [discussion: 748–9].

42. Holty JE, Guilleminault C. Maxillomandibular advancement for the treatment of obstructive sleep apnea: a systematic review and meta-analysis. Sleep Med Rev 2010;14(5):287–97.

43. Fee WE Jr, Ward PH. Permanent tracheostomy: a new surgical technique. Ann Otol Rhinol Laryngol 1977;86(5 Pt 1):635–8.

44. Eliashar R, Goldfarb A, Gross M, et al. A perment tube-free tracheostomy in a mobrbidly obese patient with severe obstructive sleep apnea syndrome. Isr Med Assoc J 2002;4(12):1156–7.

45. Akst LM, Eliachar I. Long-term, tube-free (permanent) tracheostomy in morbidly obese patients. Laryngoscope 2004;114(8):1511–2 [author reply: 1512–3].

46. Rapoport DM, Garay SM, Epstein H, et al. Hypercapnia in the obstructive sleep apnea syndrome. A reevaluation of the "Pickwickian syndrome". Chest 1986;89(5):627–35.

47. Sher AE. Upper airway surgery for OSA. Sleep Med Rev 2002;6(3):195–212.

Overview of Oral Appliance Therapy for the Management of Obstructive Sleep Apnea

Leopoldo P. Correa, BDS, MS

KEYWORDS

- Obstructive sleep apnea • Oral appliance therapy • Continuous positive airway pressure
- Multidisciplinary approach

KEY POINTS

- Oral appliances are increasingly used in dental practices, and are indicated for the management of mild to moderate obstructive sleep apnea (OSA) and sometimes for patients with severe OSA who cannot tolerate continuous positive airway pressure therapy.
- Short-term and long-term follow-up is necessary to assess the efficacy of the device from subjective and objective measurements.
- A multidisciplinary approach involving a sleep physician, a dentist, an ear/nose/throat specialist, and a primary care physician is imperative for a better treatment outcome.
- Short-term and long-term side effects may occur with appliance therapy; it is recommended that dentists offering oral appliance therapy be educated and gain knowledge about the diagnosis, prevention, and management of common side effects, including temporomandibular disorders that occur with the use of such devices.

INTRODUCTION

Obstructive sleep apnea (OSA) is a common disorder in the general population, with an estimated prevalence of 4% in men and 2% in women aged between 30 and 60 years.[1] OSA is a condition characterized by frequent episodes of upper airway obstruction that occurs during sleep, resulting in reduction of blood oxygen saturation and arousals from sleep.[2] It is a common disease that is largely underdiagnosed and untreated, resulting in significant implications for cardiovascular disease,[3] mortality,[4] and economic impact.[5] Affected patients have neurocognitive and neurobehavioral impairment.[6] Population-based epidemiologic studies have estimated the prevalence and severity spectrum of undiagnosed OSA, and have found that even mild severity is associated with significant morbidity.[1]

Common symptoms reported by patients include excessive daytime sleepiness, snoring, and gastroesophageal reflux.[7] Snoring is commonly reported in these patients; the complaint of snoring precedes the complaint of daytime sleepiness, and the intensity of both increases with weight gain and alcohol intake.[8] Retropositioning of the tongue is one of the most common features of patients with OSA. The dimension of pharyngeal lumen and the elongation of the uvula and soft palatal draping also seem to play important roles in the partial or complete obstruction of the upper airway.[9] Other anatomic features

Statement of Interest: The author declares no conflict of interest.
Department of Oral and Maxillofacial Pathology, Oral Medicine and Craniofacial Pain, Tufts University School of Dental Medicine, 1 Kneeland Street # 601, Boston, MA 02111, USA
E-mail address: leopoldo.correa@tufts.edu

Sleep Med Clin 8 (2013) 505–516
http://dx.doi.org/10.1016/j.jsmc.2013.07.007

common to those with OSA include mandibular retrognathism, inferiorly positioned hyoid bone, tonsillar hypertrophy, deviated septum, nasal polyp, and enlarged nasal turbinates.[10–14]

Because of their practice of constant examination of the maxilla, mandible, and oropharyngeal areas, dental professionals have been recognized as being part of the multidisciplinary therapeutic team for the management of OSA by helping to identify possible risk factors for the development of a narrow upper airway.[15] The updated practice parameters from the American Academy of Sleep Medicine recommend the use of oral appliances for patients with mild to moderate OSA and for those with severe OSA who cannot tolerate continuous positive airway pressure (CPAP) therapy.[16] Current guidelines also recommend face-to-face evaluation with a sleep physician as part of a diagnostic process that must take place before initiation of oral appliance therapy.

CLASSIFICATION AND MECHANISM OF ACTION

Oral appliances are classified as mandibular repositioning devices (MADs) and tongue-retainer devices (TRDs). The primary action of a MAD is to increase and stabilize the oropharyngeal and hypopharyngeal airway space by repositioning and maintaining the lower jaw in forward status during sleep (**Fig. 1**). MADs require sufficient teeth to allow retention (at least 6 teeth on each arch); various oral appliances are available whose differences rely on design, material of fabrication, size, and thickness (**Fig. 2**). The mechanism of action of a TRD is the protraction of the tongue by way of a slight negative pressure in the bulb compartment of the device; displacement of air is achieved once the tongue is placed in this compartment. TRDs do not require support of teeth for the fitting, and are

indicated in patients with compromised dentition, including insufficient teeth, or periodontal disease (**Fig. 3**).

Mandibular advancement devices are more commonly known as oral appliances. **Fig. 2** shows different oral appliances viewed from frontal, lateral, and posterior views.

Fig. 3 shows radiographic and photographic depictions of a TRD.

EFFICACY AND SIDE EFFECTS

Current practice parameters recommend the use of oral appliances for mild to moderate OSA and for patients with severe OSA who do not tolerate CPAP therapy.[16] Several studies have shown the efficacy of oral appliances on reducing apnea severity. Oral appliances appear to be used more, and were preferred over CPAP when the treatments were compared.[17–20] Several studies have shown that oral appliances are more effective in patients with the following characteristics: younger age, lower body mass index, small neck size, positional OSA, female gender, and retrognathic mandible.[21–25]

Common side effects reported are excessive salivation, bite discomfort, occlusal change, pain in teeth, and symptoms of temporomandibular disorder (TMD). Discomfort from the appliance is the major cause for discontinuation of treatment or poor compliance.[26–30]

SYMPTOMS OF TEMPOROMANDIBULAR DISORDER

TMD symptoms refers to a group of symptoms involving the muscles of mastication, neck, and the temporomandibular joint (TMJ), and represents a complex family of heterogeneous disorders influenced by genes, sex, age, and environmental and behavioral triggers.[31] The prevalence of TMD in the general population has shown high variability in

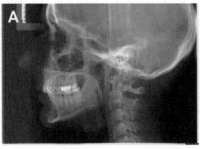
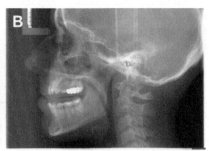

Fig. 1. Lateral radiograph. (*A*) Without mandibular repositioning device; (*B*) with mandibular repositioning device.

A Frontal view   **B** Lateral View   **C** Posterior View

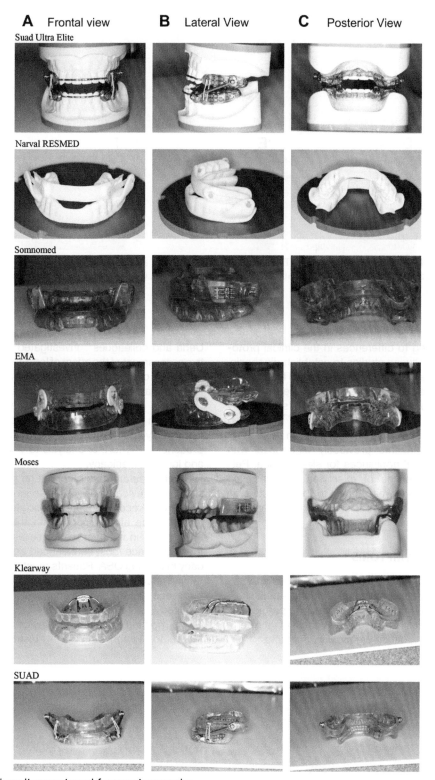

Suad Ultra Elite

Narval RESMED

Somnomed

EMA

Moses

Klearway

SUAD

Fig. 2. Oral appliances viewed from various angles.

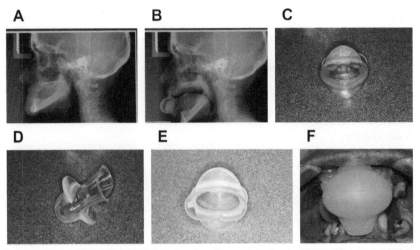

Fig. 3. Use of a tongue-retainer device (TRD). Lateral radiographs of a patient without a TRD (*A*) and with the device in place (*B*). (*C*) Frontal view. (*D*) Lateral view. (*E*) Posterior view. (*F*) Clinical photo of a patient with missing posterior teeth wearing the device.

results, owing to differences in the clinical protocols used between studies to establish diagnosis. One study reported the prevalence of TMD associated with the use of oral devices for sleep apnea as 19.8% at baseline, but decreasing significantly over time.[30] Cunali and colleagues[32] assessed the efficacy of mandibular exercises in the control of pain in patients previously diagnosed with TMD using oral appliances for sleep apnea. Performing sequences of exercises by controlled mouth opening was found to be effective in reducing pain and increasing the compliance of oral appliances.

OCCLUSAL SYMPTOMS

Occlusal changes occur in some patients after the short-term or long-term use of oral appliances, and such changes may be temporary or permanent. Several studies have shown the effect of long-term use of oral appliance on occlusal contacts.[27,33–35]

Ueda and colleagues[36] investigated the quantitative assessment of the effect of long-term oral appliance use on occlusal contact areas; the results showed that 86.7% of patients showed a significant change in occlusal contacts. Clinical techniques have been developed in an attempt to minimize occlusal symptoms (**Figs. 4** and **5**), but these approaches need further analysis to confirm validity and long-term efficacy.

Practice parameters recommend the fitting of a sleep oral device by dental personnel familiar with TMJ, dental occlusion, and associated oral structures.[16] Side effects occur with the use of oral appliances; in most cases these are minor, and the importance must be balanced against the efficacy in treating OSA. Patients must be informed of these potential side effects before initiating oral appliance therapy, and constant monitoring is required.

The morning repositioning device, designed by the author, is shown in **Fig. 4**. Instructions given

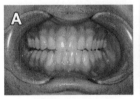
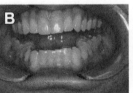
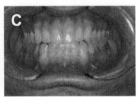

Fig. 4. Morning jaw-repositioning device. (*A*) A patient with bite change after short-term use of sleep oral appliance. (*B*) A Biocryl device of 1.5-mm thickness and vacuum press–fabricated in the office is fitted over the lower teeth, adding orthodontic resin on occlusal surfaces to allow posterior guidance of the jaw. (*C*) Bite in full closure, allowing occlusal and jaw guidance back to its natural position.

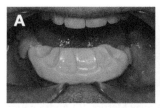
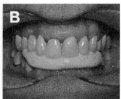
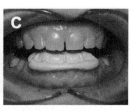

Fig. 5. Direct AM Positioner. (*A*) The patient relaxes the jaw into "centric" position and closes the mouth gently. (*B, C*) A jaw-exercise routine is performed every morning. (*Courtesy of* J. Parker, DDS, Edina, MN.)

to the patient include wearing the lower device after removal of sleep oral appliance, apply gentle face stretching exercises bilaterally while opening and closing the mouth for 2 minutes and then continue wearing the device for about 15 minutes.

The direct AM Positioner (see **Fig. 5**) is made of Thermacryl Plus (Airway Management). These heat-sensitive acrylic beads are placed over the lower anterior teeth. The patient relaxes the jaw into "centric" position and closes the mouth gently, then waits 5 to 10 minutes after removing the MAD in the morning before using the AM Positioner. Patients are given jaw exercises to do during the first 5 to 10 minutes after removing the MAD, after which they place the AM Positioner and close into it gently, and hold the teeth in it for 2 to 3 seconds before release, and repeat this 5 times per minute for 20 minutes. This routine can be performed while in the shower or when getting ready for work in the morning.

BITE REGISTRATION

Bite registration is one of the first steps in the fabrication of oral appliances, as this will record the initial jaw position that will be duplicated on the oral appliance (**Fig. 6**). Different devices are available for bite registration (**Fig. 7**). Recommendation for initial jaw protrusion varies from 50% to 75% of maximum jaw protrusion, depending on clinician expertise, TMD symptoms, and apnea severity.

CLINICAL EVALUATION

Clinical examination of the dental sleep patient includes an overview of the chief complaint, history of the present condition including past treatments, medical and medication history, review of systems, social and sleep history, and examination including nasal, maxillomandibular, oropharyngeal, and musculoskeletal areas. Appendix shows a template of a clinical evaluation form used by the author.

Nasal Obstruction

During sleep, breathing is primarily nasal, but patients with nasal obstructions favor mouth breathing, which decreases the hypopharyngeal space, leading to increased upper airway resistance and more frequent apneic and hypopneic episodes.[37] Some studies have reported a possible relationship between chronic nasal obstruction and OSA.[13,38] Nasal obstruction results in an increase in upstream airflow resistance, which predisposes the pharynx to collapse.[39] Guilleminault and Pelayo[40] reported that nasal obstruction and mouth breathing influence facial growth, which may further lead to difficulty in breathing while asleep. Nasal obstruction may be an independent etiologic factor in the pathogenesis of OSA; however, it is important to recognize patients with nasal obstruction caused by changes in mandibular angle during growth and development that further may lead to changes in the posture of the head, mandible, neck tonicity, and craniofacial morphology.[41–43] Referral of patients with

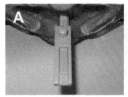
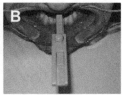
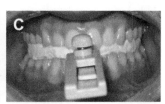

Fig. 6. Bite registration using a George gauge. Patient in habitual bite with device (*A*), with jaw protrusion (*B*), and with bite-registration material (*C*).

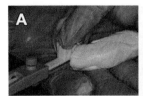
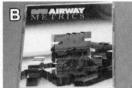
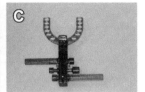

Fig. 7. Common bite-registration devices. (A) George gauge. (B) Airway Metrics. (C) Andra gauge.

nasal obstruction to an ear/nose/throat (ENT) specialist as part of a multidisciplinary approach is important for dentists to keep in mind during patient assessment.

Maxillomandibular Shape

Narrow maxillary arches are normally accompanied by high palatal vault, in many cases resulting in reduction of nasal passages (**Fig. 8**). The shape and size of maxilla play an important role, as it acts as a fence where the mandible can be neuromuscularly free or remain trapped. Mehta and colleagues[44] described the occlusal fencing concept whereby the maxilla dictates the boundaries of the mandible in final closure. If the maxilla is constricted, the mandibular teeth will crowd to accommodate to the space allowed by the maxillary teeth, creating a retrusive position of the mandible. The throat and airway space are the posterior fence; anything that restricts and displaces the mandible posteriorly will affect the airway space and change the position of the patient's head (**Fig. 9**).[45]

Oropharyngeal

Retro-positioning of the tongue is one of the most common features of patients with OSA. The dimension of pharyngeal lumen, the elongation of the uvula, and soft palatal draping also seem to

play important roles in the partial or complete obstruction of the upper airway.[9]

The tongue, in relation to the size of the oropharyngeal cavity, plays an important role in airway restriction (**Fig. 10**).

Different classifications have been developed to assess the correlation between tongue posture and airway patency; Mallampati and colleagues[46–48] developed a classification as an indicator of a relatively difficult endotracheal intubation, evaluating the relationship between the tongue and oral cavity and identifying structures visible to the clinician during tongue protrusion. Their study showed significant correlation between the ability to visualize pharyngeal structures and the ease of laryngoscopy (**Box 1**). Nuckton and colleagues[49] assessed the clinical usefulness of the Mallampati score in patients with OSA, and found it to be an independent predictor of both the presence and severity of OSA.

Friedman and colleagues[50] modified the technique described by Mallampati by examining the oropharynx of patients without protrusion of the tongue (Modified Mallampati Index) (**Box 2**). This index was part of physical findings used to predict the presence and severity of OSA. Their findings were correlated with the Respiratory Disturbance Index, resulting in statistically significant value as a reliable predictor of OSA.

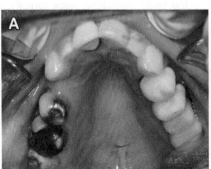
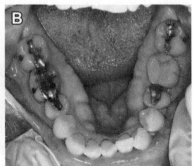

Fig. 8. (A) Narrow maxillary arch with deep palatal vault. (B) Narrow mandibular arch with lingual tori.

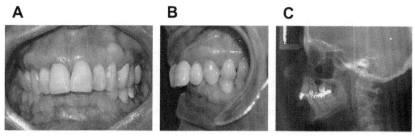

Fig. 9. (*A*) Patient showing deep occlusal overbite. (*B*) Lateral view showing significant overjet. (*C*) Lateral radiograph of the same patient showing a retrusively positioned jaw and narrow airway.

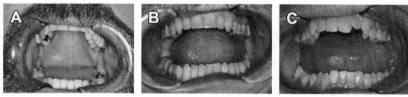

Fig. 10. (*A*) Tongue below occlusal plane. (*B*) Tongue above the occlusal plane. (*C*) Tongue occupying most of the oral cavity in a patient with narrow maxilla and mandibular arches.

Box 1
Mallampati classification

The patient is asked to open the mouth and protrude the tongue maximally. A score of 3 or 4 increases the risk of having OSA.

- Class I: Faucial pillars, soft palate, and uvula can be visualized
- Class II: Faucial pillars and soft palate can be visualized
- Class III: Only soft palate can be visualized
- Class IV: Only hard palate can be visualized

Box 2
Friedman modified Mallampati index

The patient is asked to open the mouth widely with the tongue left in place. A score of 3 or 4 increases the risk of having OSA.

- Grade I: Tonsils, pillars, and soft palate are clearly visible
- Grade II: Uvula, pillars, and upper pole are visible
- Grade III: Only part of the soft palate is visible
- Grade IV: Only the hard palate is visible

Musculoskeletal

Examination of the masticatory and neck muscles is an important step in the evaluation of the sleep apnea patient before receiving oral appliance therapy. The mechanism of action of oral appliances is to maintain the lower jaw in forward position and increase the vertical dimension of occlusion (VDO). This jaw movement creates a temporary overstretching of muscles in the face and neck. Muscle tenderness may warrant the need to review oral appliance design, or carry out possible adjustments. Ceneviz and colleagues[51] investigated the immediate effect of changing mandibular position using nonrepositioning and repositioning bite appliances on the electromyographic (EMG) activity of the masseter, temporalis, sternocleidomastoid, and trapezius muscles; their findings suggested that changes in mandibular position lowered the EMG activity of masticatory and cervical muscles. Franco and colleagues[52] evaluated the influence of an oral appliance in neutral and in 50% advanced position on morning headache and orofacial pain in nonapnea subjects; statistically significant reductions morning headache and orofacial pain intensity were observed in both positions.

Dentists using oral appliances for the management of OSA need to bear in mind the effect and potential side effects of mandibular advancement on adjacent areas including the masticatory and neck muscles, and the TMJ.

SUMMARY

Oral appliances are increasingly used in dental practices, and are indicated for the management of mild to moderate OSA and for some patients with severe OSA who cannot tolerate CPAP therapy. Short-term and long-term follow-up is necessary to assess the efficacy of the device from subjective and objective measurements. A multidisciplinary approach involving a sleep physician, a dentist, an ENT specialist, and a primary care physician is imperative for a better treatment outcome. Short-term and long-term side effects may occur while using appliance therapy, and it is recommended that dentists offering sleep oral appliance therapy are educated and gain knowledge about the diagnosis, prevention, and management of common side effects, including TMDs, occurring with the use of oral devices.

REFERENCES

1. Young T, Peppard PE, Gottlieb DJ. Epidemiology of obstructive sleep apnea: a population health perspective. Am J Respir Crit Care Med 2002; 165(9):1217–39.

2. Guilleminault C. Diagnosis, pathogenesis, and treatment of the sleep apnea syndromes. Ergeb Inn Med Kinderheilkd 1984;52:1–57.

3. Shamsuzzaman AS, Gersh BJ, Somers VK. Obstructive sleep apnea: implications for cardiac and vascular disease. JAMA 2003;290(14): 1906–14.

4. Young T, Finn L, Peppard PE, et al. Sleep disordered breathing and mortality: eighteen-year follow-up of the Wisconsin sleep cohort. Sleep 2008;31(8):1071–8.

5. AlGhanim N, Comondore VR, Fleetham J, et al. The economic impact of obstructive sleep apnea. Lung 2008;186(1):7–12.

6. Verstraeten E. Neurocognitive effects of obstructive sleep apnea syndrome. Curr Neurol Neurosci Rep 2007;7(2):161–6.

7. Wenner JB, Cheema R, Ayas NT. Clinical manifestations and consequences of obstructive sleep apnea. J Cardiopulm Rehabil Prev 2009;29(2): 76–83.

8. Berger G, Berger R, Oksenberg A. Progression of snoring and obstructive sleep apnoea: the role of increasing weight and time. Eur Respir J 2009; 33(2):338–45.

9. Abramson Z, Susarla S, August M, et al. Three-dimensional computed tomographic analysis of airway anatomy in patients with obstructive sleep apnea. J Oral Maxillofac Surg 2010; 68(2):354–62.

10. Berger RM. Mandibular retrognathia and sleep apnea. JAMA 1982;247(16):2234.

11. Bucchieri A, Mastrangelo C, Stella R, et al. Cephalometric evaluation of hyoid bone position in patients with obstructive sleep apnea. Minerva Stomatol 2004;53(1–2):33–9 [in Italian].

12. Chang SJ, Chae KY. Obstructive sleep apnea syndrome in children: epidemiology, pathophysiology, diagnosis and sequelae. Korean J Pediatr 2010; 53(10):863–71.

13. Ishii L, Godoy A, Ishman SL, et al. The nasal obstruction symptom evaluation survey as a screening tool for obstructive sleep apnea. Arch Otolaryngol Head Neck Surg 2011;137(2):119–23.

14. Mekhitarian Neto L, Fava AS, Lopes HC, et al. Epidemiological analysis of structural alterations of the nasal cavity associated with obstructive sleep apnea syndrome (OSA). Braz J Otorhinolaryngol 2005;71(4):464–6.

15. Paskow H, Paskow S. Dentistry's role in treating sleep apnea and snoring. N J Med 1991;88(11): 815–7.

16. Kushida CA, Morgenthaler TI, Littner MR, et al. Practice parameters for the treatment of snoring and obstructive sleep apnea with oral appliances: an update for 2005. Sleep 2006;29(2):240–3.

17. Lim J, Lasserson TJ, Fleetham J, et al. Oral appliances for obstructive sleep apnoea. Cochrane Database Syst Rev 2006;(1):CD004435.

18. Barnes M, McEvoy RD, Banks S, et al. Efficacy of positive airway pressure and oral appliance in mild to moderate obstructive sleep apnea. Am J Respir Crit Care Med 2004;170(6):656–64.

19. Tan YK, L'Estrange PR, Luo YM, et al. Mandibular advancement splints and continuous positive airway pressure in patients with obstructive sleep apnoea: a randomized cross-over trial. Eur J Orthod 2002;24(3):239–49.

20. Barthlen GM, Brown LK, Wiland MR, et al. Comparison of three oral appliances for treatment of severe obstructive sleep apnea syndrome. Sleep Med 2000;1(4):299–305.

21. Marklund M, Stenlund H, Franklin KA. Mandibular advancement devices in 630 men and women with obstructive sleep apnea and snoring: tolerability and predictors of treatment success. Chest 2004;125(4):1270–8.

22. Liu Y, Park YC, Lowe AA, et al. Supine cephalometric analyses of an adjustable oral appliance used in the treatment of obstructive sleep apnea. Sleep Breath 2000;4(2):59–66.

23. Otsuka R, Almeida FR, Lowe AA, et al. A comparison of responders and nonresponders to oral appliance therapy for the treatment of

obstructive sleep apnea. Am J Orthod Dentofacial Orthop 2006;129(2):222–9.

24. Yoshida K. Influence of sleep posture on response to oral appliance therapy for sleep apnea syndrome. Sleep 2001;24(5):538–44.

25. Ng AT, Darendeliler MA, Petocz P, et al. Cephalometry and prediction of oral appliance treatment outcome. Sleep Breath 2012;16(1):47–58.

26. de Almeida FR, Lowe AA, Tsuiki S, et al. Long-term compliance and side effects of oral appliances used for the treatment of snoring and obstructive sleep apnea syndrome. J Clin Sleep Med 2005; 1(2):143–52.

27. Pantin CC, Hillman DR, Tennant M. Dental side effects of an oral device to treat snoring and obstructive sleep apnea. Sleep 1999;22(2):237–40.

28. de Almeida FR, Bittencourt LR, de Almeida CI, et al. Effects of mandibular posture on obstructive sleep apnea severity and the temporomandibular joint in patients fitted with an oral appliance. Sleep 2002;25(5):507–13.

29. Giannasi LC, Almeida FR, Magini M, et al. Systematic assessment of the impact of oral appliance therapy on the temporomandibular joint during treatment of obstructive sleep apnea: long-term evaluation. Sleep Breath 2009;13(4):375–81.

30. Perez CV, de Leeuw R, Okeson JP, et al. The incidence and prevalence of temporomandibular disorders and posterior open bite in patients receiving mandibular advancement device therapy for obstructive sleep apnea. Sleep Breath 2013; 17(1):323–32.

31. Scrivani SJ, Keith DA, Kaban LB. Temporomandibular disorders. N Engl J Med 2008;359(25): 2693–705.

32. Cunali PA, Almeida FR, Santos CD, et al. Mandibular exercises improve mandibular advancement device therapy for obstructive sleep apnea. Sleep Breath 2011;15(4):717–27.

33. Almeida FR, Lowe AA, Otsuka R, et al. Long-term sequelae of oral appliance therapy in obstructive sleep apnea patients: part 2. Study-model analysis. Am J Orthod Dentofacial Orthop 2006; 129(2):205–13.

34. Rose EC, Schnegelsberg C, Staats R, et al. Occlusal side effects caused by a mandibular advancement appliance in patients with obstructive sleep apnea. Angle Orthod 2001;71(6):452–60.

35. Otsuka R, Almeida FR, Lowe AA. The effects of oral appliance therapy on occlusal function in patients with obstructive sleep apnea: a short-term prospective study. Am J Orthod Dentofacial Orthop 2007;131(2):176–83.

36. Ueda H, Almeida FR, Lowe AA, et al. Changes in occlusal contact area during oral appliance therapy assessed on study models. Angle Orthod 2008;78(5):866–72.

37. Fitzpatrick MF, McLean H, Urton AM, et al. Effect of nasal or oral breathing route on upper airway resistance during sleep. Eur Respir J 2003;22(5): 827–32.

38. Friedman M, Maley A, Kelley K, et al. Impact of nasal obstruction on obstructive sleep apnea. Otolaryngol Head Neck Surg 2011;144(6): 1000–4.

39. Ryan CM, Bradley TD. Pathogenesis of obstructive sleep apnea. J Appl Physiol 2005;99(6):2440–50.

40. Guilleminault C, Pelayo R. Sleep-disordered breathing in children. Ann Med 1998;30(4):350–6.

41. Klein JC. Nasal respiratory function and craniofacial growth. Arch Otolaryngol Head Neck Surg 1986;112(8):843–9.

42. Cuccia AM, Lotti M, Caradonna D. Oral breathing and head posture. Angle Orthod 2008;78(1):77–82.

43. Peltomaki T. The effect of mode of breathing on craniofacial growth—revisited. Eur J Orthod 2007; 29(5):426–9.

44. Mehta N, Abdallah E, Lobo-Lobo S. Three Dimensional Assessment of Dental Occlusion (Occlusal Fencing): A Clinical Technique. Inside Dentistry 2006;2(4):28–36.

45. Choi JK, Goldman M, Koyal S, et al. Effect of jaw and head position on airway resistance in obstructive sleep apnea. Sleep Breath 2000; 4(4):163–8.

46. Mallampati SR. Clinical sign to predict difficult tracheal intubation (hypothesis). Can Anaesth Soc J 1983;30(3 Pt 1):316–7.

47. Mallampati SR, Gatt SP, Gugino LD, et al. A clinical sign to predict difficult tracheal intubation: a prospective study. Can Anaesth Soc J 1985;32(4): 429–34.

48. Bins S, Koster TD, de Heij AH, et al. No evidence for diagnostic value of Mallampati score in patients suspected of having obstructive sleep apnea syndrome. Otolaryngol Head Neck Surg 2011;145(2): 199–203.

49. Nuckton TJ, Glidden DV, Browner WS, et al. Physical examination: Mallampati score as an independent predictor of obstructive sleep apnea. Sleep 2006;29(7):903–8.

50. Friedman M, Tanyeri H, La Rosa M, et al. Clinical predictors of obstructive sleep apnea. Laryngoscope 1999;109(12):1901–7.

51. Ceneviz C, Mehta NR, Forgione A, et al. The immediate effect of changing mandibular position on the EMG activity of the masseter, temporalis, sternocleidomastoid, and trapezius muscles. Cranio 2006;24(4):237–44.

52. Franco L, Rompre PH, de Grandmont P, et al. A mandibular advancement appliance reduces pain and rhythmic masticatory muscle activity in patients with morning headache. J Orofac Pain 2011;25(3):240–9.

APPENDIX: CLINICAL EVALUATION FORM

Date of Service:

Patient:
Date of Birth:
Primary Care Physician:
Sleep Physician:

REASON FOR VISIT:

CHIEF COMPLAINT (concise statement in the patient's own words):

HISTORY OF PRESENT ILLNESS / PROBLEM (chronological description of the development of the patient's present illness/ medical condition from the first sign and/or symptom or from the previous encounter to the present-Quality-Duration-severity-timing-modifying factors, associated signs and symptoms):

REVIEW OF SYSTEMS (An inventory of body systems obtained by asking a series of questions in order to identify signs and/or symptoms that the patient may be experiencing or has experienced):

- Constitutional (Unexplained weight loss, night sweats, fatigue, sleeping pattern, appetite, fever, itch/rash, recent trauma, lumps/bumps/masses, unexplained falls):

- Eyes (Visual changes, headache, eye pain, double vision, blind spots, floaters):

- Ear, Nose, Mouth, Throat: (Runny nose, frequent nose bleeds, sinus pain, stuffy ears, ear pain, ringing in ears, gingival bleeding, toothache, sore throat, pain with swallowing):

- Cardiovascular (Chest pain, shortness of breath, exercise intolerance, palpitations, faintness, loss of consciousness):

- Respiratory (Shortness of breath, cough, exercise intolerance, difficulty breathing through the nose, mouth breather):

- Gastrointestinal (Abdominal pain, changes in appetite, heartburn, indigestion, nausea, vomiting, diarrhea, constipation):

- Musculoskeletal (TMJ, neck, pain, misalignment, stiffness morning vs day long; improves/worsens with activity), joint swelling, decreased range of motion, crepitus, arthritis):

- Urinary (Incontinence, frequency, urgency, nocturia, pain):

- Skin (Pruritus, rashes, stria, lesions, wounds, incisions, nodules, tumors, eczema, excessive dryness and/or discoloration):

- Neurological (Fainting, numbness, tingling, tremors, weakness, changes in sight, smell, hearing and taste, seizures, headache, poor balance, speech problems):

- Psychiatric (Memory loss, depression, anxiety, stress, mood changes, school or work performance):

- Endocrine (Thyroid disfunction, diabetes):

- Hematologic (Anemia, bleeding disorders, excessive bleeding, blood transfusion):

- Allergic / Immunologic (Difficulty breathing or feeling of choking as a result of exposure to anything, swelling or pain swollen, allergic response (rash/itch) to materials, foods, animals; reaction to bee sting, unusual sneezing, runny nose or itchy/teary eyes; food, medication or environmental allergy):

PAST FAMILY AND SOCIAL HISTORY:

MEDICAL HISTORY (Total sum of health status prior to the presenting problem):

- General state of health (excellent, good, fair, poor):
- Medical conditions:
- Prescription medications:
- Over the counter medications:
- Supplements and herbs:
- Allergies (to medications, latex, environment, food, animals):
- Injuries (note the type and date of injury):
- Surgical procedures:
- Hospitalizations (including all surgical, medical, and psychiatric hospitalizations):

FAMILY HISTORY (Review of medical events in the patient's family):

- Father:
- Mother:
- Sister(s):
- Brother(s):

SOCIAL HISTORY (An age appropriate review of past and current activities):

- Marital status (Single, married, divorced, widow)
- Children (number, gender, and ages):
- Occupation (some occupations linked to health problems):
- Work schedule (day / night shift):
- Caffeine intake (type, amount, and duration):
- Alcohol intake (type, amount, and duration):
- History of substance abuse (type, amount, duration, and rehabilitation):
- Smoking history (type, amount, and duration):
- Diet history (balance of food, time of meals, snacks, soda intake, water intake):
- Physical exercise (type, amount, and duration):
- Psychiatric History: (Affective symptoms-Depression-anxiety-stress-suicidal ideation-domestic violence-litigation "disability"-functional impairmentents)

SLEEP HISTORY:

- Bed time schedule (weekdays and weekends):
- Time to fall asleep (activities before falling asleep-reading, watching TV, social media):
- Difficulty falling asleep:
- Difficulty maintaining asleep:
- Hours of sleep (weekdays and weekends):
- Wake up schedule (weekdays and weekends):
- Night time symptoms: (Snoring, witnessed apnea episodes, excessive movement, violent sleep behavior, sleep walking, sleep talking, frequent awakenings, clenching and grinding, headaches, TMJ pain)
- Daytime symptoms: (Excessive daytime sleepiness, fatigue, need to take naps, morning headaches
- Impairments: Drowsy driving, difficulty concentrating, memory problems)

PSG SLEEP STUDY DATA

- Sleep efficiency:
- Apnea Hypopnea Index (AHI):
- Respiratory Disturbance Index (RDI):
- # Apneas:
- # Hypopneas:
- # RERAS
- # Central Apneas:
- Minimum 02:
- Nadir O2:

EXAMINATION:

GENERAL APPEARENCE (Development – Nutrition - Deformities - Attention to grooming):

VITAL SIGNS (Blood pressure - Pulse rate- Respiratory rate- Height – Weight – Pain Level):

OROPHARYNGEAL:
Lips (Presence of sores, dryness, bleeding) :

Teeth (Missing teeth, dental work, wear facets, decay, fractures, occlusion classification, dental midline deviation):

Gums (Periodontal disease, gum recession, inflammation, frenum midline deviation):

Maxillary Arch (Arch size and shape (small-medium-large-narrow-V shape-constricted), palatal vault (deep, normal), presence of palatal tori, maxillary canting, occlusal plane/curve):

Mandibular Arch (Arch size and shape (small-medium-large-retrognatic-constricted), presence of lingual tori, occlusal plane/curve):

Maxillo-Mandibular Relationship (Point of first contact on closure, jaw shifting after point of first contact, occlusal fence I (antero-posterior restriction-incisors inclination), occlusal fence II (lateral restriction- canines inclination), occlusal fence III (Reduction of VDO- molars inclination):

Soft palate (Short-elongated) - Tongue (Size, posture related to occlusal plane (above-below), scalloped) –

Uvula (small-medium-large-absent) - Tonsils (small-medium-large-absent)- Mallampati classification (I - II – III - IV)

MUSCULOSKELETAL:
Head posture (Normal - mild - moderate - severe):

Shoulders posture (Normal – rounded):

Masticatory muscles Palpation: Tenderness / pain (mild-moderate-severe-right-left) on masseter (deep and superficial), temporal tendon, lateral and medial pterygoids, digastric, hyoid muscles (supra-infra), temporalis (anterior-medial-posterior fibers)

Neck and shoulder muscle palpation: Tenderness / pain (mild-moderate-severe-unilateral-bilateral) on sternocleidomastoid, mastoids, scalenus, trapezius, deltoids, posterior neck muscles.

Temporomandibular Joint (TMJ): Palpation (pain-tenderness), auscultation (clicking, crepitus, unilateral-bilateral-early opening-late opening), subluxation, open lock, range of motion (opening-lateral-protrusion), deviation on opening (left-right-straight).

RADIOGRAPHIC IMAGING FINDINGS:
Panoramic: / Cephalogram / CT scan

ASSESSMENT: (Diagnosis with medical codes + Summary of today's procedures)

TREATMENT PLAN (Treatment recommendations - Referrals – Prescriptions - Future plan – Next visit):

DENTIST NAME (Provider):

Signature: _____   DATE: _____

Weight Loss in the Management of Obstructive Sleep Apnea

Shirley F. Jones, MD[a], Ahmad Chebbo, MD[b]

KEYWORDS

- Obstructive sleep apnea • Obesity • Weight loss • Bariatric surgery • Weight loss medication • Diet
- Exercise • Continuous positive airway pressure

KEY POINTS

- Although obesity is one of the important risk factors for obstructive sleep apnea (OSA), the mechanism behind its causality is not well understood.
- In obese patients with OSA, weight loss should not be recommended as the sole treatment of OSA, but should be used in conjunction with other treatments such as continuous positive airway pressure.
- Although weight loss strategies vary, these can mainly be classified into surgical, pharmacologic, and lifestyle (including caloric restriction, behavioral therapy, and exercise) treatments.
- In general, weight loss may reduce the number of apneas and hypopneas, but complete remission in most patients is not to be expected.
- Additional challenges with the difficulty of sustainable weight reduction should impart close attention and follow-up to ensure continued evaluation and management of OSA.

Understanding the relationship between weight loss and obstructive sleep apnea (OSA) begins with a central understanding of the pathogenicity of weight gain on OSA. This article first focuses on obesity as a risk factor for OSA and the potential mechanisms that underscore obesity to the pathophysiology of OSA and, finally, summarizes the types of weight loss strategies, including surgical, pharmaceutical, and lifestyle interventions and their effects on OSA.

OSA is estimated to affect 2% to 4% of the general population.[1] Risk factors for OSA include family history, male gender, age, and obesity. In 2009 to 2010, more than 78 million adults and more than 12 million children in the United States were obese.[2] Men, older women, and adolescents represent populations with the highest rates. As the rates of obesity climb, so will rates of its associated diseases, specifically, diabetes,

hypertension, and OSA. Most patients with OSA are obese. Data from the Wisconsin Sleep Cohort study, a large population-based study aimed to determine the natural history of cardiopulmonary effects of sleep-disordered breathing and its prevalence, indicate that a one standard deviation increase in the body mass index (BMI) is associated with a 4-fold increase in risk for sleep-disordered breathing[1] and that each percentage change in weight is associated with an approximate mean change in the apnea hypopnea index (AHI) of 3%.[3] Hence, a person who gains 5% of body weight would be expected to increase his/her AHI by 15% compared with an individual whose weight remains stable.[3] The greatest numbers of OSA are in patients presenting for bariatric surgery and a BMI greater than 35 kg/m[2]. It is estimated that 2 of 3 women and greater than 95% of men who present for bariatric

a Pulmonary and Sleep Medicine, Scott & White Healthcare, Texas A&M HSC COM, 2401 South 31st Street, Temple, TX 76508, USA; b Division of Pulmonary and Critical Care, Maricopa Integrated Health System, 2601 East Roosevelt Street, Phoenix, AZ 85008, USA
E-mail address: shjones@sw.org

Sleep Med Clin 8 (2013) 517–525
http://dx.doi.org/10.1016/j.jsmc.2013.07.001
1556-407X/13/$ – see front matter © 2013 Elsevier Inc. All rights reserved

surgery have an AHI more than 10 events per hour.[4] Although obesity is a known risk factor for OSA, its exact mechanism is less clear. Obesity likely modulates upper airway control through mechanical effects on structure and function, ventilation, and hypoxemia.

OSA is characterized by repetitive occlusions of the upper airway, resulting in oxygen desaturation and/or arousals. Although the causal relationship between obesity and OSA is not well understood, obesity may promote occlusion of the upper airway through decreases in the size of the upper airway, which enhances its collapsibility. Obesity increases fat deposition of the trunk, abdomen, and neck, particularly in the posterior and lateral regions of the oropharynx and the soft palate,[5,6] leading to increased airway collapsibility in obese patients compared with normal patients.[7] Obesity also increases muscle and fat in the uvula and is significantly related to the severity of sleep-disordered breathing.[8] Population-based studies further support that obesity and larger neck size are associated with greater risk for sleep-disordered breathing.[1] A one standard deviation increase in neck circumference is associated with a 5-fold increase in risk for sleep-disordered breathing. Functional studies of airway critical pressure (the nasal pressure at which airflow ceases) indicates that patients with OSA have increased upper airway collapsibility with a critical pressure of 3.3 cm water,[9] in contrast to normal patients with upper airway critical pressures of −13.3 cm water.[10] Patients with OSA have higher critical pressure, lower airflow, and higher degrees of upper airway collapsibility compared with snorers and normals.[11] Use of positive airway pressure can increase the diameter of the upper airway, improve airflow, and modify the critical pressure.[9] Even small amounts of weight loss may reduce the critical pressure. In one study a 13% reduction in weight resulted in a decrease in critical pressure from 3.1 to −2.4 cm water. An additional study supports that complete resolution of OSA can occur once critical pressure falls to less than −4 cm water.[7] These studies support that upper airway collapsibility improves with weight reduction in patients with OSA.

Obesity may also affect mechanical loading of the upper airway through metabolic dysregulation and their effects on the upper airway. Leptin and adiponectin, both manufactured by adipocytes, play a role in this complex interaction on energy consumption and expenditure. Leptin functions to inhibit appetite, promote satiety, and stimulate ventilation. Antagonists of leptin such as C-reactive protein mitigate the physiologic properties of leptin.[12] On the contrary, adiponectin levels increase with weight loss and are inversely associated with overall and central adiposity.[13] Low levels of adiponectin have been associated with the development of type 2 diabetes and insulin resistance,[14] diseases commonly seen in patients with obesity and OSA.

Obesity may also affect OSA through pathways targeting ventilation and hypoxemia. Obesity hypoventilation syndrome is defined as obesity (BMI >30 kg/m^2), daytime hypoventilation with awake P_{CO_2} greater than 45 mm Hg, and sleep-disordered breathing in the absence of other causes of hypoventilation. In obesity hypoventilation, the increase in the work of breathing is related to decreased lung compliance and the efforts to displace the ribs and diaphragm,[15] generating ventilation perfusion mismatch. Muscle impairment may also play a role. Finally, patients with obesity hypoventilation have reduced response to hypoxia and hypercapnia.[16]

Data from the Wisconsin Sleep Cohort Study indicate that weight loss is associated with a reduction in the severity and likelihood sleep-disordered breathing. A 10% reduction in weight is estimated to produce a 26% decrease in the AHI.[3] Despite obvious benefits to losing weight in this population, small studies indicate that initial weight loss success is not sustainable in the long term. In 24 subjects who had cured their OSA following weight loss, regain of weight led to recurrence of OSA.[17] Currently, weight loss is not recommended as primary therapy for OSA. It is instead recommended as an adjunct to more proven strategies such as continuous positive airway pressure (CPAP). Despite the untoward and negative outcomes associated with obesity, achieving weight loss can be quite challenging. Comorbid medical illnesses associated with obesity and symptoms of OSA including hypersomnia and fatigue may affect weight loss goals and efforts. Also, patients of advanced age and with comorbid illness may be deemed less suitable for certain weight loss therapies such as surgery. Hence patients with OSA face several challenges when trying to lose weight. A variety of ways to lose weight are available and a review of the literature on weight loss strategies in patients with OSA and its effects on OSA are discussed.

SURGICAL THERAPIES

Bariatric surgery has emerged as a treatment option for morbidly obese patients who fail traditional weight loss approaches. In the Swedish Obese Subjects Study, a prospective, nonrandomized intervention trial comparing longitudinal outcomes of more than 4000 patients undergoing bariatric surgery to matched controls, patients who had surgery lost more weight (23% of BMI in the surgical group vs 0.1% in the control group). Weight loss was maintained by the tenth year (16% of BMI in the surgical group) with a lower incidence of obesity-related morbidity at 10-year follow-up.[18] Bariatric surgery induces weight loss by malabsorption, restriction, or hormonal alterations. Considerations for bariatric surgery include a BMI greater than 40 kg/m^2 or BMI greater than 35 kg/m^2 with one or more comorbid conditions, such as diabetes, dyslipidemia, coronary artery disease, hypertension, OSA, or nonalcoholic steatohepatitis.[19] One of the most common bariatric procedures is a Roux-en-y gastric bypass (RYGB), which consists of a small proximal gastric pouch anastomosed to the roux or alimentary limb of the small intestine. The small intestine is divided at 30 to 50 cm distal to the ligament of Treitz. The proximal portion of the small intestine and the remaining gastrum become the biliopancreatic limb, which transports secretions such as gastric acid once anastomosed 75 to 150 cm from the gastrojejunostomy. The gastrojejunostomy is formed by connecting the proximal gastric pouch to the more distal portion of the divided small intestine. Ninety percent of RYGB are performed laparoscopically.[20] RGYB induces weight loss by restriction (creation of a small gastric pouch), by malabsorption (by diversion of the pancreaticobiliary secretions) to a short common gut, and by affecting hormone levels via a decrease in the orexigenic hormone ghrelin secreted by the foregut.[21,22] Lengthening the roux limb can promote further malabsorption. Weight loss is rapid the first year after surgery and ranges from 62% to 70% of excess weight lost, but usually stabilizes after 2 years.[23] Another commonly performed surgery for weight loss is the laparoscopic adjustable gastric banding (LAGB). Weight loss is achieved by restriction of the upper part of the stomach by placement of a tight adjustable prosthetic band. The band is made of a locking silicone ring connected to an implanted infusion port located in the subcutaneous tissue. Infusion of saline in the port will decrease the size of the band and promote stomach restriction.[24] Although weight loss after LAGB is more gradual compared with RYGB surgery, both have similar long-term results.[25,26] Less operative mortality and reversibility are the most significant benefits of the LAGB.[27] Another form of restrictive weight loss surgery is the laparoscopic sleeve gastrectomy (LSG), which consists of creating a small tubular stomach by removing most of the greater curvature. Although initially used as a first-step procedure before

RYGB or duodenal switch surgery,[28,29] it is now widely used as an isolated bariatric procedure. Data are limited about its safety and long-term outcomes; however, a recent report examining 1-year outcomes between LAGB, LSG, and open RYGB and laparoscopic RYGB showed that reductions in BMI and morbidity associated with LSG lie between those of LAGB and RYGB, with no difference in mortality.[30] Leakage of the staple line is one of the major complications of LSG and occurs in 7% of patients.[31] Two endoscopic procedures, the intragastric balloon and the endoluminal vertical gastroplasty, have been used in clinical trials; however, additional research is needed to investigate long-term outcomes. Other types of weight loss surgery include biliopancreatic diversion and biliopancreatic diversion with duodenal switch, which rely primarily on malabsorption to facilitate weight loss, but both are rarely used because of the high incidence of complications, including protein malnutrition, diarrhea, and stomal ulceration.[32] Currently, there are no clear guidelines regarding procedure selection and the procedure largely depends on the expertise of the surgeon, the institution, and patient preference.[19] Several studies have been performed to evaluate outcomes of OSA in patients who have undergone bariatric surgery. Despite significant weight loss after bariatric surgery and improvement in the severity of OSA, it may still persist in some cases.[33] Bariatric surgery by itself is not a cure for OSA, which is defined by a normal AHI and complete discontinuation of CPAP. A meta-analysis reviewed the effect of bariatric surgery in 342 patients with OSA. Although the severity of the OSA had improved, and the AHI had decreased by 38 events from 54 to 15.8, moderate OSA was still observed.[33] This moderate degree of OSA was still present despite a significant amount of weight loss and a reduction of BMI by 17.9 kg/m^2 (55.3–37.7 kg/m^2).[33] These findings highlight that despite large amounts of weight loss and reductions in BMI, a significant portion of patients after bariatric surgery are still moderately obese at 10-years follow-up.[18] A recent randomized controlled trial comparing bariatric surgery (LAGB) to conventional weight loss in obese patients did not find any statistically significant differences in AHI reduction between groups despite greater degrees of weight loss in the bariatric surgery group.[34]

In summary, bariatric surgery as a weight loss therapy is effective in reducing obesity-related comorbidities and mortality; however, obese patients should not expect a complete cure of their OSA but could achieve improvements in severity of disease. OSA persists in many patients despite major weight loss, and use of CPAP should be anticipated.

PHARMACOLOGIC THERAPIES

Anti-obesity drugs are being used frequently to assist in achievement of weight loss by modifying fat digestion and suppressing appetite. However, the effect of these drugs with the primary focus on OSA has been studied in very few trials. Many of these trials involved sibutramine, which has been withdrawn from the market; however, existing trials using sibutramine in patients with OSA have yielded mixed results when OSA outcomes were measured. In an open uncontrolled cohort study of 87 obese subjects with OSA, at 6-month follow-up, the respiratory disturbance index and weight had decreased by 16.4 events per hour and 8.3 kg, respectively.[35] In contrast, in a randomized controlled trial examining the efficacy of sibutramine versus CPAP on sleep-disordered breathing, subjects who received sibutramine did not achieve a statistically significant reduction in OSA severity or AHI at 1 year from 41.5 to 33 events per hour. In part, this may be due to the modest reduction in weight loss of 5% compared with the Yee study in which subjects lost more weight,[36] suggesting that greater degrees of improvement in OSA may be linked to the amount of weight lost.

Orlistat inhibits pancreatic lipase, thereby decreasing dietary fat absorption. Orlistat is approved for use in the United States either by prescription (120 mg) or over the counter (60 mg).[37] In multiple randomized controlled trials and a meta-analysis, the use of orlistat compared with lifestyle changes alone was associated with greater weight loss at 4 years. Use of orlistat has also been shown to decrease the incidence of type 2 diabetes in obese patients.[38] In studies performed specifically in obese patients with sleep-disordered breathing, use of orlistat in conjunction with dietary modification was associated with an average of 3.5 kg of additional weight loss after 1 year but many patients were not able to comply with the dietary restrictions.[39] The major side effects of orlistat are flatus, fecal incontinence, and oily spotting.[40] Patients taking orlistat should be advised to take a multivitamin tablet given the risk of fat-soluble vitamin malabsorption.

Other drugs that suppress appetite include the serotonin agonists, sympathomimetics, antidepressants, and antiepileptic drugs. Their use however is limited by frequent and serious side effects, short-term use, and regain of weight after their discontinuance. Lorcaserin, a selective 5-HT2C serotonin receptor agonist, was recently approved by the Food and Drug Administration (FDA) for the treatment of obesity.[41] Data about safety and efficacy are limited to a few short-term trials that showed a significant dose-dependent weight loss compared with placebo, with headache, nausea, and dizziness being the most common side effects.[42] In a randomized controlled trial of lorcaserin versus placebo, subjects receiving lorcaserin lost 5.8% of body weight compared with 2.8% in the placebo group.[42] Sympathomimetic drugs such as phentermine stimulate the release of norepinephrine or inhibit its reuptake into nerve terminals. It activates the sympathetic nervous system, which suppresses appetite and increases resting energy expenditure. Phentermine is approved by the FDA for short-term use (12 weeks) and leads to weight loss of 5 to 6 pounds compared with placebo. The weight loss may plateau after a few months with some regain in weight after medication discontinuance. Weight loss is offset by frequent side effects and the potential risk of drug abuse as is the case with all sympathomimetic medications. Phentermine-topiramate, a new medication recently approved by the FDA, leads to significant weight loss at 1 year compared with placebo (10% vs 1.6% of baseline body weight). The most common adverse events with phentermine-topiramate are paresthesia, dry mouth, constipation, dysgeusia, and insomnia.[43] Although studies emphasize its effectiveness as a weight loss medication, long-term safety data are lacking. Its discontinuation should be gradual because of the risk of seizure with topiramate withdrawal. Although topiramate alone has been used in the management of epilepsy, its notable side effect of weight loss has led to its off-label use as a weight-loss medication. In a study be Li and colleagues,[44] patients who received topirimate lost 6.5% of total body weight. Despite positive results, for now topiramate as single therapy is not recommended to treat obesity. Bupropion, a drug used to treat depression, has been shown to produce significant weight loss.[45] A combination of bupropion and naltrexone has been studied in a large randomized, double-blind, placebo-controlled trial with more than 1700 subjects. Nearly half of the subjects randomized to receive combination sustained-release naltrexone (16 or 32 mg) with sustained-release buproprion lost weight as compared with only 16% of subjects receiving placebo. The average weight lost with the combination drug was 5% to 6% of body weight,[46] with the most frequent side effects of nausea and headache reported. Currently, there is no commercial form of the drug combination. In summary, weight loss medications can be added to diet and exercise in obese patient with BMI greater than 30, or BMI greater than 27 with comorbidities. Downsides of the use of weight-loss medications include frequent side effects, short-term benefit, and lack of long-term safety. Expected weight loss with these medications is modest and short-lived and should be combined with lifestyle changes.

LIFESTYLE INTERVENTIONS

Lifestyle interventions include diet modification, behavioral therapy, exercise, and their combinations. Surprisingly, little data exist on the efficacy of weight loss via dietary management on OSA. A Cochrane review called for more randomized controlled trial data with regard to the effectiveness of weight loss, exercise, and sleep hygiene techniques on the treatment of OSA.[47] The available studies in this area have several limitations, including small sample size, lack of a control group, and short-term follow-up. To date, only 2 randomized controlled trials have been performed using a control group. Tuomilehto and colleagues[48] reported the results of a prospective randomized controlled parallel group 1-year follow-up study in 72 patients on a very low calorie diet (VLCD) with supervised lifestyle counseling in patients with mild OSA. Subjects receiving 600 to 800 kcal/d using a commercially available weight loss product lost a mean of 10.7 kg (10.6% of the initial weight) versus −2.4 kg (2.6% of the initial weight) in controls who received lifestyle counseling only. At the end of the study period, nearly twice as many subjects in the intervention group were cured of OSA compared with the control group (61% vs 32%). Furthermore, there was a significant improvement in mean oxygen saturation and less time with oxygen saturation less than 90% during sleep in the intervention group.[48] In addition, subjects in the intervention arm lost a mean of 11.6 cm in waist circumference. A 5-cm reduction in waist circumference was associated with a decrease in AHI of 2.5 events per hour.[48] A larger randomized controlled trial comparing VLCD to controls in obese patients with moderate to severe OSA receiving CPAP showed that subjects in the intervention arm lost 18.7 kg and decreased the AHI by 25 events per hour compared with a 1.1-kg weight gain and no effect on AHI in controls at the end of a 9-week period.[49] Seventeen percent of subjects on the VLCD were cured of OSA (defined as AHI <5) and 50% of subjects were reclassified as mild OSA (AHI <15) by the end of the study period.[49] Although impressive, the major limitation of this study was its short duration; hence, the authors were unable to comment on the sustainability of weight loss beyond 9 weeks.[49] Other studies examining the effect of VLCD on OSA have shown that even modest degrees of weight loss in general reduce the AHI, but do not cure OSA. In a single study of VLCD in patients with OSA, a mean reduction of 9.2 kg led to significantly improved blood pressure and a reduction in the oxygen desaturation index from 31 to 19 events per hour.[50] Interestingly, the authors reported that in 20% of subjects OSA did not improve despite weight loss. Similar results were noted by Surratt and colleagues,[51] who examined 8 obese subjects with OSA who consumed between 400 and 800 kcal/d. Although weight loss from a VLCD led to a significant drop in the BMI (54–46 kg/m^2), it did not lead to a statistically significant improvement in the AHI probably because subjects were still morbidly obese at the termination of the trial. A study examining a combination of VLCD and exercise in a small group of obese patients with AHI greater than 10 showed significant and partially sustainable weight loss of 12.3 kg over a period of 12 months without significant improvements in the AHI.[52] In general, VLCD may produce significant degrees of weight loss in the short term with variable improvements in the degree of OSA that are not necessarily correlated with weight loss. Although such weight loss programs can be run effectively in the outpatient setting,[53] it should be stressed that several patients will still have OSA despite weight loss and that treatment of OSA may still be needed.

Behavioral therapy refers to strategies that help set and achieve weight loss goals, manage stress, and improve healthy behaviors. Behavioral therapy is effective particularly when combined with additional strategies to lose weight, such as calorie restriction or medications.[54] Unfortunately, there are very few studies that report the impact of behavioral therapy alone on weight loss in patients with OSA. The largest study to date, the Sleep AHEAD Study, included 264 subjects with OSA and type 2 diabetes mellitus, randomizing them to receive either an intensive lifestyle intervention using calorie restriction and physical activity or diabetes support and education (control). The intensive lifestyle intervention led to a mean weight loss of 10.8 kg and a reduction in AHI of 4.6 events per hour compared with a 0.6-kg weight gain and 4.8 events per hour increase in the AHI among controls.[55] Although the average change in AHI seems modest, nearly 40% of subjects in the intervention arm improved the severity of OSA. Remission rates of OSA in both arms were low at 3% to 13%.[55] Behavioral therapy was also reported to generate weight loss by Kajaste and colleagues[56] following a cognitive behavioral weight reduction program. Forty-four percent of patients decreased the oxygen desaturation index to less than 10 and decreased the oxygen desaturation index by more than 50% at 1-year follow-up. Dietary self-monitoring via food logs may be helpful for some patients in one small study to lose small amounts of weight.[57] These studies indicate that behavioral therapy seems to be most effective when used in conjunction with programs that incorporate VLCD.[48,49,52,55,58]

Exercise is considered a key component in weight loss programs. Exercise efficiently burns calories and, when combined with caloric restriction, weight loss can be achieved. Some studies have been performed examining the impact of exercise on OSA. In a small open trial of exercise in patients with moderate to severe OSA patients using CPAP, after 6 months of physical exercise, the respiratory disturbance index decreased by 9 events per hour on average and was observed even in the absence of any significant change in weight.[59] Data from 2 longitudinal studies lend additional support to these findings. Cross-sectional data from the Wisconsin Sleep Cohort Study showed an association between increased hours of exercise per week and reduced sleep-disordered breathing after adjustment for covariates.[60] Similarly, data from the Sleep Heart Health Study indicate that patients with sleep-disordered breathing perform in less vigorous physical activity compared with patients without sleep-disordered breathing, and that vigorous exercise ≥3 hours per week is associated with a respiratory disturbance index one-third less than found in sedentary patients in an unadjusted model.[61] It is not entirely understood if exercise exerts an independent positive effect on OSA, and the existing studies are inconclusive. In a randomized controlled trial comparing effects of an aerobic exercise versus stretching on AHI, subjects randomized to 12 weeks of moderate-intensity aerobic exercise decreased their AHI by 24% on average without significant change in weight.[62] Meanwhile, longitudinal data also from the Wisconsin Sleep Cohort Study indicate that exercise reduces the incidence of new onset mild or moderate sleep-disordered breathing over a follow-up period of 8 years. Although the observed effect in this study was partially mediated by the change in weight, there also seemed to be some protective effect independent of body habitus.[63] Exercise may affect OSA by increasing in upper airway muscle tone, changing body fat distribution of body fat, and/or altering control of breathing and arousal.[63]

CONTINUOUS POSITIVE AIRWAY PRESSURE

CPAP itself may mediate an effect on weight loss through sleep. Daytime sleepiness and fatigue are commonly reported in patients with OSA and can be both motivational and empowerment barriers to weight loss. CPAP can improve fatigue and reduce sleepiness in OSA and theoretically could reduce some challenges of weight loss. Unfortunately few studies have been published in this area. In patients using a VLCD and cognitive behavioral weight loss program, the use of CPAP did not result in any additional weight loss.[58] Similarly, a retrospective study found that CPAP use of ≥4 hours per night ≥70% of nights was not associated with weight loss. There were no significant differences in weight loss between adherent and nonadherant users.[64] Interestingly, women CPAP users gained weight. It is important to recognize that in the Redenius study, sleep duration was not monitored, a significant covariate linked to weight gain.[65] On the contrary, a small study of 32 obese or overweight patients with OSA on CPAP reported that CPAP adherent users were more likely to lose weight than nonadherent users.[66] More studies examining OSA as a risk factor for obesity, accounting for significant covariates, are needed and also whether CPAP adherence has an independent effect. At this point, CPAP alone cannot be recommended as the sole weight loss strategy for obese patients with OSA.

SUMMARY

Although obesity is one of the important risk factors for OSA, the mechanism behind its causality is not well understood. In obese patients with OSA, weight loss should not be recommended as the sole treatment of OSA, but should be used in conjunction with other treatments such as CPAP. Although weight loss strategies vary, these can mainly be classified into surgical, pharmacologic, and lifestyle (including caloric restriction, behavioral therapy, and exercise) treatments. In general, weight loss may reduce the number of apneas and hypopneas, but complete remission in most patients is not to be expected. Furthermore, additional challenges with the difficulty of sustainable weight reduction should impart close attention and follow-up to ensure continued evaluation and management of OSA.

REFERENCES

1. Young T, Palta M, Dempsey J, et al. The occurrence of sleep disordered breathing among middle-aged adults. N Engl J Med 1993;328: 1230–5.

2. Ogden CL, Carroll MD, Kit BK, et al. Prevalence of obesity in the United States, 2009-2010. NCHS Data Brief. 2012 Jan;(82):1–8.

3. Peppard PE, Young T, Palta M, et al. Longitudinal study of moderate weight change and sleep disordered breathing. JAMA 2000;284:3015–21.

4. Schwartz AR, Patil SP, Laffan AM, et al. Obesity and obstructive sleep apnea: pathogenic mechanisms and therapeutic approaches. Proc Am Thorac Soc 2008;5:185–92.

5. Horner RL, Mohiadden RH, Lowell DG, et al. Sites and sizes of fat deposits around the pharynx in obese patients with obstructive sleep apnea and weight matched controls. Eur Respir J 1989;2:613–22.

6. Schwab RJ, Gupta KB, Gefter WB, et al. Upper airway and soft tissue anatomy in normal subjects and patients with sleep disordered breathing. Significance of the lateral pharyngeal walls. Am J Respir Crit Care Med 1995;152:1673–89.

7. Schwartz AR, Gold AR, Schubert N, et al. Effect of weight loss on upper airway collapsibility in obstructive sleep apnea. Am Rev Respir Dis 1991;144:494–8.

8. Stauffer JL, Buick MK, Bixler EO, et al. Morphology of the uvula in obstructive sleep apnea. Am Rev Respir Dis 1989;140(3):724–8.

9. Smith PL, Wise RA, Gold AR, et al. Upper airway pressure flow-relationships in obstructive sleep apnea. J Appl Physiol 1988;64(2):789–95.

10. Schwartz AR, Smith PL, Wise RA, et al. Induction of upper airway occlusion in sleeping individuals with subatmospheric nasal pressure. J Appl Physiol 1988;64:535–42.

11. Gleadhill EC, Schwartz AR, Schubert N, et al. Upper airway collapsibility in snorers and in patients with obstructive hypopnea and apnea. Am Rev Respir Dis 1991;143(6):1300–3.

12. Chen K, Li F, Li J, et al. Induction of leptin resistance through direct interaction of C-reactive protein with leptin. Nat Med 2006;14:425–32.

13. Gavrila A. Serum adiponectin levels are inversely associated with overall and central fat distribution but are not directly regulated by acute fasting or leptin administration in humans: cross-sectional and interventional studies. J Clin Endocrinol Metab 2003;88:4823–31.

14. Shrestha C, He H, Liu Y, et al. Changes in adipokines following laparoscopic Roux-en-Y gastric bypass surgery in Chinese individuals with type 2 diabetes mellitus and BMI of 22-30 kg•m(-2.). Int J Endocrinol 2013;2013:240971.

15. Rochester DF, Arora NS. Respiratory failure from obesity. In: Mancini M, Lewis B, Contaldo F, editors. Medical complications of obesity. London: Academic Press; 1980. p. 183.

16. Sampson MG, Grassino K. Neuromechanical properties in obese patients during carbon dioxide rebreathing. Am J Med 1983;75(1):81–90.

17. Sampol G, Muñox X, Sagalés MT, et al. Long-term efficacy of dietary weight loss in sleep apnoea/hypopnea syndrome. Eur Respir J 1998;12:1156–9.

18. Sjöström L, Lindroos AK, Peltonen M, et al. Lifestyle, diabetes, and cardiovascular risk factors 10 years after bariatric surgery. N Engl J Med 2004;351(26):2683–93.

19. Mechanick JI, Kushner RF, Sugerman HJ, et al. American Association of Clinical Endocrinologists, The Obesity Society, and American Society for Metabolic & Bariatric Surgery medical guidelines for clinical practice for the perioperative nutritional, metabolic, and nonsurgical support of the bariatric surgery patient. Endocr Pract 2008;14(Suppl 1):1–83.

20. Nguyen NT, Masoomi H, Magno CP, et al. Trends in use of bariatric surgery, 2003-2008. J Am Coll Surg 2011;213(2):261–6.

21. Cummings DE, Weigle DS, Frayo RS, et al. Plasma ghrelin levels after diet-induced weight loss or gastric bypass surgery. N Engl J Med 2002;346(21):1623–30.

22. Roth CL, Reinehr T, Schernthaner GH, et al. Ghrelin and obestatin levels in severely obese women before and after weight loss after Roux-en-Y gastric bypass surgery. Obes Surg 2009;19(1):29–35.

23. MacLean LD, Rhode BM, Sampalis J, et al. Results of the surgical treatment of obesity. Am J Surg 1993;165(1):155–60.

24. Jones DB, Schneider BE, Olbers T. Atlas of metabolic and weight loss surgery. North Woodbury (CT): Cine-Med; 2010.

25. Ren CJ, Horgan S, Ponce J. US experience with the LAP-BAND system. Am J Surg 2002;184(6B):46S.

26. Spivak H, Anwar F, Burton S, et al. The Lap-Band system in the United States: one surgeon's experience with 271 patients. Surg Endosc 2004;18(2):198.

27. O'Brien PE, Dixon JB. Lap-band: outcomes and results. J Laparoendosc Adv Surg Tech A 2003;13(4):265–70.

28. Almogy G, Crookes PF, Anthone GJ. Longitudinal gastrectomy as a treatment for the high-risk super-obese patient. Obes Surg 2004;14(4):492.

29. Regan JP, Inabnet WB, Gagner M, et al. Early experience with two-stage laparoscopic Roux-en-Y gastric bypass as an alternative in the super-super obese patient. Obes Surg 2003;13(6):861.

30. Hutter MM, Schirmer BD, Jones DB, et al. First report from the American College of Surgeons Bariatric Surgery Center Network: laparoscopic sleeve

gastrectomy has morbidity and effectiveness positioned between the band and the bypass. Ann Surg 2011;254(3):410–20.

31. Sammour T, Hill AG, Singh P, et al. Laparoscopic sleeve gastrectomy as a single-stage bariatric procedure. Obes Surg 2010;20(3):271–5.

32. Marceau P, Hould FS, Simard S, et al. Biliopancreatic diversion with duodenal switch. World J Surg 1998;22(9):947–54.

33. Greenburg DL, Lettieri CJ, Eliasson AH. Effects of surgical weight loss on measures of obstructive sleep apnea: a meta-analysis. Am J Med 2009; 122(6):535–42.

34. Dixon JB, Schachter LM, O'Brien PE, et al. Surgical vs. conventional therapy for weight loss treatment of obstructive sleep apnea: a randomized controlled trial. JAMA 2012;308(11):1142–9.

35. Yee BJ, Phillips CL, Banerjee D, et al. The effect of sibutramine-assisted weight loss in men with obstructive sleep apnoea. Int J Obes (Lond) 2007;31(1):161–8.

36. Ferland A, Poirier P, Sériès F. Sibutramine versus continuous positive airway pressure in obese obstructive sleep apnoea patients. Eur Respir J 2009;34(3):694–701.

37. Heck AM, Yanovski JA, Calis KA. Orlistat, a new lipase inhibitor for the management of obesity. Pharmacotherapy 2000;20(3):270–9.

38. Torgerson JS, Hauptman J, Boldrin MN, et al. XENical in the prevention of diabetes in obese subjects (XENDOS) study: a randomized study of orlistat as an adjunct to lifestyle changes for the prevention of type 2 diabetes in obese patients. Diabetes Care 2004;27(1):155–61.

39. Svendsen M, Tonstad S. Orlistat after initial dietary/behavioural treatment: changes in body weight and dietary maintenance in subjects with sleep related breathing disorders. Nutr J 2011;10:21.

40. Hollander PA, Elbein SC, Hirsch IB, et al. Role of orlistat in the treatment of obese patients with type 2 diabetes. A 1-year randomized double-blind study. Diabetes Care 1998;21(8):1288–94.

41. Goldenberg MM. Pharmaceutical approval update. P T 2012;37(9):499–502.

42. Fidler MC, Sanchez M, Raether B, et al. A one-year randomized trial of lorcaserin for weight loss in obese and overweight adults: the BLOSSOM trial. J Clin Endocrinol Metab 2011;96(10):3067–77.

43. Allison DB, Gadde KM, Garvey WT, et al. Controlled-release phentermine/topiramate in severely obese adults: a randomized controlled trial (EQUIP). Obesity (Silver Spring) 2012;20(2):330–42.

44. Li Z, Maglione M, Tu W, et al. Meta-analysis: pharmacologic treatment of obesity. Ann Intern Med 2005;142(7):532.

45. Anderson JW, Greenway FL, Fujioka K, et al. Bupropion SR enhances weight loss: a 48-week double-blind, placebo- controlled trial. Obes Res 2002;10(7):633–41.

46. Greenway FL, Fujioka K, Plodkowski RA, et al. Effect of naltrexone plus bupropion on weight loss in overweight and obese adults (COR-I): a multicentre, randomised, double-blind, placebo-controlled, phase 3 trial. Lancet 2010;376(9741): 595–605.

47. Shneerson J, Wright JJ. Lifestyle modification for obstructive sleep apnoea. Cochrane Database Syst Rev 2001;(1):CD002875.

48. Tuomilehto HP, Seppä JM, Partinen MM, et al. Lifestyle intervention with weight reduction. First-line treatment with mild obstructive sleep apnoea. Am J Respir Crit Care Med 2009;179:320–7.

49. Johansson K, Neovius M, Lagerro YT, et al. Effect of a very low energy diet on moderate and severe obstructive sleep apnoea in obese men: a randomized controlled trial. BMJ 2009;339: b4609.

50. Kansanem M, Vanninen E, Tuunainem A, et al. The effect of a very low-calorie diet-induced weight loss on the severity of obstructive sleep apnoea and autonomic nervous function in obese patients with obstructive sleep apnoea syndrome. Clin Physiol 1998;4:377–85.

51. Surratt PM, McTier RF, Findley LJ, et al. Effect of very-low-calorie diets with weight loss on obstructive sleep apnea. Am J Clin Nutr 1992; 56:182S–4S.

52. Barnes M, Goldsworthy UR, Care BA, et al. A diet and exercise program to improve clinical outcomes in patients with obstructive sleep apnea—a feasibility study. J Clin Sleep Med 2009;5:409–15.

53. Lojander J, Mustajoki P, Rönkä S, et al. A nurse-managed weight reduction programme for obstructive sleep apnoea syndrome. J Intern Med 1998;244:251–5.

54. Foster GD, Makris AP, Bailer BA. Behavioral treatment of obesity. Am J Clin Nutr 2005;82(Suppl): 230S–5S.

55. Foster GD, Borradaile KE, Sanders MH, et al. A randomized study on the effect of weight loss on obstructive sleep apnea among obese patients with type 2 diabetes. Arch Intern Med 2009; 169(17):1619–26.

56. Kajaste S, Telakivi T, Mustajoki P, et al. Effect of a cognitive-behavioural weight loss programme on overweight obstructive sleep apnea patients. J Sleep Res 1994;3:245–9.

57. Hood MM, Corsica J, Cventros J, et al. Impact of a brief dietary self-monitoring intervention on weight change and CPAP adherence with obstructive sleep apnea. J Psychosom Res 2013;74:170–4.

58. Kajaste S, Brander PE, Telakivi T, et al. A cognitive-behavioral weight reduction program in the treatment of obstructive sleep apnea syndrome with

or without initial nasal CPAP: a randomized study. Sleep Med 2004;5:125–31.

59. Giebelhaus V, Strohl KP, Lormes W, et al. Physical exercise as an adjunct therapy in sleep apnea—an open trial. Sleep Breath 2000;4:173–6.

60. Peppard PE, Young TY. Exercise and sleep-disordered breathing: an association independent of body habitus. Sleep 2004;27:480–4.

61. Quan S, O'Connor GT, Quan JS, et al. Association of physical activity with sleep-disordered breathing. Sleep Breath 2007;11:149–57.

62. Kline CE, Crowley EP, Ewing GB, et al. The effect of exercise training on obstructive sleep apnea and sleep quality: a randomized controlled trial. Sleep 2011;34:1631–40.

63. Awad KM, Malhotra A, Barnet JH, et al. Exercise is associated with a reduced incidence of sleep-disordered breathing. Am J Med 2012;125: 485–90.

64. Redenius R, Murphy C, O'Neill E, et al. Does CPAP lead to change in BMI? J Clin Sleep Med 2008;4: 205–9.

65. Patel SR, Malhotra A, White DP, et al. Association between reduced sleep and weight gain in women. Am J Epidemiol 2006;164:947–54.

66. Loube DI, Loube AA, Erman MK. Continuous positive airway pressure treatment results in weight loss in obese and overweight patients with obstructive sleep apnea. J Am Diet Assoc 1997;97: 896–7.

Pharmacologic Therapy for Obstructive Sleep Apnea

Vivien C. Abad, MD, MBA

KEYWORDS

- Obstructive sleep apnea • Pharmacologic • Treatment • Review • Targets

KEY POINTS

- Current pharmacotherapy for sleep apnea is adjunctive, but its role can be transformed as we learn more about the various risk factors and interrelated pathology underlying the pathophysiology of sleep apnea.
- Because obesity is present in two-thirds of patients with documented sleep apnea, novel antiobesity medications may help in weight control and may secondarily improve breathing abnormalities.
- Medications addressing endothelial dysfunction, combined with positive airway pressure therapy, may help prevent hypoxemic sequelae of sleep apnea.
- New medications that can increase upper airway muscle tone and target fibrillin to improve connective-tissue laxity may also be useful.
- Determining the molecular signatures of sleep apnea may help identify diagnostic, prognostic, and surrogate markers for obstructive sleep apnea, and identify markers for drug-response phenotypes.

INTRODUCTION

Obstructive sleep apnea (OSA) is a major health hazard that is estimated to affect 12 million Americans. Up to 5% of adults in Western countries remain undiagnosed.[1] Severity of OSA is defined by the number of apneic and hypopneic events per hour of sleep, also known as the apnea-hypopnea index (AHI). Among Americans between the ages of 30 and 60 years, 24% of men and 9% of women have mild OSA (AHI ≥5), and 9% of men and 4% of women have at least moderate OSA (AHI ≥15).[1]

Sleep apnea is multifactorial in origin. Obesity, craniofacial abnormalities, age, gender, congenital and acquired conditions, and environmental factors may increase collapsibility of the upper airway during inspiration; combined with insufficient neuromuscular compensation, these factors may lead to failure to keep the airway patent. Ventilatory instability, pharyngeal neuropathy, and fluid shifts toward the pharynx have been implicated in the pathophysiology of OSA. OSA has been associated with accidents, hypertension, ischemic heart disease, strokes, insulin resistance, and increased mortality.[2–4]

Primary treatment modalities attempt to prevent upper airway collapse through a positive airway pressure (PAP) device, an oral appliance (OA), or surgical modification of the upper airway. However, at least 8% to 9% of new OSA patients decline continuous PAP (CPAP),[5] and adherence rates vary from 30% to 60%.[6] Dropout rates in OA users vary from 0% to 38% because of lack of efficacy or side effects.[7] A review of placebo-controlled crossover trials of OAs reported that the AHI decreased from 25 to 14 in 64% of OSA patients.[8] Adjustable OAs are preferable over fixed OA devices.[9] In a group of 602 OSA patients, mean AHI decreased from a baseline of 30 to fewer than 5 events per hour in 57% of individuals with an adjustable OA, compared with 47%

Division of Sleep Medicine, Department of Psychiatry and Behavioral Science, Stanford Medicine Center, 450 Broadway Street, Pavilion B, 2nd Floor Redwood City, CA 94063, USA
E-mail address: vcabad@yahoo.com

Sleep Med Clin 8 (2013) 527–542
http://dx.doi.org/10.1016/j.jsmc.2013.07.002
1556-407X/13/$ – see front matter © 2013 Elsevier Inc. All rights reserved.

fixed-OA subjects.[9] Surgical success rates for OSA vary depending on the procedure. A review compared the percent reduction in mean AHI postoperatively relative to baseline mean AHI: maxilla-mandibular advancement, 87%; uvulopalatopharyngoplasty, 33%; laser uvuloplasty, 18%; radiofrequency to the soft palate, base of the tongue, or multilevel treatment, 34%; and soft-palate implants, 26%.[10] Adjunctive surgeries for OSA include nasal procedures to relieve nasal obstruction or bariatric surgery to address obesity.

Medical therapy for sleep apnea includes weight reduction, positional therapy, supplemental oxygen therapy, and pharmacotherapy. Drugs can potentially improve OSA by maintaining patency of the upper airway during sleep, increasing respiratory drive, reducing the proportion of rapid eye movement (REM) sleep, facilitating cholinergic tone during sleep, or reducing upper airway resistance/surface tension. Unfortunately, agents that have been investigated have inadequately prevented upper airway collapse or have improved AHI insufficiently to warrant their use as primary therapy. Pharmacotherapy in OSA remains in a secondary or adjunctive role. This article discusses current pharmacotherapy and the treatment goals for sleep apnea.

PHARMACOTHERAPEUTIC AGENTS
Medications that Promote Alertness in Treated OSA Patients

Residual excessive sleepiness (RES) can persist in all categories of OSA-treated patients.[11–14] Reported RES prevalence (defined subjectively) among CPAP users varies from 207 of 4129 (5%)[11] to 60 of 502 (12%),[12] and up to as many as 106 of 149 (71%) individuals.[13]

Modafinil and armodafinil use in CPAP users with RES

For patients with RES on CPAP therapy, it is important to objectively verify hours of use per night (the prevalence of Epworth Sleepiness Scale [ESS] score <10 is higher with more usage hour per night),[13] monitor adequacy of pressure settings based on AHI from device data, and reevaluate and treat coexisting comorbid psychiatric illnesses, medical conditions, and other primary sleep disorders.[11,12] The value of treating RES in these patients has been questioned[15] because the percentage of sleepy subjects (ESS >10) among 572 CPAP users (mean body mass index [BMI] 35 kg/m^2) at 16% did not significantly differ from a "normal" control group of 525 subjects (mean BMI 27 kg/m^2) at 14%.[15] In the usual clinical setting, however, OSA-treated patients with

unexplained hypersomnolence are considered for supplemental stimulant therapy to improve their quality of life and reduce their risk of accidents.

Modafinil and armodafinil are the main stimulants used to address RES in treated OSA. Modafinil is metabolized into the R and S enantiomers, whereas armodafinil is the R and longer-lasting enantiomer of modafinil. Modafinil induces wakefulness by inhibiting dopamine and noradrenaline reuptake transporters. Peak plasma absorption (fasting state) occurs at 2 to 4 hours for modafinil and 2 hours for armodafinil. Both drugs have an elimination half-life of 13 hours, with similar mean maximum plasma drug concentration.[16] Compared with modafinil on a milligram-to-milligram basis, armodafinil achieves higher plasma concentrations late in the day.[16] There are no head-to-head studies comparing the efficacy of modafinil with that of armodafinil in reducing sleepiness in OSA subjects.

Modafinil is started at either 100 mg or 200 mg each morning and titrated upwards to 300 to 400 mg if needed. Split dosing (AM and mid-afternoon) is an alternative if mid-afternoon sleepiness occurs. Armodafinil is started at 150 mg in the morning and is increased after 1 week to 250 mg if needed. Both drugs are metabolized by the liver, with renal excretion of metabolites. Interactions with other drugs are due to their effect on cytochrome P450 enzymes. The most frequent side effects are headache, nausea, anorexia, dry mouth, and diarrhea. Serious rashes, including Stevens-Johnson syndrome and toxic epidermal necrolysis, have been reported with modafinil. Patients should be advised to discontinue modafinil or armodafinil if rash develops. Caution should be exercised in prescribing either medication to patients with a history of heart disease (particularly left ventricular dysfunction and mitral valve prolapse) or arrhythmias, because palpitations and electrocardiographic T-wave ischemic changes have been reported with modafinil. Users should be informed that the efficacy of birth-control tablets may be reduced, and advised to consider alternative/supplemental contraception.

Modafinil does not reduce AHI, but does improve vigilance and quality of life.[17–19] In 2 randomized, double-blind, placebo-controlled trials of modafinil (4 weeks,[17] 12 weeks[18]), ESS scores improved,[17,18] with normalization (ESS <10) in 51% of modafinil-treated subjects, compared with 27% in the placebo group.[17] Multiple Sleep Latency Test (MSLT) sleep-onset latencies did not improve.[17] ESS and sleep-related functional status continued to improve over a 12-week open-label trial of modafinil in 125 moderate to severe OSA patients who had previously completed a 4-week double-blind trial.[19] A 2-week double-blind randomized crossover study of CPAP-treated OSA patients who received modafinil or placebo reported that modafinil did not significantly improve ESS scores or MSLT sleep-onset latency; Maintenance of Wakefulness Test (MWT) sleep-onset latency marginally improved, indicating improved ability to stay awake despite lack of subjective improvement.[20] The lack of improvement in ESS scores in this study may be partially due to fewer hours of CPAP usage per night in the modafinil group compared with the placebo group.[20]

Armodafinil improves wakefulness, as shown in 2 (12-week, randomized, double-blind, placebo-controlled) trials of CPAP-treated sleepy OSA subjects (N = 395,[21] N = 259[22]). MWT sleep latency increased from baseline by 2.3 minutes in the armodafinil (150 mg) group, whereas the placebo group's mean sleep latency decreased by 1.3 minutes.[22] With the combined armodafinil groups (150, 250 mg), mean MWT sleep latency increased from baseline by 1.9 minutes, whereas the placebo group decreased by 1.7 minutes.[21] With armodafinil, ESS scores and fatigue scores improved, and episodic secondary memory and patient-estimated wakefulness also improved.[21,22]

Possible long-term use of stimulant therapy in sleepy OSA patients

Armodafinil improved subjective sleepiness in 474 OSA patients, with mean baseline ESS of 16 decreasing by 6.4 in a 12-week multicenter open-label trial.[23] Fifty-eight percent of these patients had completed 12 months of armodafinil use. By the end of the trial, 55% had an ESS lower than 10, and the Clinical Global Impression of Change (CGI-C) substantially improved in 65% of OSA subjects.[23] Thirteen percent discontinued medication because of mild to moderate adverse events: headache (25%), nasopharyngitis (17%), and insomnia (14%). Armodafinil seems to be well tolerated and appears to sustain improvement in daytime sleepiness even after a year's usage.

Possible role of stimulants in acute withdrawal from CPAP

In a randomized, double-blind, placebo-controlled crossover trial in 21 severe OSA patients (mean AHI 49) on CPAP therapy (mean use 7 hours/night), 200 mg of modafinil prevented decline in simulated driving performance (reduced steering variability), improved neurocognitive performance (reduced mean number of lapses and mean reciprocal reaction time) on psychomotor vigilance test (PVT), and reduced subjective sleepiness.[24] This study needs additional confirmation, but suggests

that on a short-term basis modafinil therapy may help mitigate sleepiness and neurocognitive dysfunction associated with short-term withdrawal of CPAP therapy.

Stimulants in OSA and major depression

Comorbidity with OSA ranges from 7% to 63% for depression and 11% to 70% for anxiety disorders.[25] A 12-week randomized, double-blind, parallel-group study in 249 sleepy (ESS >10) patients with OSA and either major depression or dysthymia compared armodafinil 250 mg/d (n = 125) with placebo (n = 124).[26] Mean CGI-C score for sleepiness significantly improved with armodafinil use (69% vs 53%), although mean ESS change was minimal (−6 vs −5). MWT sleep latency did not significantly improve (2.6 vs 1.1 minutes). There was no significant effect on depression in either group.[26] In summary, stimulants improve subjective daytime sleepiness in depressed OSA patients but do not improve depression.

Other stimulants (caffeine, amphetamine, methamphetamine, methylphenidate)

Caffeine content varies from 36 to 71 mg in 12-oz sodas, 5 to 175 mg in a cup of coffee, and 42 to 141 mg in a can of energy drink.[27] Caffeine plasma levels peak between 30 and 75 minutes, and half-life varies from 3 to 7 hours. There are no published studies documenting the efficacy of caffeine use in sleep apnea in adults. Data from the Sleep Heart Health Study indicates that consumption of caffeinated soda, but not tea or coffee, is independently associated with severity of sleep apnea in women.[28] In men, the association with caffeine intake was present only with severe sleep-disordered breathing (SDB). The SDB-caffeine association was not affected by age and was not explained by sleepiness.[28]

There may be a role for intravenous caffeine in children with OSA who are undergoing tonsillectomy. A randomized, double-blind, placebo-controlled study of children (N = 72) undergoing tonsillectomy for presumed OSA (diagnosis was based on history alone or history and polysomnography) reported that the overall incidence of adverse postoperative respiratory events (laryngospasm, upper airway obstruction, desaturation, and/or need for reintubation) was lower in the caffeine group (11 of 36, 31%) than in the placebo group (21 of 36, 58%).[29] Preoperative mean AHI in the caffeine group (n = 14) was 10, compared with 13 in the placebo group (n = 17).[29]

Amphetamine, methamphetamine, and methylphenidate are highly potent stimulants more commonly used to treat attention-deficit/hyperactivity disorder or to improve alertness in patients with narcolepsy. Clinical trials have not been performed using these agents in the setting of OSA. These agents have greater potential risk for dependency and abuse because they produce intensified feelings of contentment, relaxation, and euphoria even at low doses.[30] Given the potential for cardiovascular risk[31] and neurotoxicity[32] with these agents and their dependency/abuse potential, they are not recommended for the treatment of RES in sleep apnea.

In summary, the role of caffeine in maintaining alertness in adult OSA patients is unproven. More studies are needed to confirm the efficacy of caffeine administration in the preoperative setting (tonsillectomy) for pediatric patients with OSA to reduce complications. The use of amphetamine, methamphetamine, or methylphenidate for OSA patients is not recommended.

Pharmacologic Agents that Reduce Nasal Air Resistance and Congestion

Nasal steroid sprays, leukotriene inhibitors, decongestants, domperidone

Eleven percent of OSA patients have associated allergic rhinitis.[33] Nasal obstruction increases nasal airway resistance (NAR), which contributes to upper airway collapse. In a double-blind, placebo-controlled, crossover study of 23 patients (n = 13 moderate OSA, n = 10 snorers), fluticasone nasal spray significantly lowered AHI and NAR, and improved daytime alertness and nasal congestion, but snoring persisted.[34] Another placebo-controlled, triple-blind, parallel-group study (N = 25 children with OSA and allergic rhinitis) reported that mean AHI decreased in the fluticasone group from 11 to 6 but increased from 11 to 13 in the placebo group. Respiratory movements/arousals and frequency of desaturations of blood oxygen also decreased in the fluticasone group, although OSA scores and tonsil sizes did not significantly change.[35] Intranasal budesonide improved AHI and reduced median oxygen desaturation of hemoglobin index in an open-label study of 27 children with mild SDB,[36] and improved polysomnographic measures of sleep quality, AHI, respiratory arousal index, nadir pulse oxygen saturation, and adenoidal size in 48 children who completed a randomized, double-blind, placebo-controlled trial.[37] In both studies, benefits persisted after discontinuation of budesonide (several months,[36] 8 weeks[37]).

Leukotrienes, which are anti-inflammatory markers, are increased in sleep apnea. Tonsils of children with SDB have increased expression of cysteinyl leukotriene receptors in T lymphocytes in comparison with tonsils of controls (children with recurrent tonsillitis). Montelukast, a leukotriene receptor antagonist, at a dose of 4 or 5 mg (based on age), was administered to 24 children with mild SDB in a 16-week, open-label, parallel-group study. Montelukast decreased their obstructive AHI, peak end-tidal CO_2, and respiratory arousal index, and also reduced adenoidal size.[38] In a double-blind, placebo-controlled trial of montelukast (N = 23), the mean obstructive apnea index (AI; number of apneic episodes per hour) significantly decreased and the mean AHI trended downward, but sleep parameters were unchanged.[39]

Intranasal budesonide and montelukast (4 or 5 mg based on age) were administered to 22 children with residual SDB (1 < AHI < 5) following tonsillectomy and adenoidectomy, in a comparison with 14 children with residual SDB who did not receive drug therapy.[40] Mean AHI significantly decreased from 3.9 to 0.3 in the treated group, whereas mean AHI increased from 3.6 to 4.7 in the nontreated group. Nadir for blood oxygen saturation (SpO$_2$) also improved from 87.3% to 92.5% in the treated group; sleep parameters were unchanged except for decreased stage 1 non-REM (NREM) sleep in the treated group.[40]

Xylometazoline did not improve AHI, ESS, or sleep quality in 12 OSA patients with chronic nasal congestion who participated in a randomized, placebo-controlled, crossover trial.[41] In a randomized, placebo-controlled, sham-controlled trial of oxymetazoline plus nasal strip in 10 OSA patients, respiratory disturbance index (RDI; the average number of episodes of apnea, hypopnea, and respiratory event–related arousal per hour of sleep) decreased by 12 on average, but only 1 of 10 patients achieved AHI lower than 15. Mean AHI decreased from 40 to 30 with treatment.[42] Sleep parameters (sleep efficiency; percentages of slow-wave sleep and REM sleep) improved, and percentage of mouth breathing during the night normalized from 39% to 8% of the night.[42]

Domperidone has peripheral antidopaminergic activity and prokinetic effects. It also increases hypercapnic ventilatory response and peripheral chemosensitivity.[43] Pseudoephedrine, an α-adrenergic agonist, is a commonly used decongestant. In an unblinded, uncontrolled study in 23 sleepy snorers with probable OSA, domperidone (10–20 mg) and pseudoephedrine (60 mg) significantly improved the oxygen desaturation index (ODI; the number of times per hour of sleep that the blood oxygen level drops by 3% or more from baseline), mean SpO$_2$, and ESS. Following treatment, mean SpO$_2$ improved from 92.2% to 94.2% and mean ODI improved from 42.5 to 25.9. Mean ESS decreased from 14 to 4. Sixteen of 23 patients had complete resolution of snoring.[44]

In summary, some adult and pediatric OSA patients may benefit from treating nasal congestion with nasal steroids. Children with residual sleep apnea following tonsillectomy and adenoidectomy may benefit from leukotriene antagonist therapy, but duration of optimum therapy has not yet been established. Nasal decongestant sprays do not appear to improve sleep apnea in adult patients. Short-term use of nasal decongestant sprays with a nasal strip may reduce oral breathing and improve nasal congestion and sleep quality, although additional studies are needed to show benefit for conditions with increased nasal congestion (such as acute exacerbation of nasal allergies). Additional studies (randomized, placebo-controlled) are needed to evaluate the role of domperidone (alone or with pseudoephedrine) in treating OSA patients and snorers.

Pharmacotherapeutic Agents that Stimulate Ventilation

Acetazolamide

Acetazolamide (AZM), a carbonic anhydrase inhibitor, stimulates ventilation by inducing metabolic acidosis. However, it also attenuates the increase in ventilation following spontaneous arousal from sleep, which may reduce the ventilatory instability during sleep-wake transitions. Results are variable, but side effects are frequent and include nausea, paresthesias, dysgeusia, polyuria, nausea, and tinnitus.

AZM reduced median NREM AHI from 50 to 24 in comparison with baseline levels in 13 OSA subjects.[45] With AZM, median loop gain decreased by 41%, primarily because of reduced plant gain; there was no significant change in pharyngeal anatomy/collapsibility, upper airway gain, or arousal threshold.[45]

In a placebo-controlled study, use of AZM (250 mg daily × 3) in 45 OSA subjects (median AHI = 49) slightly improved oxyhemoglobin saturation in comparison with the placebo group (87% vs 85% at 1860 m and 85% vs 80% at 2590 m) during ascent from a baseline of 490 m. Obstructive AHI slightly decreased but remained in the severe category at all elevations with AZM therapy. Central apnea indices increased for both groups, worsening with each elevation, but were more pronounced in the placebo group.[46] AZM subjects had longer total sleep time and better sleep efficiency at all elevations.[46]

A randomized, placebo-controlled trial in symptomatic OSA subjects with baseline AHI of 15 or greater compared AZM (250 mg daily × 4) with protriptyline (20 mg daily) for 14 days.[47] Mean AHI significantly decreased to 26 in the AZM

group, compared with 50 in the placebo group. Arterial saturations were not different, but 4% ODI was lower (19 vs 29) in the AZM group. The protriptyline-treated group did not show a significant change in either mean AHI or 4% ODI. Nadir Spo_2 was unchanged for all groups and OSA symptoms did not improve for either treatment group in comparison with placebo.[47]

In another study, 45% of 75 subjects treated with AZM had AHI reduced by 50% or less compared with pretreatment values; the responders tended to have lower BMI and milder sleep apnea.[48] Similarly, AZM significantly reduced the AI and percentage of apnea time in 14 of 20 subjects.[49]

In summary, AZM should not be used as primary therapy for OSA because its benefits are mild, results are mixed, and the side effects are frequent. AZM may be used as adjunctive therapy in combination with CPAP in OSA subjects who ascend to high altitude.

There may also be a subset of OSA patients who may respond better to AZM (those who benefit from reductions in loop gain alone), but further studies are needed to confirm this.

Methylxanthine derivatives (theophylline, aminophylline)

Theophylline and aminophylline block adenosine receptors, thereby stimulating ventilatory drive. In a double-blind, placebo-controlled, crossover trial in 12 OSA subjects using 800 mg oral theophylline per night, obstructive AHI decreased from 49 to 40, which was statistically but not clinically significant. Oxygen desaturations of more than 4% were fewer, but mean Spo_2 was unchanged and sleep quality was significantly worse with theophylline.[50] In an observational study of 13 patients with sleep apnea, theophylline disturbed sleep (reduced total sleep time and sleep efficiency) but did not normalize AHI or the desaturation index.[51] Similarly, aminophylline infusion increased sleep fragmentation and reduced sleep efficiency, and did not improve AI, mean Spo_2, and Spo_2 nadir in a randomized, placebo-controlled, crossover study of 10 OSA subjects with baseline apnea index of greater than 15.[52]

In summary, methylxanthine derivatives (theophylline, aminophylline) are not recommended for OSA because of their clinically insignificant benefit in sleep apnea parameters while significantly disrupting sleep.

Nicotinic agents

Nicotine potentially promotes ventilation via excitatory input to hypoglossal motor neurons or by increasing genioglossus and diaphragmatic activity. However, nicotine can also constrict the rostral tracheal segment. Randomized trials using nicotine patches in a small number of OSA subjects and snorers showed reduction in sleep efficiency, prolonged sleep-onset latency, and reduced percentage of REM sleep; AHI did not improve even when salivary levels of nicotine were high.[53,54] In a trial of nicotine plasters in 8 subjects with moderate OSA, mean oxyhemoglobin saturation slightly increased, but there was no improvement in mean apneas or hypopneas or duration of these events, nor was there any improvement in minimum oxyhemoglobin saturation.[55]

In summary, nicotinic agents are not effective and are not recommended for use in OSA.

Glutamate antagonists

Sabeluzole, a benzthiazole derivative, slightly improved SpO_2 nadir and slightly reduced the ODI, but did not improve OSA symptoms in 13 subjects with moderate to severe OSA.[56] SDB can be associated with hypoxia and neuronal damage, and apoptosis during hypoxemia has been linked to the N-methyl-D-aspartate (NMDA) receptor subtype of glutamate. In a randomized, double-blind, placebo-controlled, single-dose, crossover study, infusion of the NMDA receptor antagonist AR-R15896AR in 15 male patients with moderate to severe SDB did not improve AHI, minimum oxyhemoglobin saturation, or ODI.[57] Sleep parameters worsened, with reduced total sleep time and sleep efficiency, prolonged sleep onset and REM sleep latencies, and impaired sleep architecture. Side effects included nightmares, hallucinations, and vivid dreams.[57]

In summary, sabeluzole minimally improves oxyhemoglobin saturation, impairs sleep architecture, and is not recommended for use in OSA. NMDA antagonists do not improve sleep apnea, but impair sleep and produce nightmares, hallucinations, and vivid dreams.

Doxapram

Doxapram is a respiratory stimulant that acts through peripheral carotid chemoreceptors. Intravenous infusion of doxapram in 4 subjects with OSA improved average oxyhemoglobin desaturation during apneic and hypopneic episodes and decreased the average apnea length, but did not change the average number of oxyhemoglobin desaturations per hour of sleep.[58]

Postoperative respiratory complications were fewer (2% vs 29%) and postoperative sedation scores, mean stay in the recovery room, and postoperative hospital stay were significantly shorter in a group of 62 patients who received doxapram as part of perioperative anesthesia during elective laparoscopic gastric bypass surgery when compared with a similar group (n = 62) who did not receive doxapram.[59]

In summary, doxapram is not recommended as primary therapy for OSA because of its clinically insignificant benefit demonstrated in a very small number of OSA subjects. Additional randomized, placebo-controlled studies are needed to confirm the benefit of doxapram in the perioperative anesthetic care of OSA patients undergoing bariatric surgery.

Opioid antagonists

Opioid antagonists promote ventilation by competitive inhibition with endorphins at receptor sites, or by stimulating the cortex. Naloxone, an opiate antagonist, did not improve AHI and only minimally reduced ODI in 10 obese sleep-apnea patients with median AHI of 58.[60] In another group of 10 obese OSA subjects, naloxone infusion reduced the percentage of REM sleep by 80% in comparison with saline infusion. The average maximal desaturation index decreased by 21%, probably because of less REM sleep–related atonia; apnea frequency and severity did not improve.[61] In another trial of naloxone with 12 OSA patients, AI and frequency and duration of hypoxic events all improved; clinical improvement was present acutely and after 3 months.[62] In a double-blind crossover study of naltrexone versus placebo, naltrexone significantly improved blood-gas patterns (transcutaneous partial pressure of oxygen and carbon dioxide) and metabolic suffering index (defined as product of the number, duration, and magnitude of hypoxic and hypercapnic events) for the duration of hypoxic and hypercapnic events.[63] However, naltrexone impaired sleep, with significantly reduced total sleep time, slow-wave sleep, and REM sleep; increased the number of awakenings; and prolonged total wake time.[63]

In summary, opioid antagonists are not recommended for OSA. Although they improve oxyhemoglobin saturation, they cause significant sleep disruption.

Acetylcholinesterase inhibitors

Physostigmine, a cholinesterase inhibitor, was administered in a randomized crossover trial to 10 men with moderate to severe OSA: mean AHI decreased from 54 to 41, with most of the reduction occurring during REM sleep.[64]

Donezepil, another cholinesterase inhibitor, significantly decreased mean obstructive AHI from 19 to 9, significantly increased SpO_2 nadir from 81% to 86%, and significantly reduced the microarousal index from 11 to 5 events per hour in 23 patients with OSA and mild to moderate Alzheimer disease who were enrolled in a randomized, double-blind, placebo-controlled study.[65] There were no significant changes in total sleep time, sleep efficiency, sleep-onset latency, REM sleep latency, or awakenings after sleep onset. Mean percentage of REM sleep significantly increased from 7% to 16%, but mean REM AHI decreased from 25 to 8. Postulated factors for the reduced REM AHI included excitatory effects on medullary respiratory motor neurons, effects on the central chemosensitivity drive of the respiratory control system, increased hypoglossal nerve activity, and increased carotid-body sensitivity to hypoxia.[65] A similar randomized, double-blind study of 21 male non-Alzheimer subjects compared donepezil with placebo. Donepezil decreased obstructive AHI from 42 to 33, reduced ODI from 33 to 17, improved oxyhemoglobin saturation nadir from 79% to 83%, and improved ESS scores, although sleep efficiency decreased from 87% to 80%.[66]

In summary, although these 2 donepezil trials showed improvement in OSA parameters, larger controlled trials with clinical outcomes are needed.

Serotonergic agents and REM suppressants

Depending on receptor subtype, serotonergic agents either excite ($5-HT_{2A}$ and $5-HT_{2C}$) or inhibit ($5-HT_{1A}$, $5-HT_{1B}$) upper airway dilator activity and/or central respiratory drive. Selective serotonin reuptake inhibitors (SSRI) may exert differential responses in subsets of patients, owing to variable responsiveness of the upper airway dilator muscles.

Ondansetron, a $5-HT_3$ antagonist, did not improve AHI or desaturations higher than 4% in 10 subjects with moderate OSA.[67] In a randomized, placebo-controlled, parallel-group, 28-day trial of OSA subjects (N = 35), the subgroup (n = 10) of patients taking higher doses of ondansetron (24 mg daily) and fluoxetine (10 mg daily) noted a 40% reduction in AHI compared with placebo; combined therapy with lower doses of ondansetron (12 mg) and fluoxetine (5 mg) reduced AHI by only 9%. Ondansetron alone produced no benefit and showed a trend toward worsening AHI.[68]

Paroxetine (20 mg daily) mildly reduced the AI by 35% during NREM sleep only, did not change hypopnea indices, and did not improve daytime sleepiness, concentration, memory impairment, or depressed mood in a double-blind, placebo-controlled trial in 20 OSA subjects.[69] In another randomized placebo-controlled trial in 8 subjects, paroxetine (40 mg daily) augmented peak inspiratory genioglossus muscle activity but did not reduce the AHI.[70]

Protriptyline, a tricyclic agent, is a potent REM suppressant. When compared with AZM or placebo, protriptyline (20 mg) did not significantly improve frequency of apneas, hypopneas, or desaturations in 10 OSA subjects.[47] In 2 trials of OSA subjects (N = 5,[71] N = 12[72]), protriptyline reduced REM-related apneas (16 per hour to 3 per hour), although the overall AI changed minimally (64 per hour to 60 per hour)[71]; significantly reduced the percentage of time spent at saturations lower than 85%[71]; reduced peak decrease in oxygen saturation from 16% to 9% during NREM sleep[72]; and significantly decreased apnea as a percentage of disordered breathing time from 61% to 36%.[72] During REM sleep, there was no change in the frequency or duration of peak decrease in oxygen saturation with protriptyline use.[72]

Mirtazapine, a $5-HT_1$ agonist and $5-HT_2$ and $5-HT_3$ antagonist, also affects noradrenergic and histaminergic receptors that could enhance central respiratory drive. Low doses of mirtazapine enhance genioglossal activity, whereas higher doses decrease such activity.[73] In a randomized, double-blind, 3-way crossover study of mirtazapine (4.5 mg, 15 mg, and placebo) in 12 OSA patients, sleep fragmentation decreased, and AHI decreased by 52% in 11 of 12 patients on 4.5-mg dose and by 46% in 12 of 12 patients on 15-mg dose.[74] However, these findings were not confirmed in subsequent randomized, double-blind, placebo-controlled trials in 20 subjects (trial 1) or 65 subjects (trial 2).[75] In these trials, mirtazapine did not improve sleep apnea parameters at any of the doses used (7.5, 15, 30, and 45 mg); at doses of 15 and 30 mg, AHI worsened compared with baseline, and significant side effects included weight gain and sedation.[75]

Clonidine, an $\alpha2$-adrenergic agonist, is a potent REM suppressant. In an observational study of 8 OSA subjects, 0.2 mg of clonidine suppressed REM sleep (totally in 2 of 8, partially in 6 of 8) but did not change mean AHI.[76] Clonidine had no effect on NREM AHI, mean apnea duration, or mean lowest Spo_2. In 4 of 8 subjects, upper airway obstruction resolved and oxyhemoglobin saturation remained higher than 90% during REM sleep. During REM sleep in 2 of 8 subjects, repetitive obstructive hypopneas with persistent hypoxemia transformed to short-duration apneas and cyclical hypoxemia. The 2 of 8 subjects with total REM suppression had clinically insignificant reduction in AHI.[76] Premedication with oral clonidine before elective surgery for sleep apnea reduced the propofol dosages needed for induction and surgical anesthesia, and also reduced piritamide consumption (opioid-sparing effect) in the clonidine group (n = 15) when compared with placebo.[77] Apnea and desaturation indices were not different between the groups.[77]

Trazodone is an antidepressant that is widely used to induce sleep. To test whether trazodone can improve sleep apnea by raising the arousal threshold, a randomized, double-blind, placebo-controlled study of 9 patients with OSA (mean AHI 52) on CPAP therapy used 100 mg of trazodone daily.[78] With trazodone, subjects tolerated higher respiratory effort before arousal when the arousal was induced by increased CO_2 levels, but not when it was induced by drops in CPAP.[78]

In summary, combination therapy with higher doses of ondansetron and fluoxetine may reduce SDB, but this needs confirmation in larger trials. Paroxetine and protriptyline have clinically insignificant benefits on SDB, and neither is indicated as primary therapy for sleep apnea. Mirtazapine has significant side effects with equivocal benefit; it should not be used for sleep apnea therapy. Although not indicated as a primary treatment for OSA, clonidine may have an adjunctive role in the perioperative management of OSA patients. Additional studies are needed to determine the effects of trazodone on the arousal threshold, and whether a subset of OSA patients may benefit from its use in combination with PAP therapy.

Endocrinologic Disorders and Sleep Apnea

Acromegaly
Acromegaly is associated with soft-tissue hypertrophy of the upper airway, predisposing to obstruction during sleep. The prevalence of sleep apnea associated with acromegaly varies from 56% to 97%.[79,80] In acromegalic subjects, the prevalence of sleep apnea (AHI >5) is 97%, and 60% have severe sleep apnea (AHI >30).[80]

In a trial of 52 acromegalic patients, 30 (58%) had polysomnographically confirmed sleep apnea: 25 had obstructive sleep apnea, 3 had central sleep apnea, and 2 had mixed obstructive/central sleep apnea.[81] Fifty-three percent of the patients with sleep apnea had moderate to severe OSA. In this study, RDI correlated positively with disease activity, but not with duration of disease or levels of growth hormone (GH).[81]

Twelve overweight patients with mild to severe OSA and poorly controlled acromegaly on octreotide were treated for 6 months with the GH receptor antagonist pegvisomant (10–30 mg).[82] Pegvisomant significantly decreased tongue volume; mean AHI slightly decreased, from 23 to 18, and there was no significant change in Spo_2.[82]

Fourteen acromegalic OSA subjects were treated with octreotide acetate. After treatment, 50% of the subjects had normal tongue volume and insulin-like growth factor (IGF), but minimum Spo_2 did not significantly change. Although RDI

decreased in 64% of subjects, only 8% had resolution of sleep apnea. The improvement was likely due to weight change, because RDI did not correlate with the decrease in IGF or GH levels but correlated positively with BMI and age.[83]

In summary, treatment of underlying acromegaly reduces tongue volume but does not significantly improve sleep apnea.

Hypothyroidism
In the United States population, the estimated prevalence of overt hypothyroidism is less than 1% while the prevalence of subclinical hypothyroidism is 4%. Anecdotal reports have suggested a higher incidence of hypothyroidism in patients with sleep apnea, leading some to propose routine thyroid testing in OSA patients.

Should all patients with OSA be screened for thyroid dysfunction? Results from the following studies suggest that routine thyroid testing in all OSA patients is not warranted. Of 1000 consecutive patients who presented with snoring or symptoms of sleep apnea, 834 underwent routine thyroid testing. Of these patients, only 10 (1.2%) had previously undiagnosed hypothyroidism; 4 of these patients had confirmed sleep apnea.[84] In another study, 3 of 124 (2.4%) patients diagnosed polysomnographically with sleep apnea had previously undiagnosed hypothyroidism.[85]

Does treatment of hypothyroidism improve sleep apnea? Two studies investigating the use of thyroxine did not show any benefit in sleep apnea parameters, although improvement has been reported in other studies. The 10 aforementioned newly diagnosed hypothyroid patients were treated with thyroid hormone until euthyroid; however, repeat polysomnographic testing showed no improvement in sleep apnea parameters compared with baseline.[84] In another study, 108 subjects with OSA were divided into 3 groups: euthyroid without medication (n = 63), treated with levothyroxine, and hypothyroid not on levothyroxine.[86] RDI and percentage of apneas/hypopneas by total sleep time with less than 90% O_2 saturation were similar among the groups. Sleep propensity was greater in the hypothyroid untreated group.[86]

By contrast, 3 studies showed improvement in sleep apnea with thyroxine therapy.[85,87,88] The 3 hypothyroid patients already mentioned had complete resolution of sleep apnea after treatment with thyroxine.[85] In 50 newly diagnosed, untreated symptomatic patients with primary hypothyroidism, 15 (30%) had sleep apnea.[87] After treatment, 12 of 15 had repeat polysomnography, with complete resolution of OSA in 10 of these 12 patients;

in 2 of 12 patients, OSA persisted. In the patients whose OSA resolved, mean BMI decreased from 28 to 26 kg/m^2; the 2 nonresponders did not lose weight.[87] Another study showed that 3% of 65 OSA subjects had hypothyroidism and that 25% of 20 hypothyroid subjects had sleep apnea.[88] Treatment with thyroid hormone resolved SDB parameters, but snoring took up to a year to resolve.[88]

In summary, these studies show variable results from hypothyroidism treatment on sleep apnea parameters. Some of the improvement noted in these studies may be related to weight loss. The current consensus is to treat symptomatic hypothyroid patients, treat nonpregnant subclinical hypothyroid patients with thyroid-stimulating hormone, and treat all pregnant women who are hypothyroid.

Should female patients with severe OSA be screened for Hashimoto thyroiditis? A recent study described Hashimoto thyroiditis (HT) in 47% of OSA subjects versus 32% in normal controls.[89] Among these subjects with sleep apnea, women with severe OSA had the highest prevalence of HT (73%), even before the development of hypothyroidism. This study highlights the need for further investigation into the relationship between autoimmune thyroiditis and OSA, and whether screening for HT is indicated in women with severe OSA.[89]

Progesterone, estrogen, androgens, and androgen blockade

Menopause is an independent risk factor for the development of sleep apnea. Progesterone and estrogen enhance ventilatory chemosensitivity, and changes in these levels during the menopause may influence breathing. Menopause is an independent risk factor for the development of sleep apnea. An observational study of 2852 women older than 50 years reported that among hormonal replacement therapy (HRT) users, 7% taking only estrogen and 6% taking both estrogen and progesterone had an AHI greater than 15, compared with 15% not on HRT.[90] A study of 5 women treated with estrogen alone and then with combined estradiol plus medroxyprogesterone acetate showed that both interventions significantly reduced RDI, but combination therapy was more effective.[91] Estrogen also significantly improved the Spo$_2$ nadir from 74% to 82%.[91] In a separate study in 6 women with mild to moderate OSA, estrogen monotherapy significantly reduced AHI from 23 to 12.[92] Two other studies (N = 6,[92] N = 15[93]) showed that a combination of estrogen and progesterone reduced AHI, but the reduction was clinically insignificant.

Low testosterone concentrations in male patients with sleep apnea may be due to hypoxia, sleep fragmentation, obesity, and advanced age. A randomized, double-blind, placebo-controlled, parallel-group trial in 67 obese men with AHI greater than 10 showed that testosterone worsened ODI by 10 events/hour and worsened nocturnal hypoxemia (sleep time with O$_2$ saturation <90%) by 6% at 7 weeks; however, by 18 weeks there was no difference in these parameters when compared with placebo.[94] In another study, high-dose testosterone for 3 weeks shortened total sleep time (both NREM and REM) by 1 hour, increased duration of hypoxemia by 5 minutes, and increased RDI by 7 in 17 elderly men.[95]

In summary, the benefit from HRT with estrogen and/or progesterone therapy is equivocal, and the studies reported are small in size and do not have placebo controls. Such therapy increases the risk for ischemic strokes, breast cancer, venous thromboembolism, and cholecystitis; these risks outweigh the equivocal benefits demonstrated in these small studies. Patients who undergo testosterone therapy, particularly obese individuals, should be monitored for development of sleep apnea symptoms.

γ-Aminobutyric acid agonists

Baclofen, a γ-aminobutyric acid (GABA) agonist, is a centrally acting antispasmodic agent. In 10 subjects with moderate OSA and snoring enrolled in a double-blind, placebo-controlled study, oral baclofen (25 mg) increased total sleep time and duration of NREM sleep (stages 1, 2) and REM sleep, and reduced wake after sleep onset, but did not affect sleep efficiency, sleep latency, or frequency of arousals.[96] Changes in sleep apnea parameters (RDI, Spo$_2$) were insignificant.[96] In a study of 10 subjects with spasticity, intrathecal baclofen administered by bolus significantly increased RDI from 11 to 37 when compared with continuous infusion, which increased RDI from 11 to 21.[97] The percentage of time at Spo$_2$ below 90% was also greater with bolus infusion. Central apnea and apnea indices also increased and were worse with bolus infusion, probably because of direct effects of baclofen on ventilatory drive. This study demonstrates worsening of SDB with use of intrathecal baclofen, but continuous infusion may have fewer deleterious effects than bolus infusions.[97]

Medications for Comorbid Conditions (Heart Failure, Hypertension, Dyslipidemia, Obesity)

Endothelial dysfunction and inflammation are important mediators of accelerated atherogenesis. SDB is associated with repetitive hypoxia/reoxygenation, which in turn results in endothelial damage. Xanthine oxidase has been implicated in causing endothelial dysfunction in sleep apnea, owing to increased oxidative stress and increased formation of superoxide free radicals. In 12 patients with moderate to severe OSA enrolled in a randomized, double-blind, placebo-controlled study, sleep apnea severity and time spent with SpO_2 lower than 90% correlated significantly with baseline flow-mediated vasodilation (FMD).[98] Allopurinol, a xanthine oxidase inhibitor, reduced oxidative stress, as shown by the significant increase in FMD and reduction in levels of plasma malondialdehyde.[98] In another study, endothelial dysfunction was confirmed with FMD in the brachial artery of 10 OSA patients. Injection of 0.5 g of vitamin C, an antioxidant, increased FMD in OSA patients but had no effect on control subjects.[99]

Drug-resistant hypertension is a comorbid complication of OSA. Sleep apnea is more prevalent with hyperaldosteronism (84%) than with normal aldosterone levels (74%), although BMI and neck circumferences do not differ between the two groups.[100] In 12 obese patients with resistant hypertension and OSA, spironolactone (25 and 50 mg) significantly reduced mean AHI values from 40 to 22 and the hypoxic index from 14 to 6 events per hour; weight and blood pressure were also reduced.[101]

Metabolic syndrome, or syndrome X, affects 6% of adolescents and 24% of adults.[102] Associated major risk factors include obesity, elevated fasting triglycerides, increased fasting plasma insulin, impaired glucose tolerance, hypertension, and cardiovascular disease.[102] All-cause mortality and cardiovascular mortality increase with the metabolic syndrome. C-Reactive protein (CRP), an inflammatory marker, is increased in patients with OSA. Patients with sleep apnea with elevated CRP levels and heart disease in the intermediate risk category (Framingham Risk Score of 10%–20%) may be candidates for statin therapy. Based on the Jupiter Study results, the Canadian Cardiovascular Society recommends prophylactic statins for women older than 60 and men older than 50 years with a CRP level of greater than 2 mg/dL and intermediate risk of heart disease.[103]

Medications currently approved by the Food and Drug Administration (FDA) for the long-term management of obesity are orlistat (a reversible gastrointestinal lipase inhibitor), lorcaserin (a selective 5-HT$_{2C}$ agonist), and Qsymia (phentermine and topiramate, extended-release). However, lorcaserin is not currently available, pending final Drug Enforcement Administration scheduling classification. Potential future antiobesity drugs include cetilestat, tesofenine, metreleptin, peripheral cannabinoid-1 antagonists, gut hormones, and drug combinations.[104]

Medications to Avoid/Monitor in Patients with OSA (Benzodiazepines, Barbiturates, Narcotics, Anesthetics)

Upper airway stability during sleep can be altered by agents that depress the central nervous system, including benzodiazepines, barbiturates, narcotics, and anesthetics.

Benzodiazepines and barbiturates

Benzodiazepines and barbiturates are frequently prescribed to treat insomnia. Equivocal effects have been reported in patients with mild sleep apnea or upper airway resistance syndrome: temazepam (15, 30 mg) did not change RDI; flurazepam (30 mg) increased apneas and desaturation; triazolam (0.25 mg) and flunitrazepam (2 mg) increased upper airway resistance.[105–107] A randomized, double-blind, placebo-controlled study using nitrazepam (5, 10 mg) in 11 patients with OSA showed reduced average AI on 10 mg, slightly increased average AI on 5 mg, and no change in mean SpO_2; in 3 of 11 subjects, AI markedly increased in comparison with placebo.[108]

Phenotyping individuals with OSA who are at risk for respiratory depression is potentially useful when considering barbiturate prescriptions. A randomized, placebo-controlled study using temazepam in 20 patients with mild to moderate OSA reported that baseline awake central chemosensitivity correlated significantly with both the change in SpO_2 nadir between temazepam and placebo and the ODI, but not with the change in AHI. Peripheral chemosensitivity and ventilatory recruitment threshold did not correlate with the change in SpO_2 nadir, ODI, or AHI.[109]

Opioids

Opioids exacerbate OSA, but there are few long-term studies that address this aspect.[110–114] Long-term opioid use is associated with hypoxia and prolongation of apnea duration during NREM sleep, ataxic or Biot respiration, prolonged obstructive hypoventilation, and severe hypoxemia.[110] In 2 studies of patients on chronic opioid analgesia for at least 6 months for nonmalignant pain (N = 147,[113] N = 98[114]), OSA prevalence was 36% to 39%, central sleep apnea was 24%, mixed sleep apnea was 8% to 21%, and the remainder were considered indeterminate.[113,114] AHI correlated with the daily dose of methadone, but not with the other round-the-clock opioids.[113] In a study of 23 patients treated with methadone for 1 year, AHI did not significantly change in comparison with baseline in 18; in 5 patients the AHI increased from 4 to 30, but these patients had gained 25% or more of their entry weight.[115] Among 7 patients with restless legs syndrome treated with opioids for slightly longer than 7 years, 3 developed mild to moderate OSA, and sleep apnea progressed from moderate to severe in 1 patient; changes were not related to weight gain.[112] Results from these studies suggest that patients who are on chronic opioid therapy should be monitored for the development or worsening of sleep apnea.

Anesthetic agents

Patients undergoing procedures or surgery should inform their surgeon and anesthesiologist regarding their sleep apnea so that appropriate precautions can be taken.[116–122] Perioperative anesthetic risks in adults and children have been reviewed previously, in addition to proposed strategies for postoperative analgesia for obese OSA patients.[117,120,123] In general, drugs with central and respiratory depressant effects, including opioids, should be avoided if possible. Dexmedetomidine, an α2 agonist, may be considered in OSA patients because it is not associated with respiratory depression. When AHI is higher than 70 and the Spo_2 nadir is less than 80%, upper airway surgery has a higher perioperative risk.[120] Pentothal, propofol, nitrous oxide, opioids, and barbiturates can decrease pharyngeal muscle tone with increased collapsibility of the upper airway, and should be used cautiously.[120]

Children with OSA have greater blunting of the respiratory drive in response to opioid and benzodiazepine administration, and are at risk for upper airway obstruction.[121] Fentanyl should be used cautiously, because 46% of children with OSA who were breathing spontaneously following inhalational anesthesia developed apneas following a single dose of 0.5 μg/kg fentanyl.[122] If presedation with benzodiazepines or opioids before surgery is indicated, appropriate monitoring should be observed and an experienced airway management team should be present. The FDA issued a cautionary bulletin regarding codeine use for postoperative analgesia in children following tonsillectomy and adenoidectomy for sleep apnea.[124] The lowest effective dose should be prescribed and administered on an as-needed basis only, and caregivers should monitor the child for signs of toxicity. Three deaths and a case of severe respiratory depression have been reported in these children (2–5 years of age), the deaths being linked to ultrarapid metabolism of codeine.

SUMMARY

Because obesity is present in two-thirds of patients with documented sleep apnea, novel anti-obesity medications may help in weight control and may secondarily improve breathing abnormalities. Medications addressing endothelial dysfunction, combined with PAP therapy, may help prevent hypoxemic sequelae of sleep apnea. Because hypoxemia in OSA is associated with abnormalities in neuropeptides and inflammatory cytokines, the role of anti-inflammatory agents targeting these could be explored. New medications that can increase upper airway muscle tone and target fibrillin to improve connective tissue laxity may also be useful.

Current pharmacotherapy for sleep apnea is adjunctive, but its role can be transformed as we learn more about the various risk factors and interrelated pathology underlying the pathophysiology of sleep apnea. Because the genetic component of sleep apnea has been estimated at 40%, genome-wide association studies may further our understanding of OSA and help suggest potential therapies.[125] Determining the molecular signatures of sleep apnea may help identify diagnostic, prognostic, and surrogate markers for OSA, and identify markers for drug-response phenotypes.

REFERENCES

1. Young T, Peppard P, Gottlieb D. Epidemiology of obstructive sleep apnea: a population health perspective. Am J Respir Crit Care Med 2002; 165:1217–39.
2. Tregear S, Reston J, Schoelles K, et al. Continuous positive airway pressure reduces risk of motor vehicle crash among drivers with obstructive sleep apnea: systematic review and meta-analysis. Sleep 2010;33(10):1373–80.
3. Kato M, Adachi T, Koshino Y, et al. Obstructive sleep apnea and cardiovascular disease. Circ J 2009;73(8):1363–70.
4. Trombetta IC, Somers VK, Maki-Nunes C, et al. Consequences of comorbid sleep apnea in the metabolic syndrome—implications for cardiovascular risk. Sleep 2010;33(9):1193–9.
5. Krieger J. Long-term compliance with nasal continuous positive airway pressure (CPAP) in obstructive sleep apnea patients and non-apneic snorers. Sleep 1992;15:S42–6.
6. Weaver TE, Sawyer AM. Adherence to continuous positive airway pressure treatment for obstructive sleep apnea: implications for future interventions. Indian J Med Res 2010; 131:245–58.

7. Kushida CA, Morgenthaler TI, Littner MR, et al. Practice parameters for the treatment of snoring and obstructive sleep apnea with oral appliances: an update for 2005. Sleep 2006;29:240–3.

8. Hoffstein V. Review of oral appliances for treatment of sleep-disordered breathing. Sleep Breath 2007; 11(1):1–22.

9. Lettieri CJ, Paolino N, Eliasson AH, et al. Comparison of adjustable and fixed oral appliances for the treatment of obstructive sleep apnea. J Clin Sleep Med 2011;7(5):439–45.

10. Caples SM, Rowley JA, Prinsell JR, et al. Surgical modifications of the upper airway for obstructive sleep apnea in adults: a systematic review and meta-analysis. Sleep 2010;33(10): 1396–407.

11. Guilleminault C, Philip P. Tiredness and somnolence despite initial treatment of obstructive sleep apnea syndrome (what to do when an OSAS patient stays hypersomnolent despite treatment). Sleep 1996;19(Suppl 9):S117–22.

12. Pépin JL, Viot-Blanc V, Escourrou P, et al. Prevalence of residual excessive sleepiness in CPAP-treated sleep apnoea patients: the French multicentre study. Eur Respir J 2009;33(5):1062–7.

13. Weaver TE, Maislin G, Dinges DF, et al. Relationship between hours of CPAP use and achieving normal levels of sleepiness and daily functioning. Sleep 2007;30:711–9.

14. Weaver TE, Mancini C, Maislin G, et al. Continuous positive airway pressure treatment of sleepy patients with milder obstructive sleep apnea: results of the CPAP Apnea Trial North American Program (CATNAP) randomized clinical trial. Am J Respir Crit Care Med 2012;186(7):677–83.

15. Stradling JR, Smith D, Crosby J. Post-CPAP sleepiness—a specific syndrome? J Sleep Res 2007; 16(4):436–8.

16. Darwish M, Kirby M, Hellriegel ET, et al. Armodafinil and modafinil have substantially different pharmacokinetic profiles despite having the same terminal half-lives: analysis of data from three randomized, single-dose, pharmacokinetic studies. Clin Drug Investig 2009;29(9):613–23.

17. Pack AI, Black JE, Schwartz HR, et al. Modafinil as adjunct therapy for daytime sleepiness in obstructive sleep apnea. Am J Respir Crit Care Med 2001; 164:1675–81.

18. Black JE, Hirshkowitz M. Modafinil for treatment of residual excessive sleepiness in nasal continuous positive airway pressure-treated obstructive sleep apnea/hypopnea syndrome. Sleep 2005;28: 464–71.

19. Schwartz JR, Hirshkowitz M, Erman MK, et al. Modafinil as adjunct therapy for daytime sleepiness in obstructive sleep apnea: a 12-week, open-label study. Chest 2003;124:2192–9.

20. Kingshott RN, Vennelle M, Coleman EL, et al. Randomized, double-blind, placebo-controlled crossover trial of modafinil in the treatment of residual excessive daytime sleepiness in the sleep apnea/hypopnea syndrome. Am J Respir Crit Care Med 2001;163:918–23.

21. Roth T, White D, Schmidt-Nowara W, et al. Effects of armodafinil in the treatment of residual excessive sleepiness associated with obstructive sleep apnea/hypopnea syndrome: a 12-week, multicenter, double-blind, randomized, placebo-controlled study in CPAP-adherent adults. Clin Ther 2006; 28(5):689–706.

22. Hirshkowitz M, Black JE, Wesnes K, et al. Adjunct armodafinil improves wakefulness and memory in obstructive sleep apnea/hypopnea syndrome. Respir Med 2007;101:616–27.

23. Black JE, Hull SG, Tiller J, et al. The long-term tolerability and efficacy of armodafinil in patients with excessive sleepiness associated with treated obstructive sleep apnea, shift work disorder, or narcolepsy: an open-label extension study. J Clin Sleep Med 2010;6(5):458–66.

24. Williams SC, Marshall NS, Kennerson M, et al. Modafinil effects during acute continuous positive airway pressure withdrawal: a randomized crossover double-blind placebo-controlled trial. Am J Respir Crit Care Med 2010;181(8): 825–31.

25. Saunamäki T, Jehkonen M. Depression and anxiety in obstructive sleep apnea syndrome: a review. Acta Neurol Scand 2007;116(5):277–88.

26. Krystal AD, Harsh JR, Yang R, et al. A double-blind, placebo-controlled study of armodafinil for excessive sleepiness in patients with treated obstructive sleep apnea and comorbid depression. J Clin Psychiatry 2010;71(1):32–40.

27. Roehrs T, Roth T. Caffeine: sleep and daytime sleepiness [review]. Sleep Med Rev 2008;12(2): 153–62.

28. Aurora RN, Crainiceanu C, Caffo B, et al. Sleep-disordered breathing and caffeine consumption: results of a community-based study. Chest 2012; 142(3):631–8.

29. Khalil SN, Maposa D, Ghelber O, et al. Caffeine in children with obstructive sleep apnea. Middle East J Anesthesiol 2008;19(4):885–99.

30. Banerjee D, Vitiello MV, Grunstein RR. Pharmacotherapy for excessive daytime sleepiness. Sleep Med Rev 2004;8(5):339–54.

31. Westover AN, Halm EA. Do prescription stimulants increase the risk of adverse cardiovascular events? A systematic review. BMC Cardiovasc Disord 2012;12:41.

32. Berman SM, Kuczenski R, McCracken JT, et al. Potential adverse effects of amphetamine treatment on brain and behavior: a review. Mol Psychiatry

2009;14(2):123–42 [Erratum in: Mol Psychiatry. 2010 Nov;15(11):1121].

33. Canova CR, Downs SH, Knoblauch A, et al. Increased prevalence of perennial allergic rhinitis in patients with obstructive sleep apnea. Respiration 2004;71:138–43.

34. Kiely JL, Nolan P, Mchicholas WT. Intranasal corticosteroid therapy for obstructive sleep apnea in patients with co-existing rhinitis. Thorax 2004;59:50–5.

35. Brouillette RT, Manoukian JJ, Ducharme FM, et al. Efficacy of fluticasone nasal spray for pediatric obstructive sleep apnea. J Pediatr 2001;138:838–44.

36. Alexopoulos EI, Kaditis AG, Kalampouka E, et al. Nasal corticosteroids for children with snoring. Pediatr Pulmonol 2004;38:161–7.

37. Kheirandish-Gozal L, Gozal D. Intranasal budesonide treatment for children with mild obstructive sleep apnea syndrome. Pediatrics 2008;122(1):e149–55.

38. Goldbart AD, Goldman JL, Veling MC, et al. Leukotriene modifier therapy for mild sleep-disordered breathing in children. Am J Respir Crit Care Med 2005;172(3):364–70.

39. Goldbart AD, Greenberg-Dotan S, Tal A. Montelukast for children with obstructive sleep apnea: a double-blind, placebo-controlled study. Pediatrics 2012;130(3):e575–80.

40. Kheirandish L, Goldbart AD, Gozal D. Intranasal steroids and oral leukotriene modifier therapy in residual sleep-disordered breathing after tonsillectomy and adenoidectomy in children. Pediatrics 2006;117:e61–6.

41. Clarenbach CF, Kohler M, Senn O, et al. Does nasal decongestion improve obstructive sleep apnea? J Sleep Res 2008;17(4):444–9.

42. McLean HA, Urton AM, Driver HS, et al. Effect of treating severe nasal obstruction on the severity of obstructive sleep apnoea. Eur Respir J 2005;25(3):521–7.

43. Osanai S, Akiba Y, Fujiuchi S, et al. Depression of peripheral chemosensitivity by a dopaminergic mechanism in patients with obstructive sleep apnea syndrome. Eur Respir J 1999;13:418–23.

44. Larrain A, Kapur VK, Gooley TA, et al. Pharmacological treatment of obstructive sleep apnea with a combination of pseudoephedrine and domperidone. J Clin Sleep Med 2010;6(2):117–23.

45. Edwards BA, Sands SA, Eckert DJ, et al. Acetazolamide improves loop gain but not the other physiological traits causing obstructive sleep apnoea. J Physiol 2012;590(Pt 5):1199–211.

46. Nussbaumer-Ochsner Y, Latshang TD, Ulrich S, et al. Patients with obstructive sleep apnea syndrome benefit from acetazolamide during an altitude sojourn: a randomized, placebo-controlled, double-blind trial. Chest 2012;141(1):131–8. http://dx.doi.org/10.1378/chest.11-0375.

47. Whyte KF, Gould GA, Airlie MA, et al. Role of protriptyline and acetazolamide in the sleep apnea/hypopnea syndrome. Sleep 1988;11:463–72.

48. Inoue Y, Takata K, Sakamoto I, et al. Clinical efficacy and indication of acetazolamide treatment on sleep apnea syndrome. Psychiatry Clin Neurosci 1999;53:321–2.

49. Sakamoto T, Nakazawa Y, Hashizume Y, et al. Effects of acetazolamide on the sleep apnea syndrome and its therapeutic mechanism. Psychiatry Clin Neurosci 1995;49(1):59–64.

50. Mulloy E, McNicholas W. Theophylline in obstructive sleep apnea. A double-blind evaluation. Chest 1992;101:753.

51. Saletu B, Oberndorfer S, Anderer P, et al. Efficiency of continuous positive airway pressure versus theophylline therapy in sleep apnea: comparative sleep laboratory studies on objective and subjective sleep and awakening quality. Neuropsychobiology 1999;39(3):151–9.

52. Espinoza H, Antic R, Thornton AT, et al. The effects of aminophylline on sleep and sleep-disordered breathing in patients with obstructive sleep apnea syndrome. Am Rev Respir Dis 1987;136(1):80–4.

53. Zevin S, Swed E, Cahan C. Clinical effects of locally delivered nicotine in obstructive sleep apnea syndrome. Am J Ther 2003;10(3):170–5.

54. Davila DG, Hurt RD, Offord KP, et al. Acute effects of transdermal nicotine on sleep architecture, snoring, and sleep-disordered breathing in nonsmokers. Am J Respir Crit Care Med 1994;150:469–74.

55. Hein H, Kirsten D, Jugert C, et al. Nicotine as therapy of obstructive sleep apnea? Pneumologie 1995;49(Suppl 1):185–6.

56. Hedner J, Grunstein R, Eriksson B, et al. A double-blind, randomized trial of sabeluzole—a putative glutamate antagonist—in obstructive sleep apnea. Sleep 1996;19:287–9.

57. Torvaldsson S, Grote L, Peker Y, et al. A randomized placebo-controlled trial of an NMDA receptor antagonist in sleep-disordered breathing. J Sleep Res 2005;14:149–55.

58. Suratt PM, Wilhoit SC, Brown ED, et al. Effect of doxapram on obstructive sleep apnea. Bull Eur Physiopathol Respir 1986;22:127–31.

59. Bamgbade OA. Advantages of doxapram for postanesthesia recovery and outcomes in bariatric surgery patients with obstructive sleep apnea. Eur J Anaesthesiol 2011;28:387–91.

60. Guilleminault C, Hayes B. Naloxone, theophylline, bromocriptine, and obstructive sleep apnea. Negative results. Bull Eur Physiopathol Respir 1983;19:632–4.

61. Atkinson RL, Suratt PM, Wilhoit SC, et al. Naloxone improves sleep apnea in obese humans. Int J Obes 1985;9(4):233–9.

62. Ferber C, Sanchez P, Lemoine P, et al. Efficacy of the treatment of sleep apnea using naltrexone. A clinical, polygraphic and gasometric study. C R Acad Sci III 1988;307(12):695–700.

63. Ferber C, Duclaux R, Mouret J. Naltrexone improves blood gas patterns in obstructive sleep apnoea syndrome through its influence on sleep. J Sleep Res 1993;2(3):149–55.

64. Hedner J, Kraiczi H, Peker Y, et al. Reduction of sleep-disordered breathing after physostigmine. Am J Respir Crit Care Med 2003;168(10):1246–51.

65. Moraes W, Poyares D, Sukys-Claudino L, et al. Donepezil improves obstructive sleep apnea in Alzheimer disease: a double-blind, placebo-controlled study. Chest 2008;133(3):677–83. http://dx.doi.org/10.1378/chest.07-1446.

66. Sukys-Claudino L, Moraes W, Guilleminault C, et al. Beneficial effect of donepezil on obstructive sleep apnea: a double-blind, placebo-controlled clinical trial. Sleep Med 2012;13(3):290–6.

67. Stradling J, Smith D, Radulovacki M, et al. Effect of ondansetron on moderate obstructive sleep apnoea, a single night, placebo-controlled trial. J Sleep Res 2003;12(2):169–70.

68. Prasad B, Radulovacki M, Olopade C, et al. Prospective trial of efficacy and safety of ondansetron and fluoxetine in patients with obstructive sleep apnea syndrome. Sleep 2010;33(7):982–9.

69. Kraiczi H, Hedner J, Dahlof P, et al. Effect of serotonin uptake inhibition on breathing during sleep and daytime symptoms in obstructive sleep apnea. Sleep 1999;22:61–7.

70. Berry RB, Yamaura EM, Gill K, et al. Acute effects of paroxetine on genioglossus activity in obstructive sleep apnea. Sleep 1999;22:1087–92.

71. Brownell LG, West P, Sweatman P, et al. Protriptyline in obstructive sleep apnea: a double blind trial. N Engl J Med 1982;307:1037–42.

72. Smith PL, Haponik EF, Allen RP, et al. The effects of protriptyline in sleep-disordered breathing. Am Rev Respir Dis 1983;127:8–13.

73. Castillo JL, Menendez P, Segovia L, et al. Effectiveness of mirtazapine in the treatment of sleep apnea/hypopnea syndrome (SAHS). Sleep Med 2004;5:507–8.

74. Carley DW, Olopade C, Ruigt GS, et al. Efficacy of mirtazapine in obstructive sleep apnea syndrome. Sleep 2007;30(1):35–41.

75. Marshall NS, Yee BJ, Desai AV, et al. Two randomized placebo-controlled trials to evaluate the efficacy and tolerability of mirtazapine for the treatment of obstructive sleep apnea. Sleep 2008;31(6):824–31.

76. Issa FG. Effect of clonidine in obstructive sleep apnea. Am Rev Respir Dis 1992;145:435–9.

77. Pawlik MT, Hansen E, Waldhauser D, et al. Clonidine premedication in patients with sleep apnea syndrome: a randomized, double-blind, placebo-controlled study. Anesth Analg 2005;101:1374–80.

78. Heinzer RC, White DP, Jordan AS, et al. Trazodone increases arousal threshold in obstructive sleep apnoea. Eur Respir J 2008;31(6):1308–12.

79. Vannucci L, Luciani P, Gagliardi E, et al. Assessment of sleep apnea syndrome in treated acromegalic patients and correlation of its severity with clinical and laboratory parameters. J Endocrinol Invest 2012;36(4):237–42.

80. Hernández-Gordillo D, Ortega-Gómez Mdel R, Galicia-Polo L, et al. Sleep apnea in patients with acromegaly. Frequency, characterization and positive pressure titration. Open Respir Med J 2012;6:28–33.

81. Roemmler J, Gutt B, Fischer R, et al. Elevated incidence of sleep apnoea in acromegaly-correlation to disease activity. Sleep Breath 2012;16(4):1247–53.

82. Berg C, Wessendorf TE, Mortsch F, et al. Influence of disease control with pegvisomant on sleep apnoea and tongue volume in patients with active acromegaly. Eur J Endocrinol 2009;161(6):829–35.

83. Herrmann BL, Wessendorf TE, Ajaj W, et al. Effects of octreotide on sleep apnoea and tongue volume (magnetic resonance imaging) in patients with acromegaly. Eur J Endocrinol 2004;151(3):309–15.

84. Mickelson S, Lian T. Thyroid testing and thyroid hormone replacement in patients with sleep disordered breathing. Ear Nose Throat J 1999;78(10):768.

85. Skjodt NM, Atkar R, Easton PA. Screening for hypothyroidism in sleep apnea. Am J Respir Crit Care Med 1999;160(2):732–5.

86. Resta O, Carratù P, Carpagnano GE, et al. Influence of subclinical hypothyroidism and T4 treatment on the prevalence and severity of obstructive sleep apnoea syndrome (OSAS). J Endocrinol Invest 2005;28(10):893–8.

87. Jha A, Sharma S, Tandon N, et al. Thyroxine replacement therapy reverses sleep-disordered breathing in patients with primary hypothyroidism. Sleep Med 2006;7(1):55–61.

88. Lin CC, Tsan KW, Chen PJ. The relationship between sleep apnea syndrome and hypothyroidism. Chest 1992;102(6):1663–7.

89. Bozkurt NC, Karbek B, Cakal E, et al. The association between severity of obstructive sleep apnea and prevalence of Hashimoto's thyroiditis. Endocr J 2012;59(11):981–8.

90. Shahar E, Redline S, Young T, et al. Hormone replacement therapy and sleep-disordered

breathing. Am J Respir Crit Care Med 2003;167(9): 1186–92.

91. Keefe DL, Watson R, Naftolin F. Hormone replacement therapy may alleviate sleep apnea in menopausal women: a pilot study. Menopause 1999; 6(3):196–200.

92. Manber R, Kuo TF, Cataldo N, et al. The effects of hormone replacement therapy on sleep-disordered breathing in postmenopausal women: a pilot study. Sleep 2003;26:163–8.

93. Cistulli PA, Barnes DJ, Grunstein RR, et al. Effect of short-term hormone replacement in the treatment of obstructive sleep apnea in postmenopausal women. Thorax 1994;49:699–702.

94. Hoyos CM, Killick R, Yee BJ, et al. Effects of testosterone therapy on sleep and breathing in obese men with severe obstructive sleep apnoea: a randomized placebo-controlled trial. Clin Endocrinol (Oxf) 2012;77(4):599–607.

95. Liu PY, Yee B, Wishart SM, et al. The short-term effects of high-dose testosterone on sleep, breathing, and function in older men. J Clin Endocrinol Metab 2003;88(8):3605–13.

96. Finnimore AJ, Roebuck M, Sajkov D, et al. The effects of the GABA agonist, baclofen, on sleep and breathing. Eur Respir J 1995;8:230–4.

97. Bensmail D, Marquer A, Roche N, et al. Pilot study assessing the intrathecal baclofen administration mode on sleep-related parameters. Arch Phys Med Rehabil 2012;93:96–9.

98. El-Solh AA, Saliba R, Bosinski T, et al. Allopurinol improves endothelial function in sleep apnoea: a randomised controlled study. Eur Respir J 2006; 27(5):997–1002.

99. Grebe M, Eisele HJ, Weissmann N, et al. Antioxidant vitamin C improves endothelial function in obstructive sleep apnea. Am J Respir Crit Care Med 2006;173(8):897–901.

100. Gonzaga CC, Gaddam KK, Ahmed MI. Severity of obstructive sleep apnea is related to aldosterone status in subjects with resistant hypertension. J Clin Sleep Med 2010;6:363–8.

101. Gaddam KK, Pimenta E, Thomas SJ. Spironolactone reduces severity of obstructive sleep apnea in patients with resistant hypertension: a preliminary report. J Hum Hypertens 2010;24: 532–7.

102. Duncan G, Li S, Zhou X. Prevalence and trends of a metabolic syndrome phenotype among US adolescents: 1999-2000. Diabetes Care 2004;27: 2438–43.

103. Genest J, McPherson R, Fohlich J, et al. 2009 Canadian Cardiovascular Society/Canadian guidelines for the diagnosis and treatment of dyslipidemia and prevention of disease in the adult-2009 recommendations. Can J Cardiol 2009;25:567–79.

104. Hainer V, Hainerová IA. Do we need anti-obesity drugs? Diabetes Metab Res Rev 2012;28(Suppl 2):8–20.

105. Camacho ME, Morin CM. The effect of temazepam on respiration in elderly insomniacs with mild sleep apnea. Sleep 1995;18:644–5.

106. Schneider H, Grote L, Peter JH, et al. The effect of triazolam and flunitrazepam—two benzodiazepines with different half-lives—on breathing during sleep. Chest 1996;109:909–15.

107. Berry RB, Kouchi K, Bower J, et al. Triazolam in patients with obstructive sleep apnea. Am J Respir Crit Care Med 1995;151(2 Pt 1):450–4.

108. Hoijer U, Hedner J, Einell H, et al. Nitrazepam in patients with sleep apnea: a double-blind placebo-controlled study. Eur Respir J 1994;7(11): 2011–5.

109. Wang D, Marshal NS, Duffin J, et al. Phenotyping interindividual variability in obstructive sleep apnoea response to temazepam using ventilatory chemoreflexes during wakefulness. J Sleep Res 2011;20(4):526–32.

110. Farney R, Walker J, Cloward T, et al. Sleep-disordered breathing associated with long-term opioid therapy. Chest 2003;123:632–9.

111. Wang D, Teichtahl H, Drummer O, et al. Central sleep apnea in stable methadone maintenance treatment patients. Chest 2005;128:1348–56.

112. Walters AS, Winkelmann J, Trenkwalder C, et al. Long-term follow-up on restless legs syndrome patients treated with opioids. Mov Disord 2001;16: 1105–9.

113. Webster LR, Choi Y, Desai H, et al. Sleep-disordered breathing and chronic opioid therapy. Pain Med 2008;9(4):425–32.

114. Mogri M, Desai H, Webster L, et al. Hypoxemia in patients on chronic opiate therapy with and without sleep apnea. Sleep Breath 2009;13(1): 49–57.

115. Peles E, Schreiber S, Hamburger RB, et al. No change of sleep after 6 and 12 months of methadone maintenance treatment. J Addict Med 2011; 5(2):141–7.

116. Gross JB, Bachenberg JL, Benumof JL, et al. Practice guidelines for the perioperative management of patients with obstructive sleep apnea: a report by the American Society of Anesthesiologists Task Force on peri-operative management of patients with obstructive sleep apnea. Anesthesiology 2006;104:1081–93.

117. Chung SA, Yuan H, Chung F. A systemic review of obstructive sleep apnea and its implications for anesthesiologists. Anesth Analg 2008;107: 1543–63.

118. Passanante A, Rock P. Anesthetic management of patients with obesity and sleep apnea. Anesthesiol Clin North America 2005;23:479–91.

119. Adesanya AO, Lee W, Greilich NB, et al. Perioperative management of obstructive sleep apnea. Chest 2010;138:1489–98.

120. Schwengel DA, Sterni LM, Tunkel DE, et al. Perioperative management of children with obstructive sleep apnea. Anesth Analg 2009;109(1): 60–75.

121. Bandla P, Brooks LJ, Trimarchi T, et al. Obstructive sleep apnea syndrome in children. Anesthesiol Clin North America 2005;23:535–49.

122. Waters KA, McBrien F, Stewart P, et al. Effects of OSA, inhalational anesthesia, and fentanyl on the airway and ventilation of children. J Appl Physiol 2002;92:1987–94.

123. Porhomayon J, Leissner KB, El-Solh AA, et al. Strategies in postoperative analgesia in the obese obstructive sleep apnea patient. Clin J Pain 2013. http://dx.doi.org/10.1097/AJP.0b013e31827c7bc7. [Epub ahead of print].

124. FDA Drug Safety Communication. Codeine use in certain children after tonsillectomy and/or adenoidectomy may lead to rare, but life-threatening adverse events or death. Available at: http://www.fda.gov/Drugs/DrugSafety/ucm339112.htm. Accessed February 24, 2013.

125. Sleiman P, Hakonarson H. Genetic underpinnings of obstructive sleep apnea: are we making progress? Sleep 2011;34(11):1449–52.

Alternative Therapies for Obstructive Sleep Apnea

Amer Tfaili, MD[a,b], James A. Barker, MD, CPE, FACP, FCCP, FAASM[d,*],
Ahmad Chebbo, MD[c]

KEYWORDS

- Obstructive sleep apnea • Alternative apnea therapy • Positional therapy • Acupuncture
- Hypoglossal nerve stimulation • Didgeridoo playing

KEY POINTS

- Patients are interested in a wide variety of alternative therapies and a common disorder such as obstructive sleep apnea is approached by many as an opportunity to pursue these.
- The search for an alternative to continuous positive airway pressure (CPAP) has produced promising results.
- Some of these alternatives are effective in patients with certain categories of OSA, although further tailoring and refining are required.
- These alternatives should be entertained in selected patients with OSA who are intolerant of CPAP because CPAP is likely to remain first-line therapy in the near future.
- We predict that alternatives to CPAP will become mainstream over the next 2 decades.

INTRODUCTION

Patients are interested and actively involved in alternative medicines and therapies, and many of them do not stay with continuous positive airway pressure (CPAP) therapy over the long term even if they do not lose weight. Compliance with CPAP therapy has been well recognized by researchers and practicing physicians as a common hurdle in the treatment of obstructive sleep apnea (OSA). A wide range of compliance has been reported in the literature, ranging from 46% to 85%.[1] CPAP compliance has also been shown to decrease with time. Abdelghani and colleagues[2] followed 72 patients with OSA started on CPAP for a mean duration of 22 ± 15 months. CPAP compliance was 92% at 6 months, 83% at 12 months, and 59.9% at 3 years. In the compliant patients, the CPAP was used for a mean of 4.5 hours. Studies such as these prompted a search for CPAP alternatives for the treatment of OSA.

This article reviews these alternatives in depth and focuses on studies that measure clinically meaningful outcomes such as apnea/hypopnea index (AHI), oxygen desaturation during sleep, and measured daytime sleepiness such as the Epworth Sleepiness Scale (ESS). Literature that could shed the light onto the pathophysiologic plausibility of these alternatives is also reviewed. In the studies reviewed, continuous variables were usually reported as the mean of the value ± standard deviation or as median with its range (x to y). Categorical variables were usually reported as odds ratios with 95% confidence intervals (CIs). A 2-tailed P value was reported with most of these variables.

NASAL RESISTIVE DEVICES

Multiple imaging studies have been done on the upper airway in patients with OSA to evaluate the site of obstruction, its timing in the respiratory

a Aurora St. Luke's Medical Center in Milwaukee, Milwaukee, WI, USA; b Aurora Medical Center in Grafton, Grafton, WI, USA; c Division of Pulmonary and Critical Care, Maricopa Integrated Health System, Phoenix, AZ, USA; d Pulmonary, Critical Care, and Sleep Disorders, Texas A&M School of Medicine, Scott & White Healthcare, Scott & White Health Plan, 2401 South 31st, Temple, TX 76508, USA
* Corresponding author.
E-mail address: JABARKER@sw.org

Sleep Med Clin 8 (2013) 543–556
http://dx.doi.org/10.1016/j.jsmc.2013.07.013
1556-407X/13/$ – see front matter © 2013 Elsevier Inc. All rights reserved.

cycle, and the response to different therapeutic modalities. These imaging modalities include nasopharyngoscopy, fluoroscopy, cephalometric radiography, computed tomography (CT), magnetic resonance imaging, echo imaging, and computer fluid dynamics (CFD).[3,4] Schwab and colleagues[5] used dynamic CT imaging to evaluate the airways of 42 individuals: 15 normal controls, 14 snorers/mildly apneic patients, and 13 patients with OSA with a respiratory disturbance index (RDI) greater than 15 events/h. This study revealed that little airway narrowing occurred during inspiration even in patients with OSA and that the airway narrowed significantly at the end of the expiration, especially in patients with OSA. The investigators explained the absence of obstruction in inspiration despite the negative airway pressure at that time to be secondary to a balancing increase in upper airway dilator muscle activity, and they suspected that expiration was passive such that the loss of positive intraluminal pressure generated by the expired air led to the worst airway narrowing at the end of expiration. These findings prompted the testing of CPAP alternatives to maintain a positive intraluminal pressure at end-expiration to maintain the airway patency.

In a pilot study involving 24 patients with OSA and 6 primary snorers, Colrain and colleagues[6] evaluated the use of an expiratory resistance device (made by Ventus Medical) consisting of 2 nasal valves mounted over a nasal cannula that monitored the airflow. The valves had negligible resistance in inspiration and a resistance of 60 to 90 cm $H_2O/s/L$ at a flow of 100 mL/s during expiration. The device use had a favorable response: average AHI decreased (from 24.8 ± 22.1 to 14.2 ± 22.1, $P<.001$), the oxygen desaturation index (ODI) decreased (from 14.6 ± 16.9 to 9.9 ± 15.2, $P<.01$), and percentage of total sleep time (TST) with snoring decreased (from $26.9\% \pm 19\%$ to $9.4\% \pm 10.7\%$, $P<.001$). The device was well tolerated, with only 2 subjects describing it as very uncomfortable. Only 1 of the 11 patients who had previously used CPAP considered the device to be somewhat less comfortable than CPAP, whereas the rest found CPAP to be much less comfortable than the device.

Rosenthal and colleagues[7] reexamined the same expiratory resistance device on 34 patients with OSA. Patients underwent 4 polysomnograms (PSGs): 1 baseline control PSG and 3 PSGs using the device with 3 different resistances (50, 80, and 110 cm $H_2O/s/L$). This was followed with a final PSG after 30 days of using the device with the most effective resistance. Twenty-eight patients completed the study protocol and intent-to-treat analysis revealed a decrease in average AHI from 24.5 ± 23.6 on control PSG to 13.6 ± 19.6 with the 50 cm $H_2O/s/L$ resistance, 12.5 ± 18.8 with the 80 cm $H_2O/s/L$ resistance, and 14.4 ± 19.7 with the 110 cm $H_2O/s/L$ resistance. Thirty days after using the device with the most effective resistance, the final PSG revealed an average AHI of 15.5 ± 18.9 ($P = .001$). Also at 30 days, the percentage of sleep time snoring also decreased (from $27.5\% \pm 23.2\%$ to $14.6\% \pm 20.6\%$, $P = .013$), ESS decreased (from 8.7 ± 4.0 to 6.9 ± 4.4, $P<.001$), and the Pittsburgh Sleep Quality Index (PSQI) improved (from 7.4 ± 3.3 to 6.5 ± 3.6, $P = .042$). The device was well tolerated and worn on 94% of the 30 nights.

Further encouraged by these results, Berry and colleagues[8] conducted a prospective, multicenter, sham-controlled, parallel-group, randomized, double-blinded trial on 250 patients with OSA (AHI$\geq$10) using a new expiratory positive airway pressure (EPAP) nasal device. This Ventus Provent was a single-use nasal valve inserted into each nostril and sealed with adhesive. The Provent valve had negligible inspiratory resistance and an expiratory resistance of 80 cm $H_2O/s/L$ at a flow of 100 mL/s. The sham device looked similar to the active device but had negligible inspiratory and expiratory resistance. At 1 week, median AHI with the active device decreased (from 13.8 to 5.0, $P<.0001$) but not with the sham device (from 11.6 to 11.1, $P = $ not significant [NS]). Similar results were observed at 3 months with median AHI decreasing with the active device (from 14.4 to 5.6, $P<.0001$) and not with the sham device (from 10.2 to 8.3, $P = $ NS). At 3 months, ESS decreased with both devices: from 9.9 ± 4.7 to 7.2 ± 4.2 ($P<.0001$) in the EPAP group and from 9.6 ± 4.9 to 8.3 ± 5.1 ($P = .001$) in the sham device group. However, the Provent group had a significantly bigger decrease in ESS than the sham group ($P = .04$). The active device also showed improvement in the ODI and percent TST with oxygen saturations greater than 90%. The Provent success rate (success defined as AHI decrease $\geq$50% or AHI decrease to <10) was 62% at 1 week and 50.7% at 3 months. Reported adherence to Provent was at 88.2% versus 92.3% for the sham device ($P = .02$).

Long-term use of the Ventus Provent EPAP device was evaluated by Kyger and colleagues[9] in a prospective, single-arm, open-label extension of the AERO trial. Responders from the AERO trial (response defined as AHI decrease $\geq$50% or AHI decrease to <10) who used the device for 4 hours or more per night and 5 nights or more per week were eligible. Forty-one of 51 eligible patients chose to participate and, after 7 early terminations,

34 patients finished the study. Compared with baseline data collected in the AERO trial, the Provent device at 12 months still had a favorable response: median AHI decreased from 15.7 to 4.7 ($P<.001$), median ODI decreased from 12.6 to 7.6 ($P = .08$), percent TST snoring decreased by a median of 74.4% ($P<.001$), and average ESS improved from 11.1 ± 4.2 to 6.0 ± 3.2 ($P<.001$). The device was reported to be worn on 89.3% of nights. Forty-two percent of all Provent users (17/41) reported adverse events, including difficulty exhaling, nasal discomfort, dry mouth, headache, and insomnia.

Patel and colleagues[10] evaluated the Provent valve in 20 patients with OSA (AHI>5) and found similar results. In the 19 patients who tolerated the device, RDI decreased (from 49 ± 28 to 27 ± 29 events/h, $P<.001$), with 50% of patients having adequate response (defined as RDI decrease of >50% to <20 events/h). No significant predictor of response could be elucidated.

In another trial, by Walsh and colleagues,[11] 59 patients with OSA (AHI>15 or AHI>10 with OSA symptoms) who had not tolerated CPAP therapy were single-blindedly offered Provent EPAP devices with 2 different resistances (50 cm H_2O/s/L [R50] and 80 cm H_2O/s/L [R80] at a flow of 100 mL/s). Patients were allowed to chose a preferred device after trying both (24 patients chose R50 and 15 patients chose R80) or were assigned a device if they had no preference. Forty-seven patients (80%) tolerated the EPAP trial and completed a screening/baseline PSG (PSG1). Forty-three of these patients met all inclusion criteria and proceeded to get a second PSG (PSG2) to assess the efficacy of the device within 10 days of PSG1. Efficacy was defined as greater than a 50% reduction in AHI from PSG1, or AHI less than 10, or greater than 30% decrease in AHI associated with a decrease in ESS greater than 2 from a baseline less than 12. Twenty-four patients fulfilled the efficacy criteria and proceeded with a third PSG (PSG3) done about 5 weeks after continued use of the device. In these 24 patients, average AHI was 31.9 ± 19.8 at PSG1, 11.0 ± 7.9 at PSG2, and 16.4 ± 12.2 at PSG3 ($P<.001$ compared with PSG1 and $P = .023$ compared with PSG2). The investigators attributed the increase in AHI in PSG3 compared with PSG2 to the regression to the mean statistical phenomenon. ESS also improved in this group (from 11.1 ± 5.1 at PSG1 to 8.7 ± 4.4 at PSG3, $P = .03$). Reported compliance was greater than 92%. Predictors of efficacy were a Mallampati score of less than 4, a lower baseline AHI, and a lower baseline percentage of TST spent with oxygen saturation less than 90%.

EPAP nasal resistive devices show promising results, as shown by the review of the published literature. The mechanism of action has a clear and proven pathophysiologic explanation and its simplicity is appealing. However, these devices are difficult to tailor to the individual patient because they have fixed resistances, and this can explain the partial response in some patients. This partial response could be solved by using a device with variable adjustable resistance in the sleep laboratory to determine the optimal resistance, and then prescribing an EPAP nasal device with a matching resistance.

POSITIONAL THERAPY

The effect of sleep position on the OSA has been well established. Positional OSA has been defined as OSA with AHI in the supine position that is at least double the AHI in a nonsupine position.[12(pp189)]

Oksenberg and colleagues[13] retrospectively reviewed the PSG data of 666 patients diagnosed with OSA (defined as RDI>10) and selected 547 patients (RDI>10, age>20 years, body mass index [BMI] >20 kg/m², and >30 minutes of either sleep position) for analysis to compare positional patients (PP) with nonpositional patients (NPP), and 55.9% of patients had positional sleep apnea. Compared with NPP, the PP group were 2 years younger (age, 52.9 vs 54.9 years, $P = .02$), thinner (BMI, 29.4 vs 31.9 kg/m², $P = .001$), and had milder disease: lower apnea index (AI) (13.7 vs 26.5 events/h, $P = .001$), lower RDI (27.8 vs 44.0 events/h, $P = .001$), and higher oxygen saturation (Sao_2) nadirs (rapid eye movement [REM] sleep, 81.1% vs 72.7%, $P = .001$; and non-REM [NREM] sleep, 84.7% vs 81.5%, $P = .001$).

Similar differences between PP and NPP were observed by Soga and colleagues[14] in 31 patient with OSA (AHI>15), notably younger age (43.0 vs 51.6 years), lower AHI (21.1 vs 50.9 events/h), and lower BMI (26.4 vs 28.4 kg/m²), but none of these differences were statistically significant. This finding could be explained by the small sample size compared with the study by Oksenberg and colleagues[13] mentioned earlier. For the site of obstruction in PP versus NPP, Ravesloot and de Vries[15] performed drug-induced sleep endoscopy (DISE) on 100 patients with OSA and noted a trend toward more obstruction to occur in the base of tongue and epiglottis in PP ($P = .058$).

Probably the first reported attempt at positional therapy came from the wife of a patient who described in a letter to her doctor how she "sewed a pocket into the back of a T-shirt and inserted a hollow, light-weight plastic ball" into the pocket, resulting in the resolution of her husband's snoring and daytime sleepiness within about 2 days of use.[16]

Maurer and colleagues[17] tested a vest with a half-cylindrical piece of hard foam in its dorsal part on 12 men with positional OSA and compared the PSGs with the baseline PSGs done the night before. Adequate response was defined as a reduction in AHI of greater than 50% to a value of less than 10 events/h. With the vest, AHI decreased (26.5 ± 12.0 to 7.6 ± 5.11 events/h, $P<.005$), Sao_2 nadir increased (80% ± 7.2% to 85% ± 7.8%, $P<.05$), and percentage of TST with Sao_2 less than 90% decreased (11.7% ± 11.3% to 1.5% ± 2.1%, $P<.005$). Nine patients (75%) had adequate response to the vest.

The vest was again tested by Wenzel and colleagues[18] on 14 patients with positional OSA to assess its efficacy and long-term compliance. The vest use again led to a reduction in AHI (31.3 ± 12.9 to 13.8 ± 9 events/h, $P<.001$), a trend to a higher Sao_2 nadir (82% ± 6.2% to 86.4% ± 4.7%, but $P = NS$), and a decrease in percentage of TST with Sao_2 less than 90% (8.2% ± 7.1% to 3.8% ± 4.5%, $P<.001$). Only 4 patients (28.6%) reported still using the vest 24 ± 28.8 months later and, in these patients, the ESS decreased (from 8.5 ± 3.2 to 6.5 ± 2.9, $P<.05$). Discomfort was reported to be the reason for the poor compliance.

Oksenberg and colleagues[19] offered a different form of positional therapy, the tennis ball technique (TBT), to 78 patients with positional OSA after the patients declined CPAP therapy. The patients purchased, for US$7.5, a wide cloth belt that had a pocket that was later stuffed with a tennis ball. The belt was worn around the chest with the pocket to the back, thus preventing a supine sleep position. A questionnaire was sent to the patients 6 months after starting the intervention. Fifty patients (64.1%) returned the questionnaire. Nineteen patients (38%) reported continued use of the technique and had better self-reported sleep quality ($P<.005$), improved daytime alertness ($P<.046$), and decreased snoring loudness ($P<.001$). Discomfort was the most common reason behind noncompliance. In the same study, the efficacy of the technique was shown in 12 other patients: AHI decreased (46.5 ± 19.9 vs 17.5 ± 19.4 events/h, $P<.002$) and Sao_2 nadir increased (REM, 81.3% ± 9.9% vs 90.3% ± 4.7%, $P<.009$; and NREM, 85.1% ± 5.6% vs 89.9% ± 3.9%, $P<.009$). Long-term compliance was also studied by Bignold and colleagues,[20] who sent questionnaires to 108 patient 2.5 ± 1.0 years after starting TBT. Sixty-seven patients responded and

responders had similar demographic and clinical characteristics to the nonresponders. Only 4 patients (6%) reported continued TBT use.

A slightly modified TBT was also compared with nasal CPAP (nCPAP) in a randomized crossover study of 20 patients with positional OSA (mean AHI, 22.7 ± 12.0). A thoracic antisupine band (TASB) was wrapped around the anterior chest and shoulder, intersecting on the back in the interscapular area at the level of the sixth vertebra where a ball was inserted. One month later, the TASB effectiveness was inferior to CPAP, with mean AHI of 12.0 ± 14.5 with the band versus 4.8 ± 3.9 with nCPAP ($P = .02$). Successful outcome (defined as AHI<10) was reached in 72% of patients with the TASB versus 89% with nCPAP ($P = .004$). However, patient-reported adequate adherence to therapy (defined as use for ≥4 h/night on ≥70% of nights) was better for the TASB (95%) than nCPAP (45%), with $P<.001$. There was no significant difference in ESS between the two treatments.[21]

In another study involving 16 patients with positional OSA, Heinzer and colleagues[22] reported a more objective assessment of compliance with a further modification of the TBT. The modified device used a firm plastic piece over the back instead of a ball and added shoulder straps to the belt to prevent sideways movement of the plastic piece. An actigraphic recorder in the device monitored its use and, at 3 months, the device was used 73.7% ± 29.3% of the time for an average of 8.0% ± 2.0 h/night.

Other forms of positional therapy devices have been used. Loord and colleagues[23] used The Positioner on 23 patients with positional OSA (AHI>15 in supine and AHI<5 events/h in lateral position). The device consisted of a vest attached to a board with Velcro fasteners and a pillow placed at the head of the board. The design allowed turning between lateral positions but not the supine position. Five patients could not tolerate the device and 18 patients completed the study. PSGs were done at baseline and at 6.8 ± 3.2 months. Thirteen of the 18 patients had a decrease in AHI with 11 patients (61%) having second AHI less than 10 events/h, with mean AHI decreasing from 21.8 to 14.3 ($P = .02$). ESS also decreased from 11.8 to 10.2 ($P = .02$). Another device, the Zzoma Positional Sleeper, was compared with CPAP on 38 patients with positional OSA (nonsupine AHI<5). This device consisted of a backpack-type foam attached over an elastic band that was wrapped around the chest. The foam was bulky and wedge-shaped to secure the patient in a lateral position. With the device, there was no time spent in the supine position.

Median AHI decreased from 11 to 2 events/h with the device and to 0 events/h with CPAP (P<.001). Fifty percent of the patients preferred the device, whereas 34% preferred CPAP and the rest were undecided.[24]

To overcome the poor compliance caused by the discomfort causing frequent awakenings with other devices, Van Maanen and colleagues[25] instead used a small battery-operated vibrating device (3 × 3 × 1 cm) on 30 patients with OSA. The device had a position sensor and vibrations started 10 seconds after the supine position was assumed and increased in intensity until the patient changed position. With the device on, mean AHI decreased (from 27.7 ± 2.4 to 12.8 ± 2.2 events/h, P = .00) with 7 patients (23%) achieving an AHI of fewer than 5 events/h. Percentage of TST in the supine position decreased (40% ± 3.5% to 19.0% ± 4.1%, P = .00) without an increase in the number of awakenings. Encouraged by these results, Van Maanen and colleagues[26] tested the Sleep Position Trainer (SPT; a small device in a pocket of a neoprene strap worn around the chest) on 31 patients with positional OSA. The device had a USB port to communicate more than 90 days' worth of position data to a computer and to charge the device. With the device, median AHI decreased (from 16.4 to 5.2 events/h, P<.001), Sao_2 nadir increased (85.4 ± 4.1 to 88.4 ± 3.6, P<.001), and median ESS score decreased (from 11 to 9, P = .004). There was no increase in awakenings and median compliance with the device use was 92.7% (range, 62%–100%).[26] The SPT (by NightBalance BV) is now available by prescription in some European countries.[27]

An adaptation of the SPT is now available as an Android phone application under the name of Apnea Sleep Position Trailer, which records the sleep position, causes the phone to vibrate if the supine position is detected, and sounds an alarm if the person does not respond by changing position.[28] The application can be downloaded from Google Play for US$2.60.[29] The Android phone is then placed in a sport belt such as the Tune Belt (by Tune Belt Inc), which is available for less than US$25.[30]

The efficacy of positional therapy for positional OSA has been shown and, until recently, patient discomfort has been the biggest obstacle to good compliance. With the advent of smarter devices, it seems the days of the bulky devices are numbered. Positional therapy device development is another example of market innovation, such as smart phone applications, bypassing the lengthy approval process of regulatory bureaucracy.

SNORE PILLOWS

In the search for alternatives to CPAP for treatment of OSA, readjustment of the head position during sleep was attempted to increase the airway caliber in the hope of preventing the obstructive apneas.

Kushida and colleagues[31] tested PillowPositive, a cervical pillow that promotes head extension, on 18 patients with mild to moderate OSA. Baseline electromyogram (EMG) was done on 2 nights, followed by a 5-night adjustment period sleeping with the cervical pillow, and then repeat EMG over 2 nights was performed with the cervical pillow. The use of the cervical pillow resulted in a reduction in the mean RDI (from 17.8 ± 6.8 to 13.6 ± 7.3, P = .003) but made no significant difference in obstructive events, oxygen saturation nadir, or subjective sleep quality.[31]

SONA Pillow, a pillow designed to prevent supine sleep positions, was tested on 22 patients with OSA. In the subgroup of patients with mild (N = 11, RDI 5–19) and moderate (N = 8, RDI 20–40) OSA, the pillow use reduced the average RDI by 17 to less than 5 (P = .001), increased Sao_2 (P = .004), and decreased or eliminated snoring (P = .017).[32] Svaticova and colleagues[33] also tried the SONA Pillow on 18 patients with recent stroke (within 14 days) and OSA in a randomized, controlled, crossover study. The pillow use resulted in a reduction in the median AHI from 39 (range 21–54) to 27 (range 22–47, P = .011). At 3 months, 4 of the 9 patients randomized to the pillow (44%) were still using the pillow every night or most nights.

A different pillow designed to achieve an elevated posture was tested on 14 patients with OSA in a randomized crossover study. The shoulder-head elevation pillow (SHEP), a foam wedge with 60° inclination, was compared with nCPAP and was significantly inferior: mean AHI decreased from 27 ± 12 to 21 ± 17 with the SHEP versus 5 ± 3 with nCPAP (P = .008 comparing the two treatments).[34]

It is difficult to consider the aforementioned pillows as CPAP alternatives, but there is probably a role for them as adjunct treatments for OSA.

HYPOGLOSSAL NERVE STIMULATION

Multiple studies examined the site of obstruction in the upper airway in patients with OSA during both wakefulness and sleep. Different methods were used including physiologic measurements of pressure and resistance, flextube reflectometry using acoustic reflection, fiberoptic visualization, and different imaging modalities including cephalometric roentgenograms, fluoroscopy, CT, and magnetic resonance imaging.[35] Patients had one or more site of obstruction with the retropalatal site dominating followed by the retrolingual site, with the site of obstruction affected by sleep phase but not by sleep position.[36]

Submental electric stimulation was initially attempted and decreased AHI, longest apnea duration, lowest Sao_2, and time spent with Sao_2 less than 85%.[37,38] Videoradiography during submental electric stimulation in a patient showed a forward movement of the tongue breaking the obstructive apnea without evident arousal of the patient.[39] In a subsequent study of 8 patients with positional and nonpositional OSA, submental and transhyoidal transcutaneous electric stimulation led to protrusion of the tongue with increased cross-sectional area of the orohypopharyngeal segment of the upper airway, but it failed to decrease the AHI. In this study, a cutoff of AHI greater than or equal to 40/h was used to define OSA.[40]

After more mixed results obtained with submental stimulation,[41,42] Schwartz and colleagues[43] tried soft palate electric stimulation on 7 patients and successfully treated snoring but not OSA. Selective stimulation of the genioglossus muscle was later shown to improve airway patency.[44] Eisele and colleagues[45] then showed that stimulation of the branch of the hypoglossal nerve, which contracts the genioglossus muscle, produced protrusion and contralateral deviation of the tongue, whereas stimulating the nerve led to retrusion and ipsilateral deviation of the tongue. The genioglossus muscle is an extrinsic muscle of the tongue that attaches to the superior genial tubercle of the mandible.[46] Although this muscle was originally thought to be the single tongue protrusor muscle, tongue protrusion is more likely produced by the combined efforts of muscle units from different tongue muscles.[47] The complexity of the tongue functional anatomy can explain the conflicting results obtained with submental stimulation.

Schwartz and colleagues[48] implanted the Medtronic Inspire I stimulating system, a unilateral hypoglossal nerve–stimulating device into 8 patients with OSA. The device consisted of a half-cuff electrode placed around the hypoglossal nerve branch innervating the genioglossus muscle of the tongue, an intrathoracic pressure sensor drilled through the superior manubrium, and an implantable pulse generator placed in the infraclavicular subcutaneous pocket. After the device was activated, mean AHI (measured in episodes per hour) decreased during NREM sleep (from 52 ± 20.4 to 22.6 ± 12.1, P<.001) and REM sleep (from 48.2 ± 30.5 to 16.6 ± 17.1, P<.001). Mean low Sao_2 also improved during NREM sleep (from 89.7% ± 2.9% to 91.7% ± 2.0%, P<.5) and REM sleep (from 88.7% ± 6.5 % to 91.6% ± 2.2%) after the device activation.

A different hypoglossal nerve stimulation device, the Apnex Medical Hypoglossal Nerve Stimulation (HGNS) system was used by Eastwood and colleagues[49] in a multicenter trial on 21 patients with moderate to severe OSA who failed multiple attempts of CPAP implementation. In addition to AHI between 20 and 100/h with at least an AHI greater than 15/h during NREM sleep, a hypopnea-driven AHI with hypopneas constituting greater than or equal to 80% of the events and a BMI less than or equal to 40 kg/m^2 were among the inclusion criteria. The new device had a stimulating lead, which was placed on the hypoglossal nerve distal to the branches that innervate the retrusor muscles of the tongue. Intraoperative fluoroscopy was used to verify proper placement yielding the desired tongue protrusion with stimulation. This stimulator lead was then tunneled under the skin and attached to an infraclavicularly implanted neurotransmitter that was also attached to 2 sensing leads that were tunneled distally along each costal margin. The sensors measured changes in bioimpedence to signal the beginning of inspiration. The patient controlled the device with a handheld controller. Patients used the device 89% ± 15% of nights for 5.8 ± 1.6 h/night. PSGs done at 6 months for 19 of these patients showed a decrease in AHI (from 43.1 ± 17.5 to 19.5 ± 16.7 events/h, P<.001) and in arousal index (from 43.8 ± 19.5 to 11.0 ± 13.8 events/h, P<.001). Patients also had symptomatic improvement with ESS decreasing from 12.1 ± 4.7 to 8.1 ± 4.4 with P<.001 over the same time period.

The Inspire II Upper Airway Stimulation (UAS) by Inspire Medical Systems, the second generation of the system studied by Schwartz and colleagues,[48] was used in a 2-part open prospective study done by Van de Heyning and colleagues.[50] The new system had the pressure-sensing lead placed in the fourth intercostal space instead of being drilled through the superior manubrium and the stimulating lead embedded in cuffs wrapping around the main hypoglossal nerve in part 1 and around the medial branch of the nerve that innervates the genioglossus muscle in part 2 of the study. In part 1 of the study, 22 patients with OSA (with AHI≥25 and BMI<35 kg/m^2) who failed or could not tolerate CPAP therapy received the device, with 20 of them completing the study (1 lost to follow-up and 1 had a device-related infection). Seven of these patients underwent a DISE procedure to evaluate the site, degree, and pattern of the upper airway collapse during sleep. The subjects were evaluated with PSG at baseline, 2, 4, and 6 months. The patients as a group did not have a significant improvement in AHI at 6 months. The patients were then divided into responders (AHI decreasing more than 50% to less than 20 events/h at 6 months) and nonresponders, and their baseline characteristics were compared. The responders had a lower baseline AHI (26.1 ± 5.0 vs 51.1 ± 16.8 events/h, $P<.01$) and a lower baseline BMI (27.8 ± 1.8 vs 30.7 ± 2.6 kg/m², $P<.05$). Analysis of the results of the DISE procedure that had been done on 7 of the 20 patients showed that the 3 patients who had complete concentric collapse at the level of the soft palate were nonresponders, whereas the other 4 patients were responders. Based on these results, the second part of the study inclusion criteria were adjusted to favor responders: BMI less than or equal to 32 kg/m², AHI between 20 and 50 events/h, and the absence of complete collapse at the level of the soft palate on DISE. A total of 9 patients were enrolled in this part, with 8 patients reaching the 6-month follow-up and included in the data analysis (1 patient excluded because of inadequate tongue response). As expected, this group was responsive to the intervention, with decreased AHI (28.9 ± 9.8 to 10 ± 11 events/h, $P<.01$) and arousal index (22.7 ± 8.2, $P<.01$). Only 1 patient was a nonresponder. Among all 28 subjects in both parts of the study, ESS significantly improved with intervention (11 ± 5.0 to 7.6 ± 4.3, $P<.01$).

The longest follow-up was 1 year, reported by Mwenge and colleagues.[51] In this pilot study, 14 patients with OSA and having intolerance to CPAP therapy were included. The aura6000 by ImThera Medical was successfully implanted in 13 of the 14 patients. This device has no sensor limb and consists of an implanted pulse generator (IPG) and a 6-electrode stimulator lead ending with a cuff that encircles the hypoglossal nerve near the middle tendon of the digastric muscle. Another distinctive feature of this device is the transcutaneously rechargeable IPG battery. At 12 months, the AHI decreased (from 45 ± 18 to 21 ± 17 events/h, $P<.001$) and so did the arousal index (from 37 ± 13 to 25 ± 14, $P<.001$). There was also an insignificant decrease in ESS (from 11 ± 7 to 8 ± 4, $P = .09$).

Encouraged by these results, 6 trials are ongoing using the 3 devices mentioned earlier (clinicaltrials.gov).[52] To date, none of these devices is approved by the US Food and Drug Administration for routine patient use in the United States, but the Apnex HGNS system has been approved for sale in Europe.[53]

ACUPUNCTURE

Acupuncture has been a mainstay of traditional Chinese medicine for thousands of years. In the West, the practice has been an integral part of alternative therapies for various diseases. Most studies comparing acupuncture with sham procedures for treatment for OSA have been reported in Chinese. The targeted body areas were in the head and neck, most notably the ear.

In an animal study, Janssens and colleagues[54] reported performing acupuncture on 84 different animals in various forms of respiratory depression. The acupuncture procedure involved mainly needling of the philtrum point VG 26 (Jen Chung), which is located in the midline of the nasolabial cleft or philtrum at the level of the lower canthus of the nostril, by inserting a needle of 25 to 28 gauge to a depth of 10 to 20 mm. Sixty nine animals (48 dogs and 21 cats) were in respiratory depression or apnea induced by general anesthesia. Respiration was restored to normal or near normal in all of these animals within 10 to 30 seconds of the needle insertion. Acupuncture also revived 3 of 7 cats and dogs with anesthesia-induced cardiopulmonary arrest after 4 to 10 minutes of needle stimulation. Despite this being an animal study, this report shows the potential of acupuncture in the stimulation of breathing.

In a study on 45 patients with sleep apnea syndrome, Wang and colleagues[55] randomly assigned 30 patients to auricular plaster therapy, a form of auricular acupuncture, and compared them with 15 patients in a control group receiving vitamin C as placebo. Statistically significant response was noted in the treatment group with improvement in AHI (from 72.4 ± 7.9 to 59.2 ± 10.6 events/h, $P<.01$) and in minimum blood oxygen saturation (from 73.3% ± 4.8% to 77.7% ± 3.8%, $P<.01$). No difference was seen in the placebo group.

In a randomized, single-blinded, placebo-controlled trial by Freire and colleagues,[56] 36 patients were randomized to 3 arms with 12 patients in each arm: a therapeutic acupuncture group, a sham acupuncture group, and a control group. The patients in the treatment group received needles in multiple acupoints in the head, face, neck, wrists, hands, legs, and ankles, whereas the sham group received needle insertions in nonacupoints. Patients in the treatment and the sham acupuncture groups received a total of 10 weekly sessions. All patients had OSA diagnosed on PSG with an AHI greater than 15/h and less than 30/h. Only 26 subjects completed the study: 10 in the treatment arm, 9 in the sham arm, and 7 in the control arm. Of the 10 patients not completing the study, 7 were excluded after randomization because of long-distance travel. Treatment was associated with improvement in ESS from 11.1 ± 3.3 to 7.5 ± 3 with $P = .29$ and AHI from 19.9 ± 4.1 to 10.1 ± 5.6 with $P = .005$. No significant change in ESS or AHI occurred in the sham or control groups. Freire and colleagues[57] later showed an immediate effect of manual acupuncture (MA) and electroacupuncture (EA) on AHI in a study involving 40 patients with moderate OSA with Apnea Hypopnea Index (AHIs) between 15 and 30/h. The patients were randomly assigned to 4 groups: MA (n = 10), EA 10 Hz (n = 10), EA 2 Hz (n = 10), and control groups. Compared with the control group, AHI decreased after MA (from 21.9 ± 8.3 to 11.2 ± 5.5, $P = .34$) and EA 10 Hz (from 20.6 ± 5.6 to 9.95 ± 5.1, $P = .01$).

Concerns have been raised about the apparent success of acupuncture, especially with the small sample sizes in the studies discussed earlier, especially in the light of the availability of more established treatments such as CPAP.[58] Nevertheless, it is possible to imagine a scenario in which the physician feels obliged to offer alternative medicine approaches such as acupuncture to the patient who fails or refuses conventional medical therapy.

SPEECH EXERCISES

Twenty or more upper airway muscles, including muscles in the soft palate, tongue, and pharynx, play a major role in keeping the upper airway patent.[59] Exercise to strengthen these muscles may help in the treatment of OSA. In a recent trial, 39 patients with moderate OSA were randomized to 3 months of daily oropharyngeal exercises (involving the tongue, soft palate, and lateral pharyngeal wall) or a daily 30 minutes of deep breathing through the nose (control group). The exercises were taught in weekly 30-minute sessions. In the exercise group (N = 16), there was a decrease in AHI (from 22.4 ± 4.8 to 13.7 ± 8.5, $P<.05$), a decrease in ESS (from 14 ± 5 to 8 ± 6, $P = .006$), and decrease in neck circumference (from 39.6 ± 3.6 to 38.5 ± 4.0 cm, $P<.05$). Snoring intensity and frequency were also significantly reduced. No improvement occurred in the control group (N = 15). Compliance with the exercises was 84% and noncompliant patients were excluded from the study.[60]

The reproducibility of these results in a typical clinical practice is difficult to ascertain, but the speech therapy was not too intensive and patient compliance was encouraging. The postintervention AHI, although reduced, did not normalize. The short duration of the study also questions whether these results can be maintained in the long term. Despite these limitations, speech exercises compare well with other CPAP alternatives and can be a viable option for the motivated patient who is intolerant of CPAP.

MUSICAL INSTRUMENTS

A didgeridoo instructor noted that he and some of his students had decreased daytime somnolence after using the instrument for several months, which prompted Puhan and colleagues[61] to test the instrument on 25 patients with moderate OSA (AHI between 15 and 30) in a randomized controlled trial. Patients in the intervention group (N = 14) received didgeridoo lessons from the instructor and practiced at home for 4 months. They practiced for an average 5.9 ± 0.86 days/wk for 25.3 ± 3.4 minutes. Compared with the control group (N = 11), the didgeridoo group had lower ESS (−3.0 [95% CI, −5.7 to −0.3], $P = .03$) and lower average AHI (−6.2 [95% CI, −12.3 to −0.1], $P = .05$) but no difference in sleep quality.

Looking for epidemiologic evidence linking OSA risk and playing wind musical instruments, Brown and colleagues[62] studied the members of the International Conference of Symphony and Opera Musicians (ICSOM). The ICSOM has 4300 active members and e-mail addresses of 3665 of them. The Berlin questionnaire assessing the OSA risk was sent via e-mail and 1111 musicians(30%) responded. There was no difference between musicians playing wind versus nonwind instruments with regard to OSA risk after adjusting for age, sex, and BMI.

Ward and colleagues[63] examined the possible epidemiologic evidence connecting OSA with playing wind instruments to establish whether the type of wind instrument made a difference. A national sample of 906 active musicians was surveyed, again using the Berlin questionnaire, to assess their risk of OSA. After correcting for BMI, playing a double-reed instrument was associated with lower risk of OSA with an odds ratio of 0.508 (95% CI 0.261–0.991, $P = .047$). Among musicians playing double-reed instruments, the OSA risk was also lower with more hours per week of instrument playing: 16.5 ± 1.2 h/wk in the low-risk musicians versus 9.1 ± 2.7 h/wk in musicians with the high OSA risk.

From the literature reviewed, it is clear that at least some wind instrument playing is associated with lower OSA risk and severity but the effect on AHI is modest and further studies are needed before such therapies can be offered as viable alternatives to CPAP therapy.

NASAL CANNULAS

A few studies have evaluated nasal cannulas in an attempt to find less burdensome alternatives to CPAP therapy.

In one of the earlier studies, Wilhoit and colleagues[64] examined the effect of using a high-flow nasal cannula (NFLOW) in 13 patients with OSA. The new device was called NFLOW and consisted of 2 fused tubes that split at the patient end in a Y shape with the two tips covered with ear wax, fitted into the nostrils, and then secured in place with an elastic band around the head. The other end of the cannula was attached to an unheated humidifier that was in turn attached to an air compressor. The flow was started at 20 L/min then increased until the obstructive apneas resolved or became rare. PSG findings with the cannula on were compared with a PSG done the night before. Four patients could not tolerate the high flow but 9 patients were able to use the cannula through the night with significant improvement of their desaturation indices: number of desaturations greater than 4% per hour and the average desaturation. Flow rates between 30 and 60 L/min were required to control the obstructive apneas. Nasal airway pressure was recorded and ranged from 1.2 to 13.2 cm H_2O on the lower end to between 7 and 20 cm H_2O on the upper end. The AHI of the group was not reported.[64]

A different and simpler nasal cannula was used in a study by McGinley and colleagues[65] in 11 adult patients with OSA. This cannula consisted of 2 fused tubes that were split to fit around the ears and the ends fused again at the nares with the nasal prongs inserted into the open nostril. This cannula was designed to decrease the noise generated by high flows (as high as 20 L/min) that were generated by the attached air compressor. The patients underwent flow titration at 0, 10, and 20 L/min in the first night and all required 20 L/min flow to relieve the airway obstruction. Patients then had PSGs done on separate nights with and without nasal insufflation at 20 L/min. AHI decreased in all patients, with the average AHI for the group decreasing from 28 ± 5 to 10 ± 3 events/h, $P<.01$. This finding represents a decrease in disordered breathing related arousals (18 ± 4 to 8 ± 2 events/h, $P<.01$) without an increase in spontaneous arousals (3 ± 1 to 3 ± 1, $P = .65$).

McGinley and colleagues[66] later showed similar benefits of the high-flow nasal cannula on 12 children (aged 10 ± 1 years; BMI 35 ± 14 kg/m²) with OSA. Treatment with nasal insufflation (TNI)

at 20 L/min was performed on one night and compared with no TNI on another night. With TNI, AHI significantly decreased (11 ± 3 vs 5 ± 2 events/h, $P<.01$). The effect of TNI was then compared with CPAP titration done earlier on 10 of the 12 patients. Two of these 10 patients (both with severe OSA with AHI>20 events/h) had a suboptimal AHI with TNI (1 required a CPAP of 20 cm H_2O and 1 could tolerate neither CPAP nor TNI). In the remaining 8 children, TNI was not inferior to CPAP (AHI 2 ± 1 vs 1 ± 1 events/h).

In an attempt to find predictors of response to TNI in OSA, Nilius and colleagues[67] studied 56 carefully selected patients with sleep-disordered breathing (SDB). Patients had to have an RDI greater than 5 events/h, have excessive daytime sleepiness, be eligible for but not on CPAP therapy, and have a CPAP pressure requirement that was less that the median pressure of each sleep laboratory (range 8–11 cm H_2O) on CPAP titration study. TNI was started at 10 L/min for comfort and automatically gradually increased to 20 L/min over 5 to 10 minutes. Response was defined as greater than or equal to 50% decrease in respiratory events with RDI less than 10 events/h. Only 3 patients (5%) had a predominance of respiratory effort–related arousals (RERA). TNI decreased RDI in the group (from 22.6 ± 15.6 to 17.2 ± 13.2 events/h, $P<.01$) but only 27% reached a therapeutic RDI. Neither the baseline RDI nor the previously prescribed CPAP pressure predicted response. Patients with a predominance of RERAs or hypopneas had a more favorable response to TNI than patients with apnea-predominant disease. None of the 8 patients who had greater than 10% central apneas at baseline responded to TNI.

A meta-analysis of 2343 patients with stroke or transient ischemic attack documented SDB with AHI greater than 5 events/h to be very frequent (72% of patients), with 38% having an AHI greater than 20 events/h. The SDB in this population is mainly obstructive with central apnea predominating in only 7% of patients.[68] Driven by the low compliance with CPAP in these patients, Haba-Rubio and colleagues[69] tried TNI with a flow of 18 L/min in 10 patients with strokes with moderate to severe SDB. TNI was tolerated in all patients, with a favorable response on AHI in 9 of them (group AHI from 40.4 ± 25.7 to 30.8 ± 25.7 events/h, $P<.001$). Martinez-Garcia and colleagues[70] showed higher adjusted mortality in patients with strokes who had AHIs greater than 20 events/h and were CPAP intolerant compared with patients with AHI less than 20 events/h, with a hazard ratio (HR) of 2.69 (95% CI 1.32–5.61, $P<.05$). In the same study, mortality was similar in CPAP-treated patients with AHIs greater than 20 events/h, those with AHI less than 20 events/h, and patients with stroke who were free of OSA.[70]

Taking these findings into account, it is reasonable to try TNI in CPAP-intolerant patients with OSA, especially if their OSAs are hypopnea predominant and they are free of any significant central apneas. However, no significant benefit is expected with TNI if the decrease in AHI is modest. In such patients, other alternatives to CPAP should be sought.

NASAL STRIPS

The role of the nose in OSA has been extensively studied. This article first reviews the studies that were designed to discern the relationship, if any, between nasal resistance and OSA, and it then examines nasal-focused therapies targeting OSA.

Early work by Blakley and Mahowald[71] examined the effect of increased nasal resistance on the severity of OSA. The hypothesis was that increased nasal resistance resulted in larger negative pressure in the nasopharynx to achieve adequate flow of air through the nose in inspiration. Such a larger negative nasopharyngeal pressure was suspected to lead to increased collapsibility to the upper airway, precipitating or worsening OSA. The study enrolled 53 men with snoring undergoing PSG to evaluate for OSA, in addition to 37 healthy volunteers with similar weight, and anterior mask rhinomanometry was performed on all the subjects. The whole group had a higher average nasal resistance than the control subgroup (0.57 ± 0.91 vs 0.34 ± 0.13 Pa/cm^3/s, $P = .01$). Linear regression in 26 subjects who were diagnosed with OSA showed that nasal resistance had no relationship with AI or with the nadir of oxygen desaturation.[71]

In another study by Atkins and colleagues,[72] 71 patients with OSA (AHI>15 events/h) and 70 antisocial snorers (ASS) (AHI<15 events/h) underwent anterior rhinomanometry measuring combined nasal resistance (CNR) and highest unilateral nasal resistance (HUNR) measured during wakefulness in a sitting position. CNR was increased in 5 of the OSA group and in 4 of the ASS group, whereas HUNR was increased in 10 of the patients with OSA and 11 of the ASS group. There was no difference in either CNR or HUNR between the two groups. There was no correlation between AHI and CNR or HUNR in either group. Miljeteig and colleagues[73] found evidence of nasal obstruction in only 4 of 54 patients with OSA and concluded that nasal obstruction was not a major contributor to OSA. The presence of unilateral or bilateral nasal obstruction had no effect on apnea or

snoring indices in an earlier study of 683 patients with snoring and suspected OSA referred to an otolaryngology clinic.

Several studies to evaluate the effect of nasal dilators were conducted. Höijer and colleagues[74] evaluated the effect of Nazovent, a plastic nasal dilator inserted into the nares, in 10 patients with snoring or witnessed apneas. PSGs revealed OSA (AHI $\geq$ 5 events/h) in 7 patients. Nasal flow increased with the device in all patients (0.7 L/s with a range of 0.55–0.81 L/s to 0.81 L/s with a range of 0.61–0.98 L/s, $P = .02$). The average AI in events per hour) for the group decreased (from 18 with a range of 1.8–60 to 6.4 with a range of 1.3–15, $P = .08$) and the minimum overnight oxygen saturation (Sao$_2$) increased (from 78% with a range of 68%–89% to 84% with a range of 76% to 88%, $P = .03$). However, there was no significant correlation between the degree of improvement in nasal flow (measured during wakefulness in a sitting position) and the improvements in AI or in minimum Sao$_2$. Snoring noise also decreased.

The Breathe Right external nasal plaster (NP) was evaluated in another study by Wenzel and colleagues[75] involving 50 patients. The patients were divided into group A, with 30 patients who had OSA (AI>10/h), and group B, with 20 snorers without OSA. Patients underwent initial PSG then cardiorespiratory polygraphy on the following 2 nights. Apart from subjective improvement in nasal breathing, the nasal plaster had neither a significant effect on AI in group A (AI was 29.1 ± 23.7 without and 26.5 ± 23.7 with the NP) nor an effect on the snoring index (SI) in group B (SI was 22.2 ± 7.3 snores/h without NP vs 25.7 ± 9.4 snores/h with NP). 90% of the patients in group A had unchanged daytime sleepiness scores but 33% of them reported better sleep quality.

Gosepath and colleagues[76] reported another trial of Breathe Right external nasal strips on 26 patients with OSA and snoring who had RDIs greater than 10 events/h. Nineteen of the 26 patients had reductions in RDI with the use of the strips. Predictors of response were nasal turbinate hypertrophy/septal deviation with or without allergic rhinitis, none or mild pharyngeal obstruction, and age less than 55 years. The positive result in this group of patients cannot be extrapolated to typical patients with OSA in whom the site of obstruction is mainly pharyngeal, in the retropalatal and retroglossal regions.[77]

A dichotomous effect of Breathe Right external nasal dilators was reported by Djupesland and colleagues[78] in 18 heavy snorers without severe OSA (defined as snoring >25% of the night and AHI<26/h). After sleeping for a week with the active nasal strip, PSG was done on the first night with the active strip and then repeated the next night with a placebo strip. In the subgroup of 6 patients who were habitual snorers with severe morning nasal obstruction (AHI<10 and combined minimal cross-sectional area [TMCA] <0.6 cm^2), the dilator showed a trend to increasing minimum sleep SaO$_2$ (from 89% [95% CI 84.5–92.6] to 93% [95% CI 89.7–96.9], P = .06) and a trend to improving AHI (from 7.4 [95% CI 3.9–10.9] to 5.4 [2.3–8.5], P = .06). In contrast, in the subgroup with TMCA greater than 0.6 cm^2, the active nasal strip led to worsening AHI (from 9.4 [95% CI 5.9–12.9] to 15.2 [95% CI 11.6–18.7], P<.05). Duration and intensity of snoring remained unchanged in either subgroup but subjective evaluation of sleep quality improved.

With these results in mind, there is a lack of evidence for any meaningful benefit for nasal dilators in patients with OSA. Subjective improvement in sleep quality was evident in some studies,[75,78,79] and this suggests a role for the strips in selected patients as an adjunct therapy but not an alternative therapy.

DIAPHRAGMATIC PACING

Diaphragm pacing has been a well established treatment of central hypoventilation and high quadriplegia.[80–82] Upper airway obstruction complicating diaphragm pacing has been well documented. In 1981, Hyland and colleagues[83] reported a case of primary alveolar hypoventilation without OSA that developed OSA after diaphragmatic pacing was initiated. The investigators attributed the obstruction to the loss of the normal temporal coordination of diaphragmatic and abductor upper airway muscle activity with diaphragmatic pacing. Upper airway obstruction was also described in a pediatric diaphragmatic pacing series and the negative airway pressure generated by the pacing was suspected to be contributing to the upper airway obstruction.[84] In a report detailing a 10-year experience with diaphragmatic pacing, Le Pimpec-Barthes and colleagues[85] discussed their reluctance to offer tracheostomy removal to their patients because of the fear of obstructive apneas.

Based on these reports, there is no role for diaphragmatic pacing for the treatment of OSA.

SUMMARY

Patients are interested in a wide variety of alternative therapies and a common disorder such as OSA is approached by many as an opportunity to pursue these. The search for a CPAP alternative has produced some promising results, as discussed in this article. Some of these alternatives are effective in certain categories of OSA, although further tailoring and refining are required. These alternatives should be entertained in selected patients with OSA who are intolerant of CPAP because CPAP is likely to remain first-line therapy in the near future. However, we predict that alternatives to CPAP will become mainstream over the next 2 decades.

REFERENCES

1. De Dios JA, Brass SD. New and unconventional treatments for obstructive sleep apnea. Neurotherapeutics 2012;9(4):702–9.
2. Abdelghani A, Slama S, Hayouni A, et al. Acceptance and long-term compliance to continuous positive airway pressure in obstructive sleep apnea. A prospective study on 72 patients treated between 2004 and 2007. Revue de pneumologie clinique 2009;65(3):147–52 [in French].
3. Sittitavornwong S, Waite PD. Imaging the upper airway in patients with sleep disordered breathing. Oral Maxillofac Surg Clin North Am 2009;21(4): 389–402.
4. Togeiro SM, Chaves CM, Palombini L, et al. Evaluation of the upper airway in obstructive sleep apnoea. Indian J Med Res 2010;131:230–5.
5. Schwab RJ, Gefter WB, Hoffman EA, et al. Dynamic upper airway imaging during awake respiration in normal subjects and patients with sleep disordered breathing. Am Rev Respir Dis 1993;148(5):1385–400.
6. Colrain IM, Brooks S, Black J. A pilot evaluation of a nasal expiratory resistance device for the treatment of obstructive sleep apnea. J Clin Sleep Med 2008; 4(5):426–33.
7. Rosenthal L, Massie CA, Dolan DC, et al. A multicenter, prospective study of a novel nasal EPAP device in the treatment of obstructive sleep apnea: efficacy and 30-day adherence. J Clin Sleep Med 2009;5(6):532–7.
8. Berry RB, Kryger MH, Massie CA. A novel nasal expiratory positive airway pressure (EPAP) device for the treatment of obstructive sleep apnea: a randomized controlled trial. Sleep 2011;34(4): 479–85.
9. Kryger MH, Berry RB, Massie C. Long-term use of a nasal expiratory positive airway pressure (EPAP) device as a treatment for obstructive sleep apnea (OSA). J Clin Sleep Med 2011;7(5):449–453B.
10. Patel AV, Hwang D, Masdeu MJ, et al. Predictors of response to a nasal expiratory resistor device and its potential mechanisms of action for treatment of obstructive sleep apnea. J Clin Sleep Med 2011; 7(1):13–22.

11. Walsh JK, Griffin KS, Forst EH, et al. A convenient expiratory positive airway pressure nasal device for the treatment of sleep apnea in patients nonadherent with continuous positive airway pressure. Sleep Med 2011;12(2):147–52.

12. Lee-Chiong T. Sleep medicine: essentials and review. In: Sleep-related breathing disorders. New York: Oxford University Press; 2008. p. 189.

13. Oksenberg A, Silverberg DS, Arons E, et al. Positional vs nonpositional obstructive sleep apnea patients: anthropomorphic, nocturnal polysomnographic, and multiple sleep latency test data. Chest 1997;112(3):629.

14. Soga T, Nakata S, Yasuma F, et al. Upper airway morphology in patients with obstructive sleep apnea syndrome: effects of lateral positioning. Auris Nasus Larynx 2009;36(3):305–9.

15. Ravesloot MJ, de Vries N. One hundred consecutive patients undergoing drug-induced sleep endoscopy: results and evaluation. Laryngoscope 2011;121(12):2710–6.

16. Editor's note Patient's wife cures his snoring. Chest 1984;85(4):582.

17. Maurer JT, Stuck BA, Hein G, et al. Treatment of obstructive sleep apnea with a new vest preventing the supine position. Dtsch Med Wochenschr 2003;128(3):71–5 [in German].

18. Wenzel S, Smith E, Leiacker R, et al. Efficacy and longterm compliance of the vest preventing the supine position in patients with obstructive sleep apnea. Laryngorhinootologie 2007;86(8):579–83 [in German].

19. Oksenberg A, Silverberg D, Offenbach D, et al. Positional therapy for obstructive sleep apnea patients: a 6-month follow-up study. Laryngoscope 2006;116(11):1995–2000.

20. Bignold JJ, Bios BS, Deans-costi G, et al. Poor long-term patient compliance with the tennis ball technique for treating positional obstructive sleep apnea. J Clin Sleep Med 2009;5(5):428–30.

21. Skinner MA, Kingshott RN, Filsell S, et al. Efficacy of the "tennis ball technique" versus nCPAP in the management of position-dependent obstructive sleep apnoea syndrome. Respirology 2008;13(5):708–15.

22. Heinzer RC, Pellaton C, Rey V, et al. Positional therapy for obstructive sleep apnea: an objective measurement of patients' usage and efficacy at home. Sleep Med 2012;13(4):425–8.

23. Loord H, Hultcrantz E. Positioner: a method for preventing sleep apnea. Acta Otolaryngol 2007;127(8):861–8.

24. Permut I, Diaz-Abad M, Chatila W, et al. Comparison of positional therapy to CPAP in patients with positional obstructive sleep apnea. J Clin Sleep Med 2010;6(3):238–43.

25. van Maanen JP, Richard W, Van Kesteren ER, et al. Evaluation of a new simple treatment for positional sleep apnoea patients. J Sleep Res 2012;21(3):322–9.

26. van Maanen JP, Meester KA, Dun LN, et al. The sleep position trainer: a new treatment for positional obstructive sleep apnoea. Sleep Breath 2013;17(2):771–9. http://dx.doi.org/10.1007/s11325-012-0764-5.

27. Night Balance. Availability. Night Balance. Available at: http://www.nightbalance.com/patients/availability. Accessed April 8, 2013.

28. Apnea. Lateral sleep position trainer. Apnea. 2012. Available at: http://www.apnea-app.net. Accessed April 8, 2013.

29. Google. Apnea lateral position trainer. Google. 2012. Available at: https://play.google.com/store/apps/details?id=m4noc.fourpone.apnea. Accessed April 8, 2013.

30. Tune Belt. 2007. Available at: https://www.tunebelt.com/domino/tunebelt/shop.nsf/parts?Openview&count=1000. Accessed April 8, 2013.

31. Kushida CA, Sherrill CM, Hong SC, et al. Cervical positioning for reduction of sleep-disordered breathing in mild-to-moderate OSAS. Sleep Breath 2001;5(2):71–8.

32. Zuberi NA, Rekab K, Nguyen HV. Sleep apnea avoidance pillow effects on obstructive sleep apnea syndrome and snoring. Sleep Breath 2004;8(4):201–7.

33. Svatikova A, Chervin RD, Wing JJ, et al. Positional therapy in ischemic stroke patients with obstructive sleep apnea. Sleep Med 2011;12(3):262–6.

34. Skinner MA, Kingshott RN, Jones DR, et al. Elevated posture for the management of obstructive sleep apnea. Sleep Breath 2004;8(4):193–200.

35. Shepard JW, Gefter WB, Guilleminault C, et al. Evaluation of the upper airway in patients with obstructive sleep apnea. Sleep 1991;14(4):361–71.

36. Shepard JW Jr, Thawley SE. Localization of upper airway collapse during sleep in patients with obstructive sleep apnea. Am Rev Respir Dis 1990;141(5 Pt 1):1350–5.

37. Miki H, Hida W, Inoue H, et al. A new treatment for obstructive sleep apnea syndrome by electrical stimulation of submental region. Tohoku J Exp Med 1988;154(1):91–2.

38. Miki H, Hida W, Chonan T, et al. Effects of submental electrical stimulation during sleep on upper airway patency in patients with obstructive sleep apnea. Am Rev Respir Dis 1989;140(5):1285–9.

39. Hillarp B, Rosen I, Wickstrom O. Videoradiography at submental electrical stimulation during apnea in obstructive sleep apnea syndrome. A case report. Acta Radiol 1991;32(3):256–9.

40. Edmonds LC, Daniels BK, Stanson AW, et al. The effects of transcutaneous electrical stimulation during wakefulness and sleep in patients with obstructive sleep apnea. Am Rev Respir Dis 1992;146(4): 1030–6.

41. Hida W, Okabe S, Miki H, et al. Effects of submental stimulation for several consecutive nights in patients with obstructive sleep apnoea. Thorax 1994;49(5):446–52.

42. Guilleminault C, Powell N, Bowman B, et al. The effect of electrical stimulation on obstructive sleep apnea syndrome. Chest 1995;107(1):67–73.

43. Schwartz RS, Salome NN, Ingmundon PT, et al. Effects of electrical stimulation to the soft palate on snoring and obstructive sleep apnea. J Prosthet Dent 1996;76(3):273–81.

44. Smith PL, Eisele DW, Podszus T, et al. Electrical stimulation of upper airway musculature. Sleep 1996;19(Suppl 10):S284–7.

45. Eisele DW, Smith PL, Alam DS, et al. Direct hypoglossal nerve stimulation in obstructive sleep apnea. Arch Otolaryngol Head Neck Surg 1997; 123(1):57–61.

46. Standring S. Upper aerodigestive tract: oral cavity. In: Standring S, editor. Grey's anatomy: the anatomical basis of clinical practice. London: Churchill Livingstone; 2008. p. 503.

47. Sokoloff AJ. Activity of tongue muscles during respiration: it takes a village? J Appl Physiol 2004;96(2):438–9.

48. Schwartz AR, Bennett ML, Smith PL, et al. Therapeutic electrical stimulation of the hypoglossal nerve in obstructive sleep apnea. Arch Otolaryngol Head Neck Surg 2001;127(10):1216–23.

49. Eastwood PR, Barnes M, Walsh JH, et al. Treating obstructive sleep apnea with hypoglossal nerve stimulation. Sleep 2011;34(11):1479–86.

50. Van de Heyning PH, Badr MS, Baskin JZ, et al. Implanted upper airway stimulation device for obstructive sleep apnea. Laryngoscope 2012; 122(7):1626–33.

51. Mwenge GB, Rombaux P, Dury M, et al. Targeted hypoglossal neurostimulation for obstructive sleep apnoea: a 1-year pilot study. Eur Respir J 2013; 41(2):360–7.

52. US National Institutes of Health. Available at: http://clinicaltrials.gov/ct2/results?term=hypoglossal+stimulation+AND+Obstructive+apnea&Search=Search. Accessed April 11, 2013.

53. American Thoracic Society News. Just approved and launched. 2012. Available at: http://news.thoracic.org/january-2012/just_approved_launched.php. Accessed April 11, 2013.

54. Janssens L, Altman S, Rogers PA. Respiratory and cardiac arrest under general anaesthesia: treatment by acupuncture of the nasal philtrum. Vet Rec 1979;105(12):273–6.

55. Wang X, Xiao L, Wang B, et al. Influence of auricular plaster therapy on sleeping structure in OSAS patients. J Tradit Chin Med 2009;29(1):3–5.

56. Freire AO, Sugai GC, Chrispin FS, et al. Treatment of moderate obstructive sleep apnea syndrome with acupuncture: a randomised, placebo-controlled pilot trial. Sleep Med 2007;8(1):43–50.

57. Freire AO, Sugai GC, Togeiro SM, et al. Immediate effect of acupuncture on the sleep pattern of patients with obstructive sleep apnoea. Acupunct Med 2010;28(3):115–9.

58. Yegneswaran B. Do sleep physicians think complementary medicine research does no harm? Sleep Med 2008;9(2):211 [author reply: 212–3].

59. Ayappa I, Rapoport DM. The upper airway in sleep: physiology of the pharynx. Sleep Med Rev 2003; 7(1):9–33.

60. Guimarães KC, Drager LF, Genta PR, et al. Effects of oropharyngeal exercises on patients with moderate obstructive sleep apnea syndrome. Am J Respir Crit Care Med 2009;179(10):962–6.

61. Puhan MA, Suarez A, Lo Cascio C, et al. Didgeridoo playing as alternative treatment for obstructive sleep apnoea syndrome: randomised controlled trial. BMJ 2006;332(7536):266–70.

62. Brown DL, Zahuranec DB, Majersik JJ, et al. Risk of sleep apnea in orchestra members. Sleep Med 2009;10(6):657–60.

63. Ward CP, York KM, McCoy JG. Risk of obstructive sleep apnea lower in double reed wind musicians. J Clin Sleep Med 2012;8(3):251–5.

64. Wilhoit SC, McTier RF, Findley LJ, et al. Treatment of obstructive sleep apnea with continuous nasal airflow. Lung 1985;163(4):233–41.

65. McGinley BM, Patil SP, Kirkness JP, et al. A nasal cannula can be used to treat obstructive sleep apnea. Am J Respir Crit Care Med 2007;176(2): 194–200.

66. McGinley B, Halbower A, Schwartz AR, et al. Effect of a high-flow open nasal cannula system on obstructive sleep apnea in children. Pediatrics 2009;124(1):179–88.

67. Nilius G, Wessendorf T, Maurer J, et al. Predictors for treating obstructive sleep apnea with an open nasal cannula system (transnasal insufflation). Chest 2010;137(3):521–8.

68. Johnson KG, Johnson DC. Frequency of sleep apnea in stroke and TIA patients: a meta-analysis. J Clin Sleep Med 2010;6(2):131–7.

69. Haba-Rubio J, Andries D, Rey V, et al. Effect of transnasal insufflation on sleep disordered breathing in acute stroke: a preliminary study. Sleep Breath 2012;16(3):759–64.

70. Martinez-Garcia MA, Soler-Cataluna JJ, Ejarque-Martinez L, et al. Continuous positive airway pressure treatment reduces mortality in patients with ischemic stroke and obstructive sleep apnea: a

5-year follow-up study. Am J Respir Crit Care Med 2009;180(1):36–41.

71. Blakley BW, Mahowald MW. Nasal resistance and sleep apnea. Laryngoscope 1987;97(6):752–4.

72. Atkins M, Taskar V, Clayton N, et al. Nasal resistance in obstructive sleep apnea. Chest 1994; 105(4):1133–5.

73. Miljeteig H, Hoffstein V, Cole P. The effect of unilateral and bilateral nasal obstruction on snoring and sleep apnea. Laryngoscope 1992;102(10):1150–2.

74. Höijer U, Ejnell H, Hedner J, et al. The effects of nasal dilation on snoring and obstructive sleep apnea. Arch Otolaryngol Head Neck Surg 1992; 118(3):281–4.

75. Wenzel M, Schonhofer B, Siemon K, et al. Nasal strips without effect on obstructive sleep apnea and snoring. Pneumologie 1997;51(12):1108–10 [in German].

76. Gosepath J, Amedee RG, Romantschuck S, et al. Breathe Right nasal strips and the respiratory disturbance index in sleep related breathing disorders. Am J Rhinol 1999;13(5):385–9.

77. Tang XL, Yi HL, Luo HP, et al. The application of CT to localize the upper airway obstruction plane in patients with OSAHS. Otolaryngol Head Neck Surg 2012;147(6):1148–53.

78. Djupesland PG, Skatvedt O, Borgersen AK. Dichotomous physiological effects of nocturnal external nasal dilation in heavy snorers: the answer to a rhinologic controversy? Am J Rhinol 2001;15(2): 95–103.

79. Todorova A, Schellenberg R, Hofmann HC, et al. Effect of the external nasal dilator Breathe Right on snoring. Eur J Med Res 1998;3(8): 367–79.

80. Dobelle WH, D'Angelo MS, Goetz BF, et al. 200 cases with a new breathing pacemaker dispel myths about diaphragm pacing. ASAIO J 1994; 40(3):M244–52.

81. Chen ML, Tablizo MA, Kun S, et al. Diaphragm pacers as a treatment for congenital central hypoventilation syndrome. Expert Rev Med Devices 2005;2(5):577–85.

82. Khong P, Lazzaro A, Mobbs R. Phrenic nerve stimulation: the Australian experience. J Clin Neurosci 2010;17(2):205–8.

83. Hyland RH, Hutcheon MA, Perl A, et al. Upper airway occlusion induced by diaphragm pacing for primary alveolar hypoventilation: implications for the pathogenesis of obstructive sleep apnea. Am Rev Respir Dis 1981;124(2):180–5.

84. Hunt CE, Brouillette RT, Weese-Mayer DE, et al. Diaphragm pacing in infants and children. Pacing Clin Electrophysiol 1988;11(11 Pt 2):2135–41.

85. Le Pimpec-Barthes F, Gonzalez-Bermejo J, Hubsch JP, et al. Intrathoracic phrenic pacing: a 10-year experience in France. J Thorac Cardiovasc Surg 2011;142(2):378–83.

Cost of Therapy

Sophia H. Kim, MD, Nancy Collop, MD*

KEYWORDS

- Obstructive sleep apnea • Polysomnography • Diagnosis of sleep apnea
- Treatment of sleep apnea • Costs of sleep apnea diagnosis and treatment

KEY POINTS

- Obstructive sleep apnea is a common disease, often unrecognized, with potential health ramifications. It is also a chronic condition often present in patients with other comorbid conditions.
- Studies have clearly shown both quality of life and health benefits from treatment and possibly mortality reduction.
- In the studies that have examined cost-benefit ratio, treatment advantages far outweigh the costs of diagnosis for most.

BACKGROUND

Obstructive sleep apnea (OSA) is characterized by "repetitive episodes of complete (apnea) or partial (hypopnea) narrowing upper airway obstruction occurring during sleep."[1] These events frequently result in recurrent hypoxic episodes and arousals. Its prevalence in the general population has been estimated to be 4% of men and 2% of women.[2] Untreated (or unrecognized), these episodes can manifest as excessive daytime sleepiness and mild neurologic compromise in the short term to myocardial infarction (MI), stroke, hypertension, diabetes, and increased mortality over the long term. Untreated, the 15-year mortality for severe OSA is approximately 30%, with adjusted mortality hazard ratios of 1.4, 1.7, and 3.8, respectively, for mild, moderate, and severe disease (P trend = .004).[3]

DIAGNOSIS

Diagnosis for OSA requires a comprehensive sleep evaluation, with those patients determined to be at high risk sent for objective diagnostic testing, not only for confirmation but also to determine severity.[4] The 2 acceptable methods of testing include attended polysomnography (PSG) in a sleep laboratory and unattended testing with portable monitors (PMs). PSG is routinely indicated for the diagnosis of sleep-related breathing disorders.[5] Testing with PMs should be done judiciously, in the setting of a comprehensive sleep evaluation for patients who have a high pretest probability of moderate to severe OSA. Additionally, it should be supervised by a practitioner who is board certified or board eligible in sleep medicine.[6]

Given the wide variety of devices, monitoring methods have been categorized based on the number of channels and the clinical information that is obtained. Briefly, type I describes a standard full-night PSG (FN-PSG) and is the only type of study to be conducted in a sleep facility, allowing for direct patient monitoring and intervention when necessary. It typically includes a minimum of 7 channels, including electrocardiogram (ECG), electroencephalogram, electro-oculogram, chin electromyography, airflow, SaO_2, and respiratory effort. Type II monitoring, also referred to as comprehensive portable PSG, also has a minimum of 7 channels, which may include those described for type I and is unattended. Type III monitoring uses a minimum of 4 channels, with at least 2 dedicated to ventilation, in addition to heart rate or ECG and SaO_2. Type IV monitoring has a minimum of 1 channel, and is referred to as continuous single-bioparameter or dual-bioparameter recording.[7]

Emory Sleep Center, Emory University, 1841 Clifton Road NE, Room 502, Atlanta, GA 30329, USA
* Corresponding author.
E-mail address: nancy.collop@emory.edu

Sleep Med Clin 8 (2013) 557–569
http://dx.doi.org/10.1016/j.jsmc.2013.07.008
1556-407X/13/$ – see front matter © 2013 Elsevier Inc. All rights reserved.

sleep.theclinics.com

The Centers for Medicare and Medicaid Services (CMS) is the governing body that funds and regulates the medical care programs for the elderly and indigent population in the United States. This body develops the National Coverage Determination (NCD) policies that regulate the coverage/reimbursement of federal insurance programs. Based on these policies, Medicare administrative contractors interpret and issue local coverage determinations (LCDs), which are usually propagated for Medicaid at the state level. In 2008, CMS revised the NCD primarily to include home sleep testing (HST) as a reimbursable diagnostic tool for OSA. Based on these policies, the following types of testing were approved for coverage: (1) type I, attended PSG conducted in a sleep facility; (2) type II or III devices with studies performed unattended in or out of a sleep facility or attended in a sleep facility; (3) type IV monitors, with 3 or more channels (including airflow), performed unattended in or out of a sleep facility, or attended in a sleep facility; and (4) sleep testing monitors with 3 or more channels (including actigraphy, pulse oximetry, and peripheral arterial tonometry), performed unattended in or out of a sleep facility, or attended in a sleep facility.[8]

Although this is an article on therapy costs, it is difficult to separate diagnosis from therapy, as the algorithms of many studies will include both diagnostic testing and therapy (continuous positive airway pressure [CPAP]). For a summary of the studies assessing diagnostic strategies, see **Table 1**. Since the development of PM, there has

been a significant amount of concern surrounding the quality of data obtained from PM versus PSG. Patients are not directly observed, and there are fewer channels of information obtained. As such, the depth and breadth of data collected can be somewhat questionable when considering the long-term morbidities with inappropriate diagnosis and subsequent treatment. There have been studies to suggest that PM and PSG are equivalent in terms of clinical outcomes and CPAP use,[9] and possibly some superiority in the PM versus PSG groups in terms of adherence and duration of use.[10] In this current state of financial turmoil and soaring costs of medical care, many insurers are directing patients to PM testing with the presumption that it is more cost-effective compared with PSG.

To summarize these studies, in the first, the New England Comparative Effectiveness Public Advisory Council[8] carried out an analysis of comparative value assessing the cost-effectiveness of 3 *diagnostic strategies* for OSA compared with standard attended PSG (type I) alone. The model was based on a hypothetical cohort of 1000 Medicaid patients with suspected OSA. The 3 strategies evaluated were the following: (1) screening based on the Berlin Questionnaire, with test-positive patients undergoing confirmatory PSG; (2) a clinical prediction algorithm based on morphometric characteristics of the head and neck, with "high-risk" patients undergoing PSG; and (3) OSA diagnosis based on type III monitors for home testing. These patients did not receive a confirmatory

Table 1
Diagnostic strategies: cost analysis studies

Source	Diagnostic Strategies	Cost or ICER (Per QALY)	Lowest Cost Strategy
Institute for Clinical and Economic Review[8]	PSG alone Berlin Questionnaire + PSG Morphometric evaluation + PSG Type III HST	$652,830 $518,066 $674,621 $200,700	Type III HST
Institute for Clinical and Economic Review[8]	HST + APAP HST + Split-night PSG + CPAP Split-night PSG + CPAP	$811,129 $1,112,731 $1,244,905	HST + APAP
Pietzsch et al,[11] 2011	Full-night PSG Split-night PSG Unattended portable home monitoring	$17,131/QALY $17,887/QALY $19,707/QALY	Full night PSG
Deutsch et al,[12] 2006	Full-night PSG Split-night PSG Unattended home partial sleep monitoring	$2092/QALY $1979/QALY $1838/QALY	Unattended home partial sleep monitoring

Abbreviations: APAP, autotitrating CPAP; CPAP, continuous positive airway pressure; HST, home sleep testing; ICER, incremental cost-effectiveness ratio; PSG, polysomnography; QALY, quality-adjusted life year.

PSG. Costs for the Berlin Questionnaire screening mode included a routine office visit, presumably during which the questionnaire was administered. The morphometric data strategy required a computed tomography scan of the sinus/maxilla/mandible with a doctor's visit to interpret results. The home monitor cost was based on the Medicare fee schedule. Costs were estimated using data from the Vermont Medicaid schedule. The total costs for the PSG-alone group were $652,830; Berlin Questionnaire + PSG, $518,066; morphometric strategy + PSG, $674,621; and type III monitoring alone to $200,700. Of the 3 screening strategies tested, the morphometric testing group had the fewest number of false positives (14 of 1000) and the home testing alone had the most (30 of 1000). Lower cost of the Questionnaire and HST groups was driven by costs of the tests themselves, as well as the Questionnaire precluding PSG in one-third of patients screened.

Similarly, Pietzsch and colleagues[11] conducted a cost-effectiveness analysis comparing 3 *diagnostic and treatment strategies*: (1) FN-PSG, (2) split-night PSG (SN-PSG), and (3) unattended portable home monitoring (UPHM) followed by treatment with CPAP. The study evaluated health-related quality of life and the impact of treatment on strokes, MIs, and motor vehicle collisions (MVCs). Cost-effectiveness was expressed through the standard metric of incremental cost-effectiveness ratio (ICER), which conveys dollar value per life year (LY) or quality-adjusted LY (QALY) gained. QALY is a measure of disease burden that takes into consideration the quantity and quality of life generated by a health care intervention. The ICER is an equation that is used to facilitate medical decision making regarding health interventions. Typically used in cost-effectiveness analyses, it demonstrates a relationship between cost (numerator) and some unit of health status (denominator), such as QALY. As a point of reference, a ratio of less than $50,000 per QALY gained is typically considered cost-effective (ie, the willingness to pay threshold). The investigators used a Markov model to evaluate the health outcomes and costs for the diagnosis and treatment of OSA over 10 years and lifetime. The study cohort consisted of 50-year-old men with moderate-to-severe OSA. Results of the study suggested that CPAP therapy reduces the 10-year risk for MVCs by 52%, expected number of MIs by 49%, and risk of stroke by 31%. Translated cost, the ICER of CPAP versus no treatment is $15,915 per QALY gained. Sensitivity analyses were performed demonstrating that results were not sensitive to gender or age. Women were noted to have a slightly higher ICER at $18,942 per QALY. Additionally, as might be expected, younger people (30 years old) had a lower ICER compared with people older than 70 years ($18,836 vs $22,348, respectively, per QALY gained). In terms of diagnostic testing approach, FN-PSG had an ICER of $17,131, SN-PSG $17,887, and UPHM $19,707 per QALY gained. The different numbers of false results, both positive and negative, caused by varying sensitivities and specificities of the diagnostic modalities evaluated, resulted in significant differences in event rates, costs, and ultimately QALY. Although FN-PSG (including a second overnight study for CPAP titration) is technologically the most expensive diagnostic modality, its superior diagnostic accuracy resulted in less expense and more health benefits compared with other approaches. Sensitivity analyses were further carried out to address populations in which the pretest probabilities of OSA were 20% and 80% as compared with the 50% presumed previously. At the 20% prevalence, FN-PSG ICER continued to remain the most cost-effective method of diagnosis. In a cohort with 80% prevalence, FN-PSG was still the most cost-effective modality in men younger than 50 years and women younger than 60 years, with ICER ranging from $16,124 to $40,513 per QALY gained. However, SN-PSG was more cost effective in older cohorts with ICER, ranging from $16,599 (50-year-old man) to $23,103 (for a 70-year-old woman) per QALY gained. The cost in the lower prevalence groups (20% and 50%) was driven by increased false-positive rates resulting in unnecessary treatment and associated costs with no health benefits. These long-term treatment costs substantially outweighed the cost of the initial diagnostic testing. In contrast, in the 80% prevalence group, the costs of the diagnostic testing mode and QALYs gained from appropriate treatment, despite treatment of false negatives, contributed significantly to the ICER. A less-expensive and thus less-sensitive testing strategy in a younger cohort is not advantageous because of the longer period at risk for an event (stroke, MI, MVC). Having said that, it should be noted that UPHM can be a cost-effective approach with an ICER of $19,707 per QALY gained versus no diagnosis. This would be most relevant in populations in which FN-PSGs or SN-PSGs are not available, there are long wait times for testing, or patients are unwilling or unable to come into the laboratory for testing. Some limitations of this study to consider are that this was a modeling study based on published estimates of OSA outcomes and treatment. Some of the studies the investigators used to develop the models admittedly had limited sample sizes. The cohort modeled was a population of men and women with average cardiovascular risk. Certainly populations outside of these parameters, such as patients with mild OSA or increased cardiovascular risk, would make these data less appropriate.

In addition to their analysis on diagnostic testing, the New England Comparative Effectiveness Public Advisory Council further evaluated strategies for testing and treatment.[8] This included (1) home monitor sleep study (HST) + autotitrating CPAP (APAP), (2) HST + SN-PSG + fixed titration CPAP, and (3) SN-PSG + fixed titration CPAP. Costs were analyzed based on 1 year of treatment. Total costs for SF-PSG + fixed titration CPAP/bilevel positive airway pressure were $1,244,905; HST + APAP were $811,129; and HST, PSG, and fixed titration CPAP were $1,112,731. The cheapest strategy (HST + APAP), although being the most cost-saving, produced 30 false positives and 14 false negatives.

Deutsch and colleagues[12] performed a similar analysis using a decision-tree model to compare cost-effectiveness of 2 alternatives to conventional FN-PSG with subsequent night for titration. Specifically, they looked at SN-PSG and unattended home partial sleep monitoring (UHPSM) with CPAP titration using an autotitrating device (APAP). The study used a hypothetical cohort of adult, mostly male, patients who had symptoms highly suggestive of OSA (daytime somnolence, persistent snoring, and witnessed apneas). A decision tree was constructed using Treeage Pro Suite software (TreeAge Software, Inc, Williamstown, MA) to simulate the steps involved in diagnosis followed by CPAP titration using FN-PSG, SN-PSG, or the combination of home studies (UHPSM + APAP). The model assumed that an apnea-hypopnea index (AHI) or respiratory disturbance index (RDI) higher than 10 was diagnostic of OSA and took into consideration patient dropout rate (eg, those who do not return for titration). Cost-effectiveness of these strategies was analyzed over 5 years, with the analysis isolated to direct health care costs from the perspective of the third-party payer. Costs were based on 2004 US dollars using Medicare-reimbursement rates to calculate the base case. All 3 strategies evaluated took into account some basic assumptions, including repeat CPAP titrations due to suboptimal procedures at a rate of 3.57%, and presumed compliance rates of 80% at 3 months, 74% at 1 year, and 71% at 5 years. With regard to office visits, patients who did not have OSA or those who declined CPAP were permitted 1 postevaluation office visit. Those who were on CPAP after

in-laboratory titration were assumed to have 1 postevaluation office visit within a month and then every 6 months thereafter. Patients who underwent home studies were assumed to have 3 monthly follow-up visits after initiation of therapy and then every 3 months for 9 months, with biannual visits thereafter. The outcomes for each of the 3 pathways were as follows: (1) OSA syndrome (OSAS) treated, (2) OSAS untreated, (3) no OSAS, and (4) no OSAS treated. Results showed expected costs for FN-PSG at $4886, SN-PSG at $4565, and home studies at $4096. The corresponding cost-effectiveness ratio was calculated at $2092 per QALY for FN-PSG, $1979 per QALY for SN-PSG, and $1838 per QALY for home studies. When compared with home studies, the ICER was $5932 per QALY gained for SN-PSG and $7383 per QALY gained for an FN-PSG. The ICER for an FN-PSG compared with an SN-PSG was $11,586 per QALY gained. These results suggest that the cost for a diagnosis of patients with OSA by way of FN-PSG is more expensive than SN-PSG, which is more expensive than home studies per QALY gained. The home studies strategy was least expensive due to substantial savings resulting from fewer patients receiving long-term treatment. This was attributed to dropout and lower rates of acceptance, leaving more patients with untreated OSAS. Additionally, the investigators did not take into consideration long-term indirect costs of nontreatment. Overall, this study showed the highest ICER was at $11,586 per QALY gained in the FN-PSG compared with SN-PSG. This value is well within the acceptable range of cost-effective health care interventions. For comparison, the ICER for diabetes screening versus routine clinical practice (no screening) in patients with hypertension at annual physical at age 55 is $44,100 per QALY. Annual screening for proteinuria and subsequent treatment with appropriate medication versus routine clinical practice (no screening) in patients with hypertension at annual physical (age 50) has an ICER of $21,880 per QALY. Aspirin versus no aspirin in combination with usual care in patients at high risk for cardiovascular disease has an ICER of $2840 per QALY.[11]

COST OF TREATMENT

When considering the cost of treatment of OSA, one needs to consider the cost of diagnosis, treatment, and long-term follow-up. Additionally, treatment failure, reevaluation, and poor patient compliance can contribute to further costs. Conversely, when considering the long-term complications associated with no treatment, health care costs can be significantly outweighed.

Cost-Effectiveness of Oral Appliances

Oral appliances (OA) are a reasonable second-line treatment for OSA in settings in which patients are unwilling or unable to tolerate CPAP. There is a dearth of literature evaluating costs associated with OA therapy. The costs to the patient would include initial cost of consultation, dental records needed to manufacture the appliance, and the appliance itself. Additional costs may include cephalometric radiographs or other dental airway imaging as part of the initial assessment. Consensus opinion regarding these costs was obtained in a review by Ferguson and colleagues,[13] who found that dental laboratory costs for custom-made devices ranged from $100 to more than $600, depending on the design and quality of the appliance. Service fees varied significantly depending on the clinical protocol, time spent caring for the patient, and geographic economic factors. Dentists surveyed for the review reported service fees ranging from $200 to $2500. This wide range was attributed to lack of standardization within the field. In 1997, Loube and Strauss[14] attempted to address this lack of data by administering a survey to 124 dentists who were members of the Academy of Dental Sleep Medicine, evaluating their clinical practices. Of the respondents, 110 (87%) were dentists, 10 (9%) were orthodontists, and 4 (3%) were maxillofacial surgeons. Among the data that were collected, most pertinent to this review was the total cost to the patient for treatment with an appliance excluding any reimbursement, which was $933 (range, $400 to $2450). Based on their personal practice patterns, 95% of practitioners stated that they performed a pretreatment nocturnal PSG (NPSG) in patients referred for OSA or snoring. Seven percent believed that subjective patient reports were an appropriate substitute for NPSG and 37% believed that nocturnal pulse oximetry was an adequate substitute. In patients with known OSA, only 18% of practitioners ordered posttreatment NPSG. Despite this, 70% of survey responders believe that patients with OSA are successfully treated with OAs.

Cost-Effectiveness of CPAP Versus OA

Sadatsafavi and colleagues[15] performed a cost-effectiveness analysis using a Markov model to calculate the ICER per QALY gained over 5 years in patients with moderate to severe OSA using 3 treatment strategies: oral appliance, CPAP, or no treatment. Potential outcomes included in the model were cardiovascular and cerebrovascular events, MVCs, and their associated morbidities and mortality rates. The cost estimates were calculated from the third-party payer perspective. Costs associated with CPAP based on the 2004 US dollar included mask ($117.64), tubing ($41.02), headgear ($37.16), and monthly rental of heated humidifier ($30.11) and CPAP ($96.99). Cost estimates associated with OA were based on survey data from the study by Loube and Strauss.[14] Costs included the "initial cost," presumably the consultation and production of the appliance ($1233) and 2.5 follow-up visits within 5 years ($59.62). The ICER was calculated for OA versus no treatment and for CPAP versus OA. The results of the analysis in terms of cost-effectiveness showed that OA compared with no treatment resulted in an ICER of $2984 per QALY. When comparing CPAP with OA, CPAP resulted in an ICER of $27,540 per QALY and CPAP versus no treatment resulted in an ICER of $13,698 per QALY. In all scenarios modeled, OA was shown to be a cost-effective strategy compared with no treatment. CPAP was cost effective versus OA in most scenarios tested. Analysis was further undertaken to evaluate the impact of 4 variables (cost of OA, relative efficacy of OA as measured by its effect on AHI and Epworth Sleepiness Scale (ESS), and adherence to OA and CPAP) in the results of the cost-effectiveness analysis. Compared with no treatment, OA became cost saving if initial costs were less than $964 and remained cost effective if initial costs were less than $5710. The cost-effectiveness of OA compared with no treatment was due to its impact on reducing MVC, MI, stroke, and quality of life. When adherence was taken into consideration, OA became the best treatment strategy if CPAP adherence was 70% and OA adherence was at least 80%. If adherence for both strategies fell below 46%, no treatment was the most cost-effective option. In terms of the third-party payer willingness to pay, if the ICER is less than $32,000 per QALY, OA was the best treatment option. Anything above this threshold amount would make CPAP the best option. No treatment was the best option when the cost fell below $6000. In virtually all scenarios modeled, OA versus no treatment and CPAP versus OA resulted in ICER lower than $50,000 per QALY. As previously discussed, therapies with an ICER of lower than $50,000 per QALY gained are considered cost effective.

To our knowledge, this is the only study that has analyzed cost-effectiveness of OA and CPAP for patients with moderate to severe Obstructive Apnea Hypopnea Syndrome (OAHS). However, as with most studies that use modeling to predict disease or treatment outcome, some intrinsic limitations exist. Specifically, many general assumptions regarding OA therapy outcomes and cost were made because of the general lack of information within the current literature. Adherence to OA was presumed to be equal to CPAP, despite there being no objective way to measure OA adherence, as most studies relied on patient self-report. Additionally, this study was based on a model population of patients with moderate to severe OSA, whereas OA is usually recommended more for the treatment of patients with mild to moderate disease. Thus, the data cannot be generalized to this key population. Furthermore, there are a wide range of OA devices currently available, such as tongue-retaining devices or mandibular advancement devices. The investigators commented that it was very difficult for them to integrate all of the evidence within the literature for the various subtypes of OA.[15] Last, cost data for OA within the model was based on a survey from 1997, which may have made included cost information outdated and potentially data not representative of the standard of care depending on who responded to the survey. These limitations may have decreased the generalizability of these data.

The New England Comparative Effectiveness Public Advisory Council[8] performed an analysis comparing costs associated with treatment using CPAP versus OA. Over a 1-year period, OA costs would include device creation, interdental fixation, and calibration. Costs were estimated using the Medicare fee schedule. Costs for CPAP included price for 1-year rental and related accessories based on data from ResMed Corp, San Diego, CA. Total costs were calculated to be $2,011,940 for OA and $1,184,150 for CPAP. Analysis showed a 30% rate of treatment success in favor of CPAP versus OA, even with compliance rates of CPAP reported to be anywhere from 30% to 60%.[16] Further analyses were carried out to determine when OA therapy would be more cost-effective versus CPAP, as CPAP therapy requires continuing costs and OA is fixed after the initial investment. Basic assumptions were made that OA had a life span of 4 years and CPAP 5 years. Additionally, they presumed that costs for CPAP beyond the first year were for replacement supplies alone. Based on this, OA was estimated to become more cost-saving after 25 months of treatment.

Costs Associated with Surgical Procedures

Most of the literature available today within the area of surgical interventions for OSA consists of case series or case reports. The randomized controlled trials (RCTs) that do exist typically compare one procedure to another and frequently lack a control group. Additionally, there is some degree of variability within the procedures

themselves, such that an evidence-based approach is difficult at best. Given this, there is an even greater paucity of data regarding the cost-effectiveness of these procedures. Kezirian and colleagues[17] performed a cross-sectional study to try to evaluate practice patterns in the United States from 2000 to 2006. They grouped procedures into 3 categories: (1) palate procedures; (2) hypopharyngeal procedures that included tongue radiofrequency or midline glossectomy, lingual tonsillectomy, genioglossus advancement, genioplasty, or tongue stabilization and hyoid suspension; and (3) maxillomandibular advancement (MMA). Both national and state-level databases were used to examine inpatient and outpatient costs associated with these procedures, as there was no globally inclusive database for the time period studied. In 2006, there were approximately 35,263 combined inpatient and outpatient OSA procedures performed in the United States. This represents fewer than 0.2% of the approximately 18 million American adults with this disorder. Most OSA procedures were performed in the outpatient setting. There was a general trend toward fewer palatal surgeries and an increase in hypopharyngeal procedures and maxillomandibular advancement from 2000 to 2006. Most of the hypopharyngeal procedures were made up of tongue radiofrequency and midline glossectomy. Only costs for inpatient procedures were available and were calculated at $5115 (95% confidence interval [CI] $4726–$5505) in 2004 and $5994 (95% CI $5507–$6482) in 2006. Costs for palate surgery alone were lower compared with hypopharyngeal procedures ($P<.001$) both in 2004 and 2006. Other trends within the cost analysis were lower costs for procedures in older patients, higher costs in Medicaid patients, and higher costs for admission in rural versus urban teaching hospitals. Some drawbacks of this study to consider are that it was a database analysis and is subject to inherent limitations common to these types of analyses. These data also do not include outpatient procedures and, as such, may not be a true reflection of procedure distribution and cost. Additional costs not included in the analysis were initial consultation visits, postsurgical follow-up visits, or any costs associated with postoperative complications.

CMS does not have an NCD for OSA-related surgical procedures. The LCD for Medicare patients in Wisconsin covers uvulopalatopharyngoplasty (UPPP) and MMA in patients with an AHI/RDI greater than 15, with documentation of failure/intolerance of CPAP or other noninvasive modalities, as well as evidence of counseling and applicable abnormal anatomy. Tracheostomy is covered as a treatment option only in patients who have been unresponsive to all other therapies. Laser-assisted uvulopalatoplasty (LAUP), palatal implants, and radiofrequency ablation are not covered. From the private payer perspective, procedures universally require prior authorization.[8]

COSTS RELATED TO LACK OF TREATMENT FOR OSA
Societal Costs of Unrecognized OSA

Certainly, the cost of treating OSA is a significant area of concern in this era of rising medical costs. Less obviously, but potentially more costly, are the expenses to society by way of medical care for patients with OSA who are untreated. A number of studies have been published that perform a cost analysis on this population, and have suggested that untreated OSA is a significantly greater economic burden on the health care system due to resulting adverse health consequences. In 1999, Kapur and colleagues[18] performed a cross-sectional analysis comparing medical costs in patients with clinically significant sleep-disordered breathing (SDB) with controls in the year before diagnosis and further examined if severity of SDB affected those costs. There were a total of 238 patients with significant SDB and 476 age-matched and sex-matched controls, which were then stratified by their Chronic Disease Score (CDS). The CDS is measure of chronic disease status based on medication use according to a pharmacy database. Cost data were obtained from the health maintenance organization's (HMO's) internal cost/utilization database and adjusted using 1996 dollars. Results of the study showed that 79% of patients were male with mean age of 51 years and body mass index (BMI) of 33. The mean AHI was 37 with a median of 25. Patients were noted to have significantly higher mean and median CDS versus age-matched controls ($P<.01$). The mean annual medical cost for patients was $2720 versus $1384 for controls. Median annual medical costs for patients versus controls were $1380 versus $539, respectively. Even after adjusting for differences in CDS, mean costs for patients were significantly higher than controls ($P<.01$). Calculations were further carried out evaluating costs of undiagnosed OSA (AHI>15). Kapur and colleagues[18] estimated that a typical person with AHI greater than 15 would have an increased medical cost of $1956 over that of a person with AHI of 3. Based on this value, and using the estimated prevalence of undiagnosed moderate to severe OSA in middle-aged individuals, the investigators calculated a potential cost burden of $3.4 billion annually for untreated OSA. This study has many

implications for the significant economic impact of untreated OSA on the health care system. However, results should be interpreted with some caution, as the study was based on an HMO sample population, which may affect the generalizability of the data. Additionally, unlike the randomly chosen controls, the patients had been referred by their primary care physicians, presumably for sleep complaints. They may represent a population of patients who may use the health care system more regularly, thus reflecting a group that may at baseline have increased medical costs. Additionally, BMI was noted to be higher in the patient versus control groups. Elevated BMI could lend itself to increased health care usage because of associated comorbidities of obesity, which can be independent of OSA.

In a similar study from Canada, Ronald and colleagues[19] evaluated health care use of patients with OSA in the 10 years before diagnosis. The study was carried out using data from Manitoba Health, a government agency responsible for rendering payment on medical claims. Patients were selected based on PSG-proven OSAS. Three or 4 controls were chosen for 181 patients, matched for age, gender, and postal code. Costs were presented in Canadian dollar amounts reflecting 1984 to 1995 dollars, with the exchange rate at the time being 1.38 Canadian per 1 US dollar. In the 10 years before diagnosis, physician claims were significantly higher for patients compared with controls ($P<.001$). Specifically, the mean cost for physician claims was $3972 per patient with 109 visits compared with a mean cost of $1969 per control with 60 visits. Costs were further analyzed on a yearly basis, and in 7 of the 10 years, patients used 1.5 to 2.4 times as much in physician resources compared with controls ($P<.05$). Additionally, patients increased physician use more in the 4 years before diagnosis compared with controls. In terms of hospitalizations over 10 years, patients spent 6.2 nights in the hospital versus controls who spent 3.7 nights. The probability of an admission was significantly higher for patients compared with controls ($P<.001$). Presuming a $1000 (Canadian) cost per night of hospital stay, and all physician claims, the 10-year expenditure for patients would total $1,804,365 versus $1,032,376 for controls. Some limitations to consider are underestimation of costs as medical expenses, such as medications, home care, laboratory testing, or outpatient visits, may not have been included due to global hospital billing. Further, potential confounding may have occurred if OSA was actually a surrogate for some other medical condition, such as obesity, which was contributing to the medical costs.

Studies such as these helped establish the significant impact of OSA on health care resources. Subsequent studies began evaluating the effect of treatment on these costs. In a retrospective observational cohort study, Albarrak and colleagues[20] evaluated health care use in patients 5 years after diagnosis and treatment of OSA. Patients had PSG-diagnosed OSA and had been using CPAP continuously for 5 years after diagnosis. Patients were matched to controls in a fashion similar to Ronald and colleagues.[19] Results showed that the number of physician visits increased in the 5 years before the diagnosis and decreased in the 5 years after CPAP. Over the span of 6 years, including the year before diagnosis and the fifth year after diagnosis, patients with OSAS had more physician visits than controls (P<.0001). Specifically related to health care use, total yearly fees of patients were higher than their matched controls over the 6-year period spanning from 1 year before diagnosis to 5 years on CPAP. Fees reached a peak in the year before diagnosis and hit a nadir in the second year on CPAP. Total yearly fees in the patients for the year before diagnosis were $372.10 ± $24.15 compared with controls, which were $152.69 ± $8.09, with a mean difference that was significant (P<.0001). In the fifth year on CPAP, the total yearly fees dropped in the patients while increasing in the controls (P<.0001). These data suggest that there is an increase in health care use by patients with OSA before their diagnosis followed by a decrease after initiation of treatment. Further, although the data were not reviewed here, it appeared that most of that decrease came at the 2-year point after initiation of therapy with increase in cost thereafter. Albarrak and colleagues[20] attributed this increase in expenditure mostly to preexisting ischemic heart disease. Some caution should be taken with regard to these data. CPAP use may have inadvertently increased interaction with the health care system. Patients who were on CPAP were more closely followed so as to increase compliance. This, in and of itself could increase the chances that preventive health matters were addressed in this cohort versus the controls. Additionally, there may have been an inherent selection bias in that those patients who would be compliant with CPAP may inherently be more vigilant about their health care in general.

In addition to direct medical costs from health care use, Sassani and colleagues[21] performed a meta-analysis of costs due to OSA-related collisions and fatalities using the attributable risk percentage (ARP) based on the Levin formula.[22] Their analyses estimated that there were 810,000 collisions and 1400 fatalities attributable to drivers with OSA in 2000, resulting in an economic cost of $15.9 billion. The economic costs included lost wages and productivity, medical expenses, administrative expenses, motor vehicle damage, and employer costs for crashes to workers. Based on their analyses, assuming a CPAP compliance of 70%, Sassani and colleagues[21] projected that 567,000 collisions and 980 fatalities per year in the United States could be prevented. The associated cost savings in terms of collisions was calculated at $11.1 billion.

Costs of Inadequate Adherence to CPAP

The 2008 CMS revision of the NCD was revised primarily to include HST as a diagnostic tool for OSA, thus allowing for initiation of positive airway pressure (PAP) treatment based on those results. However, included in this revision was a limitation on coverage for PAP therapy to an initial 12 weeks with subsequent coverage continued only to those with "proven benefit."[23] At the state level, these guidelines were translated, such that "proven benefit" was defined to include evidence of clinical improvement as well as documentation of adherence. The LCDs, as subsequently adopted by most insurance entities, now require a visit with the treating physician between the 31st and 91st day after initiation of therapy so as to document clinical improvement of OSA symptoms and objective evidence that therapy was used 4 or more hours per night on 70% of nights during a consecutive 30-day period anytime during the first 3 months of initial usage. If these criteria are not met, continued coverage of the therapy is discontinued as "not reasonable and necessary."[24] Given the significant morbidity and mortality, not to mention the long-term financial costs associated with nontreatment of OSA, one needs to consider if lack of compliance as currently defined really has no benefit. Aloia and colleagues[25] performed a retrospective chart review to specifically evaluate the effect of applying the LCD criteria for adherence on neurophysiologic outcomes and Epworth Sleepiness Scale of 150 patients with OSA. Specifically, they found that 55 subjects (37%) would be considered subadherent with CPAP use at 3 and 6 months at approximately 2 hours per night at each time point. Adherent subjects were using their CPAP approximately 5.5 hours per night for the same time points. A comprehensive neuropsychologic evaluation was performed assessing a number of dimensions as well as the Epworth Sleepiness Scale. At the 3-month evaluation, both groups showed improved performance in essentially all neurophysiologic dimensions compared with baseline.

At 6 months, only one dimension of testing continued to improve in subadherent patients. These findings suggest that despite nonadherence as defined by the LCD guidelines, patients had improvement in neurocognitive functioning similar to their adherent counterparts on most testing. Additionally, nonadherent users may benefit from a cumulative effect of treatment at the 6-month mark, when their devices would otherwise have been removed.

To our knowledge, this is the first study to specifically evaluate the effects of LCD adherence requirements on patient outcome. However, there is a significant body of literature assessing clinical outcomes and extent of PAP use (**Table 2**). Many of these studies meet current LCD requirements for adherence; however, there is significant variability, and a number of studies show clinical improvement despite less than acceptable adherence. Engleman and colleagues[26] performed a randomized placebo-controlled, crossover trial looking at subjects with sleep apnea/hypopnea syndrome and the effect of CPAP use on daytime sleepiness, symptoms, cognitive function, and mood. They found statistically significant improvement in patients on CPAP in these categories of functioning.

In a subsequent study, which was limited to patients with mild OSA, Engleman and colleagues[27] found that mean effective CPAP use per night

Table 2
Summary: studies of CPAP use and clinical outcomes

Reference	CPAP Duration	Outcome Effect	P Value
Engleman et al,[26] 1994	3.4 h/night [SE 0.4]	Daytime sleepiness (MSLT) Cognitive function Vigilance Mental flexibility Attention Mood	.03 <.01 <.05 <.05 <.05
Engleman et al,[27] 1999	2.8 h/night ± 2.1 (mean ± SD)	Symptom score Epworth Sleepiness Scale Score Depression score 2 out of 7 cognitive tasks 5 subscales of health/functional status questionnaire	<.01 <.01 <.01 <.02 ≤.03
Redline et al,[28] 1998	3.1 h/night	49% of CPAP subjects improved in at least 2 of 3 categories (mood, energy/fatigue and functional status/general health) vs 26% of controls	<.05
Faccenda et al,[29] 2001	3.3 h/night (range 0–8.1)	Diastolic BP reduced by 1.5 mm Hg Systolic BP reduced by 1.3 mm Hg Decrease in Epworth Sleepiness Scale Score Increase in 3 of 4 domains of Functional Outcomes of Sleep Questionnaire	.04 .19 <.001 .01, .0004, and .029
Meta-analysis studies on the effect of CPAP on BP			
Alajmi et al,[30] 2007		Systolic BP reduced by 1.38 mm Hg Diastolic BP reduced by 1.52 mm Hg	.23 95% CI 3.6 to −0.88 .06 95% CI 3.11 to −0.07
Bazzano et al,[31] 2007		Systolic BP reduced by 2.46 mm Hg Diastolic BP reduced by 1.83 mm Hg Mean arterial pressure reduced by 2.22 mm Hg	95% CI −4.31 to −0.62 95% CI −3.05 to −0.61 95% CI −4.38 to −0.05
Haentjens et al,[32] 2007		Pooled estimate 24-h mean BP reduced by 1.69 mm Hg	.001 95% CI −2.69 to −0.69

Abbreviations: BP, blood pressure; CI, confidence interval; CPAP, continuous positive airway pressure; MSLT, Multiple Sleep Latency Test.

was 2.8 ± 2.1 hours (mean $\pm$ SD). Even with this minimal usage, CPAP improved the symptom score ($P<.01$), Epworth Sleepiness Scale score ($P<.01$), and depression score ($P<.01$) compared with placebo. In a similar study, Redline and colleagues[28] performed a randomized placebo-controlled trial of CPAP versus conservative therapy evaluating mood, energy/fatigue, and functional status/general health. CPAP use during the trial was estimated to be 3.1 hours. Despite this minimal usage, a larger percentage of patients using CPAP demonstrated improvement in at least 2 of the 3 clinical outcome domains compared with controls ($P<.05$). Additional exploratory analyses were undertaken to assess which subsets of subjects might respond to CPAP, as they found that responders (58% $\pm$ 33%) demonstrated increased compliance compared with nonresponders (31% $\pm$ 29%); $P<.05$. The investigators found that those subjects with diabetes or hypertension ($P<.05$), as well as those who reported no history of sinus problems ($P<.01$), significantly benefited from CPAP use compared with controls. Based on these results, perhaps the LCD should take into account comorbidities of patients, rather than a strict time criteria, as these patients are the most likely to have long-term morbidity (and higher health care costs) with nontreatment compared with their healthier counterparts.

Faccenda and colleagues[29] looked at the effects of CPAP therapy on blood pressure in a randomized placebo-controlled crossover trial. Mean CPAP time was 3.3 hours per night. Over the 24-hour period, there was a significant reduction in diastolic blood pressure (DBP), but no effect on systolic pressure (SBP). A significant decrease in Epworth Sleepiness Scale ($P<.001$) and an increase in 3 of 4 domains of the Functional Outcomes of Sleep Questionnaire were also noted. Although the clinical significance of a 1.5-mm Hg improvement in diastolic BP is questionable, one may consider that increased adherence per night may have demonstrated a more significant result. However, it is somewhat notable that an average use of 3.3 hours per night had any clinical effect and reinforces that idea that in the case of CPAP therapy, perhaps some is better than none.

Several meta-analyses have been performed that evaluate the effect of CPAP on blood pressure in patients with OSA. Alajmi and colleagues[30] performed a meta-analysis reviewing RCTs. These data did not show a statistically significant reduction in SBP or DBP. Bazzano and colleagues[31] undertook a similar meta-analysis looking at RCTs. Based on the studies evaluated, the mean net changes ranged from −18.0 to 2.0 mm Hg in SBP, −9.0 to 2.0 mm Hg in DBP, and −9.5 to 1.0 mm Hg in mean arterial pressure (MAP). The pooled mean net changes due to CPAP were −2.46 mm Hg (95% CI −4.31 to −0.62) for SBP, −1.83 mm Hg (95%CI −3.05 to −0.61) and −2.22 mm Hg (95% CI −4.38 to −0.05) for MAP. Finally, Haentjens and colleagues[32] performed a meta-analysis of RCTs that showed a pooled estimate of the effect of CPAP on mean blood pressure was a net decrease of 1.69 mm Hg (95% CI −2.69 to −0.69; $P<.001$). The results of these analyses indicate a small decrease in blood pressure in patients with OSA on CPAP. Although this effect seems modest, there is some association between even 1 to 2 mm Hg decrements in blood pressure and decreased cardiovascular events and stroke.[33]

Finally, in addition to the clinical benefits shown by these studies despite minimal CPAP use, Campos-Rodriguez and colleagues[34] went a step further to evaluate how PAP compliance rates effect mortality. The retrospective chart review showed increased survival in patients with increased compliance. The cumulative survival rates at 5 years were significantly lower in the less than 1 hour per day versus more than 6 hours per day groups (85.5% [95% CI 0.78–0.92] vs 96.4% [95% CI 0.94–0.98], respectively; $P<.00005$) and less than 1 hour per day versus 1 to 6 hours per day groups (85.5% [95% CI 0.78–0.92] vs 91.3% [95% CI 0.88–0.94], respectively; $P = .01$). Based on these data, the investigators were able to demonstrate a linear trend with increasing survival with increased compliance ($P = .0004$). Of particular relevance to this review is that the minimal duration of use in the 1 to 6 hours per day group of 3.9 ± 1.4 hours per day still improved survival versus the less than 1 hour per day group. These data as a whole suggest that even a minimal amount of PAP therapy in this population may improve survival compared with none at all. Unfortunately, based on the LCD criteria, those patients who are not using the minimally required duration of therapy would have their reimbursement for CPAP stopped because it would be deemed "not reasonable and necessary."

COSTS OF NOVEL THERAPIES

Despite the significant body of evidence supporting negative long-term sequelae of nonadherence to CPAP, patient adherence continues to be an ongoing issue, with physicians exerting significant effort toward improving usage. Weaver and colleagues[35] evaluated CPAP use in patients with OSA over the first 90 days of therapy. Two distinct groups emerged, labeled "consistent users," who used CPAP more than 90% of the nights versus "intermittent users," who exhibited significant variability in usage. Consistent users used CPAP approximately 6.21 ± 1.21 hours per night versus intermittent users, who averaged 3.45 ± 1.94 hours per night. The investigators looked for potential predictors of intermittent users and noted that skipping CPAP therapy for 1 or 2 nights during the initial week of treatment was commonly seen in this subgroup. It is presumably in the consistent users that some studies have found long-term compliance rates for CPAP reported as high as 81% at 5 years and 70% at 10 years with average nightly use at 6.2 hours,[36] to as low as 68% at 5 years with average nightly use at 5.6 hours.[37] However, it would appear that even in this subgroup of committed patients, adherence is still somewhat deficient. Given these circumstances, the industry has been hard at work developing alternative therapies in hopes of achieving a level of therapeutic benefit comparable to CPAP but with increased likelihood of compliance. Two such innovations that show promise are nasal expiratory PAP (EPAP) and oral pressure therapy (OPT).

Nasal EPAP

The only nasal EPAP product that is currently cleared by the Food and Drug Administration to treat OSA is known under the brand name Provent Therapy (Ventus Medical, Inc, Belmont, CA). The device itself is a single-use, 1-way valve attached to the external aspect of the nares with a hypoallergenic adhesive. The principle behind its mechanism of action is to increase resistance on expiration, creating EPAP, which is maintained until the start of the next inspiration. The theory is that EPAP decreases the likelihood of complete airway collapse with inspiration because the end-expiratory narrowing (from the prior breath) is avoided. Berry and colleagues[38] investigated the efficacy of nasal EPAP by conducting a prospective, multicenter, sham-controlled, parallel-group, randomized double-blind clinical trial. Subjects with AHI of 10 or higher were randomized to sham or Provent. They underwent 2 PSGs: 1 with the device on and 1 with the device off. This procedure was done at baseline and at 3 months. Differences in AHI were compared between groups at both time points. At 1 week, the median AHI percent change during the device-on versus device-off night in the EPAP group was –52.7% compared with the sham group, which was –7.3% (P<.0001). At 3 months, the median percent change in the EPAP group was –42.7% versus –10.1% in the sham group (P<.001). As far as cost, currently a 30-day supply of these 1-time-use devices is $65.00. Unfortunately, as insurance coverage tends to lag behind medical innovation, there is at present only intermittent insurance coverage for this therapy.

OPT

The OPT system (Winx; ApniCure, Inc, Redwood City, CA) treats OSA by decreasing airway obstruction by creating a vacuum within the oral cavity to pull the soft palate anteriorly. The system essentially consists of 3 components: a vacuum pump, tubing, and an oral interface. The oral interface includes a mouthpiece and a lip seal, which is custom-molded to the patient's mouth. The tubing connects the mouthpiece to the bedside console, which contains the vacuum pump that generates negative pressure within the oral cavity. The suction generated pulls the soft palate forward, such that it abuts the posterior aspect of the tongue, increasing the oropharyngeal space. The patient breathes through the nose while on this therapy and thus it requires that patients be capable of closed-mouth breathing. In a feasibility study undertaken by Farid-Moayer and colleagues,[39] mean AHI dropped from 34.4 ± 28.9 (mean ± SD) to 20.7 ± 23.3 on therapy (P<.001). Despite the improvements in AHI reported, there was no mean AHI lower than 5 on therapy. As far as expense is concerned, if the patient is willing and able to pay cash for a Winx system, the costs would include the console at $800, mouthpiece at $95, and tubing at $35. Typically, the mouthpiece and tubing are replaced every 3 months with the lifetime of the console being typically about 5 years. In terms of insurance, the system is likely covered under the durable medical equipment (DME) benefit by payers. The typical DME benefit has a 20% copay that goes toward the annual maximum out-of-pocket. However, individual plans vary widely (John Cones, Sales director, ApniCure, 2012, personal communication).

Regardless of the difficulties that one may have with the applicability of these novel therapies, given the negative long-term outcomes of untreated OSA, as a field, we should continue to encourage and support these innovations. Additionally, advocating for reimbursement will ultimately benefit our patients, by giving them more affordable options for treatment.

SUMMARY

OSA is a common disease, often unrecognized, with potential health ramifications. It is also a chronic condition often present in patients with other comorbidities. Studies have clearly shown both quality of life and health benefits from treatment and possibly mortality reduction. In the studies that have examined cost-benefit ratio, treatment advantages far outweigh the costs of diagnosis for most.

REFERENCES

1. American Academy of Sleep Medicine. The international classification of sleep disorders: diagnostic and coding manual. 2nd edition. Westchester (IL): American Academy of Sleep Medicine; 2005.
2. Young T, Palta M, Dempsey J, et al. The occurrence of sleep-disordered breathing among middle-aged adults. N Engl J Med 1993;328:1230–5.
3. Young T, Finn L, Peppard PE, et al. Sleep disordered breathing and mortality: eighteen-year follow-up of the Wisconsin sleep cohort. Sleep 2008;31:1071–8.
4. Epstein LJ, Kristo D, Strollo PJ Jr, et al. Clinical guideline for the evaluation, management and long-term care of obstructive sleep apnea in adults. J Clin Sleep Med 2009;5:263–76.
5. Kushida CA, Littner MR, Morgenthaler T, et al. Practice parameters for the indications for polysomnography and related procedures: an update for 2005. Sleep 2005;28:499–521.
6. Collop NA, Anderson WM, Boehlecke B, et al. Clinical guidelines for the use of unattended portable monitors in the diagnosis of obstructive sleep apnea in adult patients. Portable Monitoring Task Force of the American Academy of Sleep Medicine. J Clin Sleep Med 2007;3:737–47.
7. Ferber R, Millman R, Coppola M, et al. Portable recording in the assessment of obstructive sleep apnea. ASDA standards of practice. Sleep 1994; 17:378–92.
8. The New England Comparative Effectiveness Public Advisory Council. Diagnosis and treatment of obstructive sleep apnea in adults. Supplementary data and analyses to the comparative effectiveness review of the Agency for Healthcare Research and Quality. The Institute for Clinical and Economic Review. Available at: http://cepac.icer-review.org/wp-content/uploads/2011/04/Final-Report_January20131.pdf. Accessed March 3, 2013.
9. Kuna ST, Gurubhagavatula I, Maislin G, et al. Noninferiority of functional outcome in ambulatory management of obstructive sleep apnea. Am J Respir Crit Care Med 2011;183:1238–44.
10. Rosen CL, Auckley D, Benca R, et al. A multisite randomized trial of portable sleep studies and positive airway pressure autotitration versus laboratory-based polysomnography for the diagnosis and treatment of obstructive sleep apnea: the HomePAP study. Sleep 2012;35:757–67.
11. Pietzsch JB, Garner A, Cipriano LE, et al. An integrated health-economic analysis of diagnostic and therapeutic strategies in the treatment of moderate-to-severe obstructive sleep apnea. Sleep 2011;34: 695–709.
12. Deutsch PA, Simmons MS, Wallace JM. Cost-effectiveness of split-night polysomnography and home studies in the evaluation of obstructive sleep apnea syndrome. J Clin Sleep Med 2006;2:145–53.
13. Ferguson KA, Cartwright R, Rogers R, et al. Oral appliances for snoring and obstructive sleep apnea: a review. Sleep 2006;29:244–62.
14. Loube MD, Strauss AM. Survey of oral appliance practice among dentists treating obstructive sleep apnea patients. Chest 1997;111:382–6.
15. Sadatsafavi M, Marra CA, Ayas NT, et al. Cost-effectiveness of oral appliances in the treatment of obstructive sleep apnoea-hypopnoea. Sleep Breath 2009;13:241–52.
16. Weaver TE, Sawyer AM. Adherence to continuous positive airway pressure treatment for obstructive sleep apnoea: implications for future interventions. Indian J Med Res 2010;131:245–58.
17. Kezirian EJ, Maselli J, Vittinghoff E, et al. Obstructive sleep apnea surgery practice patterns in the United States: 2000 to 2006. Otolaryngol Head Neck Surg 2010;143:441–7.
18. Kapur V, Blough DK, Sandblom RE, et al. The medical cost of undiagnosed sleep apnea. Sleep 1999; 22:749–55.
19. Ronald J, Delaive K, Roos L, et al. Health care utilization in the 10 years prior to diagnosis in obstructive sleep apnea syndrome patients. Sleep 1999; 22:225–9.
20. Albarrak M, Banno K, Sabbagh AA, et al. Utilization of healthcare resources in obstructive sleep apnea syndrome: a 5-year follow-up study in men using CPAP. Sleep 2005;28:1306–11.
21. Sassani A, Findley LJ, Kryger M, et al. Reducing motor-vehicle collisions, costs, and fatalities by treating obstructive sleep apnea syndrome. Sleep 2004;27:453–8.
22. Rothman KJ, Greenland S. Modern epidemiology. 2nd edition. Philadelphia: Lippincott-Raven; 1998.
23. Available at: http://www.cms.gov/Regulations-and-Guidance/Guidance/Manuals/downloads/nc103c1_Part4.pdf. Accessed March 2, 2013.
24. Available at: http://www.virtuox.net/dynadocs/Documents/LCDforPAP.pdf. Accessed March 2, 2013.
25. Aloia MS, Knoepke CE, Lee-Chiong T. The new local coverage determination criteria for adherence to positive airway pressure treatment: testing the limits? Chest 2010;138:875–9.
26. Engleman HM, Martin SE, Deary IJ, et al. Effect of continuous positive airway pressure treatment on daytime function in sleep apnoea/hypopnoea syndrome. Lancet 1994;343:572–5.
27. Engleman HM, Kingshott RN, Wraith PK, et al. Randomized placebo-controlled crossover trial of continuous positive airway pressure for mild sleep

apnea/hypopnea syndrome. Am J Respir Crit Care Med 1999;159:461–7.

28. Redline S, Adams N, Strauss ME, et al. Improvement of mild sleep-disordered breathing with CPAP compared with conservative therapy. Am J Respir Crit Care Med 1998;157:858–65.

29. Faccenda JF, Mackay TW, Boon NA, et al. Randomized placebo-controlled trial of continuous positive airway pressure on blood pressure in the sleep apnea-hypopnea syndrome. Am J Respir Crit Care Med 2001;163:344–8.

30. Alajmi M, Mulgrew AT, Fox J, et al. Impact of continuous positive airway pressure therapy on blood pressure in patients with obstructive sleep apnea hypopnea: a meta-analysis of randomized controlled trials. Lung 2007;185:67–72.

31. Bazzano LA, Khan Z, Reynolds K, et al. Effect of nocturnal nasal continuous positive airway pressure on blood pressure in obstructive sleep apnea. Hypertension 2007;50:417–23.

32. Haentjens P, Van Meerhaeghe A, Moscariello A, et al. The impact of continuous positive airway pressure on blood pressure in patients with obstructive sleep apnea syndrome: evidence from a meta-analysis of placebo-controlled randomized trials. Arch Intern Med 2007;167:757–64.

33. Turnbull F. Effects of different blood-pressure-lowering regimens on major cardiovascular events: results of prospectively-designed overviews of randomised trials. Lancet 2003;362:1527–35.

34. Campos-Rodriguez F, Pena-Grinan N, Reyes-Nunez N, et al. Mortality in obstructive sleep apnea-hypopnea patients treated with positive airway pressure. Chest 2005;128:624–33.

35. Weaver TE, Kribbs NB, Pack AI, et al. Night-to-night variability in CPAP use over the first three months of treatment. Sleep 1997;20:278–83.

36. Kohler M, Smith D, Tippett V, et al. Predictors of long-term compliance with continuous positive airway pressure. Thorax 2010;65:829–32.

37. McArdle N, Devereux G, Heidarnejad H, et al. Long-term use of CPAP therapy for sleep apnea/hypopnea syndrome. Am J Respir Crit Care Med 1999; 159:1108–14.

38. Berry RB, Kryger MH, Massie CA. A novel nasal expiratory positive airway pressure (EPAP) device for the treatment of obstructive sleep apnea: a randomized controlled trial. Sleep 2011;34:479–85.

39. Farid-Moayer M, Siegel LC, Black J. A feasibility evaluation of oral pressure therapy for the treatment of obstructive sleep apnea. Ther Adv Respir Dis 2013;7:3–12.

Residual Sleepiness in Obstructive Sleep Apnea
Differential Diagnosis, Evaluation, and Possible Causes

Carl D. Boethel, MD, DABSM[a,*], Anas Al-Sadi, MD[b],
James A. Barker, MD, CPE[c]

KEYWORDS

- Residual sleepiness • Excessive daytime sleepiness • Obstructive sleep apnea
- Continuous positive airway pressure

KEY POINTS

- There is evidence that patients with obstructive sleep apnea, although treated adequately with continuous positive airway pressure (CPAP), can have residual excessive daytime sleepiness.
- The data show that this may be related to other underlying sleep disorders such as insufficient sleep, narcolepsy, or restless legs syndrome.
- Sleep duration may be the most common cause of continued excessive daytime sleepiness.
- Given the confines of finite resources that clinicians face, finding a modality that can provide data without costing too much is the key.
- Some patients continue to have sleepiness after adequate treatment with CPAP, and until these patients can be better classified, it will be difficult to provide better treatment options.

INTRODUCTION

Excessive daytime sleepiness (EDS) is a common residual symptom of patients with obstructive sleep apnea (OSA) syndrome despite adequate treatment with continuous positive airway pressure (CPAP) therapy. Based on a multicenter trial from France, the prevalence rate of EDS is 6.0% (French multicenter study).[1] It has significant effects on daytime performance and cognitive function. Recent evidence also suggested an association with increased risk of hypertension,[2–5] insulin resistance,[6,7] and all-cause mortality.[8] EDS affects 2% of the middle-aged population who use CPAP. The approach to a patient with EDS should include a detailed medical history of the original symptoms and diagnosis, a history of compliance with CPAP treatment, and of the sequence of CPAP pressure adjustments.

Insufficient sleep and sleep hygiene must be discussed as well. Likewise, it is important to review the use of sedatives or sedating medications, and to exclude underlying medical and psychological disorders that might cause sleepiness.[9–11] Identification and correction of those factors in patients with OSA helps to improve mortality and morbidity.[2]

DEFINITION OF EDS

Sleepiness can be defined as a state of wakefulness in which an individual has an increased

---

[a] Division of Pulmonary, Critical Care, and Sleep Medicine, Scott & White Sleep Institute, Scott & White Healthcare, College of Medicine, Texas A&M Health Science Center, 2401 South 31st Street, Temple, TX 76508, USA;
[b] Department of Medicine, Scott & White Healthcare, 2401 South 31st, Temple, TX 76508, USA; [c] Pulmonary, Critical Care, and Sleep Disorders, Scott & White Health Plan, Scott & White Healthcare, Texas A&M School of Medicine, 2401 South 31st, Temple, TX 76508, USA
* Corresponding author.
E-mail address: cboethel@swmail.sw.org

Sleep Med Clin 8 (2013) 571–582
http://dx.doi.org/10.1016/j.jsmc.2013.07.003
1556-407X/13/$ – see front matter © 2013 Elsevier Inc. All rights reserved.

propensity to fall asleep.[12] OSA is often associated with EDS. Most definitions of the disorder require the presence of subjective, but not necessarily objective, sleepiness[13]; however, sleepiness is not reported by all patients with OSA, even when the condition is moderate or severe.[14] Johns defined excessive sleepiness as an interaction between sleep processes known as the homeostatic and circadian sleep drives competing with the brain's wake-processes, also known as the wakefulness drives.[14] When the balance of these two drives favors the sleep drive then the patient is more likely to fall asleep.[15,16] Sleep propensity is neither a state nor a physiologic drive but is the probability of falling asleep at a particular time. OSA syndrome can cause sleepiness, and it is one of the many complaints leading patients to seek medical attention. In an evaluation of 190 sleep clinic patients with OSA confirmed by polysomnography (PSG), their chief complaints were of lack of energy, tiredness, and fatigue. Sleepiness was less frequently reported; most often, lack of energy was the term used by patients to describe their daytime symptoms and feelings.[17] Several studies have investigated the relationship between sleepiness and fatigue in patients with sleep-disordered breathing, including OSA.

MEASURING EDS

The measurement of daytime sleepiness in patients with OSA is limited to subjective sleepiness based on patient complaints of fatigue, tiredness, and cognitive dysfunction. This measurement can be attained objectively in patients with OSA; however, this objective sleep testing does add extra expense to the patient and health care finance system. There may be separate phenotypes of OSA in which some patients with mild disease have severe daytime symptoms. However, other patients show evidence of severe sleep apnea with minimal, if any, subjective or objective complaints of daytime sleepiness, which reveals that the one-size-fits-all method of measuring sleepiness is not always effective, and patients and their sleep complaints should be judged on an individual basis. In the authors' sleep clinic, patients are seen at 4 to 6 weeks following initiation of CPAP therapy to review compliance download data and clinical outcomes.

Measuring sleepiness in patients requires both subjective and objective measures. The subjective measures usually entail patient complaints and can also be assessed using various sleep scales such as the Epworth Sleepiness Scale (ESS) and the Stanford Sleepiness Scale (SSS).[15] These scales are discussed later. Measuring sleepiness

objectively requires the use of a multiple sleep latency test (MSLT) and possibly a maintenance of wakefulness test (MWT). These tests have been validated in specific situations to aid the clinician in managing the sleepy patient.

In 2005, the American Academy of Sleep Medicine provided a practice parameter for the use of the MSLT and MWT. The practice parameter suggests that MSLT is not routinely indicated in the work-up of OSA syndrome, although it does give an objective measure of sleepiness for those patients with symptomatic EDS despite therapy. Moreover, MSLT is primarily used for the evaluation of patients with suspected narcolepsy. In addition, the MSLT is not indicated for the routine work-up of patients with disorders such as insomnia and circadian rhythm disorders.[17] The MWT is indicated for assessing patients in whom alertness and sleepiness constitute a safety issue (eg, pilots with OSA, truck drivers). In addition, it can be used in narcoleptics and patients with idiopathic hypersomnia to judge response to medication treatment. The American Academy of Sleep Medicine (AASM) does not recommend relying on the MWT as a sole measure of sleepiness because MWT results do not correlate well with the risk of accidents in real-world situations.

The MSLT involves a standardized series of naps that quantitate objectively the patient's propensity to fall asleep during the day. Patients usually complete a preceding overnight polysomnogram in which they must sleep for at least 6 hours. A urine drug screen is performed to rule out any medications that could cause a false-positive or false-negative test. It is recommended that patients discontinue all psychotropic or stimulant medications for 14 days before the test. The patient undergoes 5 naps to determine the mean sleep latency (MSL) as well to see whether there are any sleep onset rapid eye movement (REM) sleep periods. Each nap opportunity lasts at least 20 minutes. The patient is monitored for 15 minutes of clock time following the first epoch of sleep. A patient is considered to be excessively sleepy if the MSL is less than 8 minutes. In data of pooled narcoleptic studies, the MSL is 3.1 minutes, and in normal controls it is 10.5 minutes.[18]

The original studies done on the MSLT used normal healthy individuals who were exposed to sleep deprivation. These studies were performed in the 1970s and were used to help determine the so-called sleepability of the patient.[18] This test is valuable in determining ease with which a patient can fall asleep in a soporific setting; however, it does little to test the ability of a patient to stay awake under similar circumstances.

Therefore, in 1982, the MWT was developed to assess the ability of a patient to stay alert in a dark room. The MWT involves having a patient spend the night in the sleep laboratory under conditions as much like home as possible. For example, if a patient uses CPAP at home, the patient is studied using the CPAP mask at the pressure that is used in the home sleep environment. The patient then has the first monitoring period at 1.5 to 3 hours following waking. This monitoring involves the patient sitting upright in a darkened room. The patient may not vocalize or move excessively during the testing period. Repeat tests are performed every 2 hours. Patients are monitored for 20 minutes, although some protocols call for monitoring for 40 minutes. If they enter into a stage of sleep, the test is terminated. Patients are considered to have failed if they fall asleep in any of the monitored periods.

The MSLT is the gold standard for measuring sleepiness because there is no other method or test to determine the sleepiness of individuals. However, it mainly measures sleep latency. There have been a significant number of studies conducted that have examined the MSLT in OSA. Patients had a benefit in MSL from 6.8 minutes before CPAP usage to 11.6 minutes with CPAP usage. In terms of the effect of CPAP on the measurement of time in the MWT, the data show a significant improvement in MSL from 18.8 minutes to 26.3 minutes when performed using a 40-minute protocol.[18] There are data that show an improvement in sleepiness objectively when CPAP is used in patients with OSA. The practice parameters provided by the AASM do not advocate an MSLT in patients with OSA with residual daytime sleepiness (RDS). There are benefits to proceeding with an MSLT and MWT, but the added cost, inconvenience to the patient, and the possibility that it will not yield adequate data are reasons to consider avoiding this test for work-up. AASM leaves this practice parameter open to the clinician's discretion, and it can be used to give an idea of the propensity of a patient to go to sleep who is compliant with CPAP therapy.

Patients usually are asked to fill out a subjective measure of sleepiness. The most commonly used clinical device to measure daytime sleepiness is the ESS. This scale was developed at the Epworth Hospital in Melbourne, Australia, by Dr Murray Johns. This scale is a questionnaire that asks patients to rate their propensity to doze off in 8 specific situations. These situations include activities that involve sitting, lying down, being mentally active, and also being mentally relaxed. Patients rate their sleep propensity between 0 and 3. Thus, patients can score as high as 24 or as low as 0. A score of 10 or greater has been validated to suggest a high likelihood of dozing.[19] Based on research performed in Australia, the United Kingdom, and Italy, the average normal nonsleepy adult has an Epworth score of approximately 4.[19]

The ESS was superior to the MSLT and MWT at determining the level of sleepiness in comparing narcoleptic patients with normal controls.[14] ESS scores were high in patients with moderate to severe sleep apnea.[16] In patients with OSA, the mean score in Dr Johns' original study was 11.7 ± 4.6. Narcoleptics scored higher at 17.5 ± 3.5 and primary snorers scored 6.5 ± 3.[16] The ESS has been validated in patients with OSA and shows a linear increase associated with the apnea-hypopnea index (AHI). This test now represents the most widely used method of measuring subjective sleepiness in patients. It is a valuable tool to use in clinics to follow therapeutic effect on patients treated for sleep apnea.[20] In a study published in 2010, the benefit of CPAP on MWT results showed that approximately 70% of patients have normal sleep latencies when tested with the MWT. This study also showed a dose-dependent and compliance-dependent benefit in the ESS with usage of CPAP. The MWT may have merit in the work-up of patients with RDS, although further research in this area would add to the strength of this argument. At present, the Federal Aviation Administration uses the MWT to test pilots with OSA for evidence of continued sleepiness, but, based on this study, it may not be as effective a measuring true EDS.[21]

The AASM does not recommend the use of an MSLT with the initial diagnosis of OSA, but they do leave the use of the MWT to the clinician's judgment. In certain situations, it may be reasonable to use an MSLT or MWT to measure the effectiveness of CPAP treatment in the laboratory, but, based on the data mentioned earlier, clinical acumen and the ESS seem to be just as effective at determining the need for further treatment of EDS in compliant patients with OSA.

CAUSES OF RESIDUAL SLEEPINESS IN PATIENTS WITH OSA
Chronic Intermittent Hypoxia Theory

It is important to understand that OSA causes behavioral and neuropsychological deficits that lead to sleepiness in patients with RDS, but it may not be the only disorder that is responsible for a patient's sleepiness. It has been postulated that chronic intermittent hypoxia results in neuronal brain injury resulting in EDS. In a recent study from China, Feng and colleagues[22] found a correlation between intermittent hypoxia and hippocampal injury. They postulate that oxidative stress that result in inflammation and apoptosis lead to cell damage and neuronal injury. In animal models, Gozal and colleagues[23] showed an association between intermittent hypoxia and marked cellular changes over time within the cortex and hippocampus of rats. These changes were associated with substantial deterioration of behavioral performance. This finding is discussed in more detail later in this article.

OSA in Insufficient Sleep

Essential in the evaluation of patients presenting with EDS is the determination adequate sleep time, which is measured on PSG as sleep efficiency. Behaviorally induced insufficient sleep may lead to EDS in patients with OSA despite getting adequate amounts of use of the CPAP machine on a nightly basis. Medicare guidelines require a minimum of 4 hours of nightly usage to qualify for payment of the CPAP machine, but this number may not be sufficient to maintain the level of alertness needed for daytime functioning.[24] The National Sleep Foundation 2000 Omnibus Sleep in America Poll showed that only one-third (33%) of adults say that they get at least the recommended 8 hours or more of sleep per night during the workweek; and one-third (33%) of adults say that they get fewer than 6.5 hours of sleep per night during the workweek. Insufficient sleep is expected to lead to frank EDS, but the more common subjective complaints are tiredness, lack of energy, or fatigue.[25–27] Kales and colleagues[26] studied 50 patients with OSA and explored the psychosocial consequences of the disorder. Seventy-six percent of patients had mild to severe deficits in terms of thinking, perception, memory, communication, or the ability to learn new information, resulting in a greater potential for being distractible, confused, and irritable.[23]

Depression

Depression seems to be prevalent in OSA. Guilleminault and colleagues[27] reported that 24% of 25 male patients with OSA had previously seen a psychiatrist for anxiety or depression. In a study by Schwartz and colleagues,[28] 41% of patients with OSA referred for a sleep evaluation showed depressive symptoms, and 39% received antidepressant treatment, indicating an association between the two disorders.[28–31] The complex relationship between the two conditions makes it difficult to assess the underlying cause and the impact of treatment on each condition. An epidemiologic study of 18,980 subjects representative of the general population in the United Kingdom, Germany, Italy, Portugal, and Spain assessed by a cross-sectional telephone survey, found that 17.6% of subjects with a Diagnostic and Statistical Manual of Mental Disorders, Fourth Edition (DSM-IV) breathing-related sleep disorder diagnosis also presented with a major depressive disorder diagnosis, and vice versa.[32,33] Frequent snoring or stopping breathing has an association with major depression by the Personal Health Questionnaire (PHQ-9) a national sample of adults.[34,35] Symptoms other than EDS that greatly affect daytime functioning are neuropsychological symptoms such as irritability, difficulty concentrating, cognitive impairment, depressive symptoms, and other psychological disturbances.

On PSG, patients with major depression typically have a prolonged sleep latency, frequent nocturnal awakenings, and early morning awakenings. They often show a decreased amount of slow wave or stage 3 sleep. Furthermore, their polysomnographic data may reveal a shortened REM latency. In comparison, patients with OSA show fragmented sleep with a large fraction of transitional sleep stages,[36] primarily stage 1 sleep. CPAP treatment and its effect to improve depressive symptoms in patients with concomitant OSA have revealed mixed findings. One large systematic review of 26 studies on the influence of CPAP and its effect on neurobehavioral performance supported the clinical assertion that typically depressive symptoms remit together with EDS under CPAP therapy, and improvement is closely associated with compliance and duration of treatment.

Narcolepsy

The prevalence of narcolepsy is estimated to be 0.02% to 0.18% of narcolepsy-cataplexy in European countries, Japan, and the United States. The prevalence of narcolepsy without cataplexy is unknown.[37] Narcolepsy typically presents in the second or third decade of life; men and women are roughly equally affected. The disease has 4 cardinal features, namely marked daytime sleepiness, cataplexy, hypnagogic hallucinations, and sleep paralysis. Some investigators view sleep fragmentation as a fifth cardinal feature. Cataplexy is pathognomonic for narcolepsy and consists of loss of skeletal muscle tone but spares the diaphragm and external ocular muscles. Penetrance of severity can range from eyelid twitching to falling to the ground. Patients who lose all muscle tone are usually able to maintain awareness of their surroundings, although they may eventually fall asleep.[39] Narcolepsy with cataplexy may be familial in some cases, with a 1% to 2% risk for development of this disorder in first-degree relatives. An autosomal dominant pattern is seen. However, most cases are sporadic.[39] Narcolepsy with cataplexy is closely associated with the human leukocyte antigen (HLA) subtypes DR2 (DRB1*1501) and DQ (DQB1*0602). The most common HLA marker associated with narcolepsy with cataplexy is DQB1*0602, with a prevalence of 85% to 95%.[38]

Narcolepsy and OSA may coexist in the same patient, but the association between these conditions has not been determined. A few studies assessing the prevalence of OSA in narcolepsy are available, and reported results range between 2% and 68%. Sansa and colleagues[32] evaluated 33 narcoleptics with AHI greater than 10. Of these 30.3% were initially diagnosed in other sleep centers as having only OSA. Eighty percent of them had cataplexy, which was already present when patients first complained of EDS in other sleep centers. Santamaria and colleagues[5] found that OSA affected a small percentage of patients with a prior diagnosis of narcolepsy. They examined 152 narcoleptic patients between 1991 and 2006, and found an AHI greater than 10 in 21%.[40-43] The diagnosis may be confirmed by PSG, which usually shows short sleep latency and may show early REM sleep onset, followed by an MSLT, which should reveal 2 or more sleep-onset REM periods with an MSL of 8 minutes or less.[44] Patients who have atypical cataplexylike events, and in whom other sleep disorders have been excluded, require confirmatory sleep studies or cerebrospinal fluid hypocretin levels for the diagnosis. HLA testing is not a useful screening or diagnostic tool; however, it might be useful in atypical narcolepsy with cataplexy presentations.[38] The traditional treatment of EDS in narcolepsy has been with stimulants, such as methylphenidate or dextroamphetamine, but modafinil or armodafinil have recently become the first-line treatment of most patients. Treatment of cataplexy with tricyclic antidepressant agents and serotonin reuptake inhibitors (SSRIs) has been used for the treatment of cataplexy. More recently, sodium oxybate has been highly efficacious for the treatment of cataplexy in narcolepsy, and it is also effective at improving sleep quality in these patients, with resultant improvement in the patient's complaints of excessive sleepiness.

If narcolepsy is found in conjunction with OSA, caution should be used, given the sedative nature of sodium oxybate and the possibility of respiratory depression.[45]

Restless Legs Syndrome and Periodic Leg Movements in Sleep

Restless legs syndrome (RLS) is characterized by unpleasant leg sensations and an urge to move the legs when at rest. Most patients with RLS do not have EDS but rather suffer from insomnia, with resultant sleep fragmentation, and inadequate amounts of sleep. However, it is possible that RLS can result in EDS. The symptoms of RLS interfere with initiating sleep because patients want to get out of bed and move around. The discomfort may be relieved by walking or by stretching, but it returns when patients are again motionless. The interference with falling sleep reduces total sleep time, and can produce EDS. Patients with RLS have an increased incidence of depression, and many antidepressant medications, in particular SSRIs, worsen RLS symptoms.[46] Kallweit and colleagues[35] studied 27 patients with RLS on therapy to identify EDS symptoms and found improvement in ESS score with improvement in RLS symptoms.[47]

Inadequate CPAP Treatment

CPAP is an effective method in the treatment of OSA. Several studies have documented ineffective treatment of OSA as a cause of residual EDS in these patients. The consequences of residual sleep apnea could be significant because patients with OSA may be at increased risk of cardiovascular complications and motor vehicle crashes.[48] Also, suboptimal CPAP treatment has been shown to be ineffective in lowering blood pressure.[49] Patients with inadequately treated OSA report excessive daytime sleepiness; however, this symptom seems to improve with adequate CPAP retitration.[50] Therefore, it may be in the patient's best interest to have a repeat sleep study to ensure adequate CPAP pressures. Most available CPAP machines sold in the United States now require measurements of compliance and can provide evidence of residual apneas and hypopneas. These data allow the sleep physician the opportunity to review a patient's night-by-night sleep and aid in determining a cause of the continued daytime sleepiness. A recent study by Mulgrew and colleagues[50] showed that patients with a high likelihood of moderate to severe OSA had continued evidence of residual apneas and hypopneas. This evidence was seen in patients who were treated with both in-laboratory titrations and autotitrations done at home. Despite rigorous efforts to improve this disorder, many of these patients continued to have EDS. Periodic breathing and central events are prevalent in patients with residual sleep apnea, particularly in severely affected patients.[51]

Central sleep apnea can be seen in some patients who are on CPAP, with various potential causes (eg, heart failure, narcotics, prior stroke), but patients experience arousals associated with these events. Therefore, ruling out central apneas is key to insuring adequate treatment of patients with OSA with RDS. Several hypotheses have been proposed for the emergence of central apneas following the initiation of CPAP therapy. Overtitration of CPAP is thought to lead to central apneas,[51] and occasionally even the initiation of CPAP can worsen sleep quality with the onset of cyclic alternating breathing, which is a form of central apnea. In such cases, the ventilatory response to arousal can drive the $Paco_2$ to less than the CO_2 apnea threshold, resulting in central apnea during subsequent sleep. This sleep disruption at the initiation of CPAP and the associated CO_2 fluctuations also tend to resolve over time as patients habituate to the interface (mask) and the application of positive pressure.[44] This process can be seen in patients using bilevel positive airway pressure, caused by augmented tidal volumes from inspiratory positive airway pressures, which drive down arterial CO_2 tensions. If it decreases to less than the apnea threshold, then central apnea occurs.[44,52]

When central sleep apneas occur as part of Cheyne-Stokes breathing (crescendo-decrescendo pattern of breathing) after initiation of CPAP, it is called complex sleep apnea. There is debate in the literature on whether this is a true disorder or an epiphenomenon of heart failure. The authors' experience shows that patients who develop Cheyne-Stokes breathing have arousals associated with the hyperpneas as well as the apneas. This may be the cause of RDS in this patient population. Servo positive airway pressure (PAP) devices are highly effective for this disorder. However, the breathing pattern can be stabilized by retitrating CPAP for the patient with complex sleep apnea. In the case of treatment-emergent central apneas, studies showed that these events generally resolve spontaneously over time.[52] Javeheri has shown that treatment with CPAP alone can resolve these central events.[44]

Underlying Causes of Residual Sleepiness: Biomarkers, Cytokines, and Hormones

Literature over the past 20 years has shown evidence of a strong relationship between OSA and cardiovascular consequences. In addition, there are increasing data suggesting that patients with OSA are at higher risks of automobile accidents. There are fewer data showing why patients with OSA may have RDS despite adequate CPAP compliance. Unlike in the setting of a myocardial infarction, in which a troponin increase indicates cardiac damage, sleep apnea lacks a biomarker. In addition, sleepiness does not seem to have a single biomarker that may represent a test that can aid the clinician in treatment and management of the sleepy patient. The American Academy of Medicine recently published in the *Journal of Clinical Sleep Medicine* a supplement that focused on ongoing research in this area,[38] but the so-called troponin of sleep remains elusive. Despite the lack of a biomarker, new data suggest that cytokines, chemokines, and hormonal changes in the brain may play a role in EDS in patients with OSA, and there the literature shows that direct neuronal injury may be a cause of the RDS in these patients.

Based on research presented in 2011, there is evidence that patients with OSA have significant neuronal changes in the frontal lobe and hippocampus. In a study presented by O'Donoghue and colleagues,[45] from a comparison of 30 patients with severe OSA with 25 age-matched male subjects, patients were evaluated with magnetic resonance spectroscopy (MRS). This method allows the measurement of metabolites of neuronal function in specific brain areas. The 2 specific areas that were examined were the hippocampus and the frontal cortex or lobe. Certain measured metabolites suggest viable neurons, such as *N*-acetylaspartate (NAA), primarily in the frontal lobe. Other compounds, most notably choline, occur in higher concentrations when there is myelin injury, which is mainly visualized on MRS in the hippocampus. Patients with OSA had statistically significant differences in NAA and choline compared with the healthy controls. The patients were studied both before and after treatment with CPAP, and there did not seem to be any improvement in the measured NAA levels, which suggests that the frontal lobe is highly susceptible to injury from OSA. However, the differences in the NAA levels were not seen with the choline metabolites after treatment with CPAP. Choline is associated with membrane turnover, a sign of inflammation, and it seems that the hippocampus is susceptible to intermittent hypoxia, which is the mechanism that seems to affect patients. Based on these data, it seems that sleep apnea, and notably the chronic intermittent hypoxia that is seen in severe OSA, causes injury to various brain structures. The investigators focused on the two areas mentioned earlier, but this suggests that other areas of the brain could be affected. Although this may not represent the main cause of residual sleepiness in patients with OSA, there is evidence of brain injury, and theoretically the intermittent hypoxia could play a role in leading to EDS in these patients. Animal models show that subjects exposed to intermittent hypoxia have similar inflammation, and in mice there seems to be the development of spatial learning deficits.[46] The cause of this development of brain injury and residual sleepiness is most likely related to several factors. Chronic intermittent hypoxia (CIH), associated with recurrent apneas and hypopneas, incites the development of inflammation in the body, and the brain seems to be affected as well as other organs. In addition, there seems to be development of significant cytokines and adhesion molecules that affect vascular tissue and also affect the neuronal tissue. Greenberg and colleagues[47] showed that mice exposed to CIH had increased amounts of nuclear factor kB (NF-kB) activity involving cardiovascular tissue compared with mice in controlled settings. The mice showed that the aorta was more sensitive to CIH, as opposed to the heart and lungs. NF-kB is an oxidant-sensitive proinflammatory transcription factor. It is measured in neutrophils, monocytes, and vascular tissues. This transcription factor is capable of producing cytokines such as interleukin (IL)-6, IL-8, and tumor necrosis factor (TNF)-a. It is also responsible for producing adhesion molecules such as intercellular adhesion molecule 1 (ICAM-1), vascular cell adhesion molecule-1 (VCAM-1), and E-selectin. Based on the resulting levels of inflammation in the vascular bed, it can be surmised that this must affect the blood vessels throughout the body, including the brain. Having been studied in a model of OSA with CIH in mice, a study was done in humans. The study examined 22 patients with varying degrees of sleep apnea. Examining NF-kB levels and gene products such as soluble E-selectin and (VCAM-1), patients with OSA showed a 4.8-fold to 7.9-fold increase in NF-kB activity compared with control patients. The level of NF-kB activity correlated with the level of severity of the OSA. Patients were then evaluated for NF-kB activity after treatment with PAP. These patients self-reported their CPAP usage and, in the patients with severe OSA, there was a trend toward lower levels of E-selectin and VCAM-1. The weakness of this study is that there were only 5 patients in the severe range, and subjective measures of PAP compliance often overestimate usage.[53] So why is NF-kB important in OSA and inflammation? It seems that, in vitro, hypoxia that is intermittent sets off the NF-kB molecule. Other triggers can activate it as well, including infection, oxidants, free radicals, and cytokines. It seems to be a central transcription factor involved in the inflammatory cascade, with resultant adhesion molecules, cytokines, coagulation factors, and chemokines causing a proinflammatory state that can lead to atherosclerosis.[54] The cytokines (TNF-a, IL-6, and so forth) can cause a positive feedback loop with NF-kB, inciting a worsening of this cascade, which can lead to damage not only to the heart and vascular bed but to the cerebrovascular bed as well. Thus, a possible result includes lacunar infarcts and/or neuronal cell death.

TNF-a, IL-1, growth hormone–releasing hormone, adenosine, and prostaglandin D2 have been shown to induce non–rapid eye movement sleep. These substances have met criteria for consideration as a sleep regulatory substance. Criteria that investigators use to determine whether a substance plays a role in modification of sleep include the following:

1. The substance can enhance sleep if injected
2. Inhibitors of the substance can reduce sleep
3. The substance works on sleep regulatory circuits
4. The substance enhances sleepiness in abnormal states
5. The level of the substance changes based on level of sleepiness[55]

TNF-a is increased in several conditions, including rheumatoid arthritis, ankylosing spondylitis, postdialysis fatigue, and sleep apnea. IL-6 has been found to increase in patients with sleep apnea and acute and chronic sleep deprivation. IL-1 and TNF-a both seem to be responsible for the sleepiness that accompanies febrile illness. Vgontzas and colleagues[56] revealed increased concentrations of inflammatory cytokines including TNF-a and IL-6 in patients who have disorders of sleepiness. These disorders included sleep apnea, narcolepsy, and idiopathic hypersomnia. They compared 12 patients with OSA with 11 narcoleptics, 8 patients with idiopathic hypersomnia, and 10 normal controls. They also studied IL-1B because it has been implicated in causing sleepiness. Only IL-6 and TNF-a levels were statistically lower in the normal controls, but there was no difference between the IL-1B levels in the patients with EDS and the controls. Their data also revealed an association between sleep fragmentation and increased TNF-a levels in patients with high body mass index.

Etanercept, a TNF-a inhibitor, may alleviate daytime sleepiness. In a study of 8 obese male patients with moderate to severe OSA, etanercept was given twice weekly for 3 weeks. The patients were assessed by overnight PSG and multiple sleep latency testing 3 times during the research protocol. A significant improvement was seen in the MSL in the patients treated with etanercept.

The TNF-a levels were similar in treated patients as opposed to patients receiving placebo. However, the IL-6 level was significantly decreased in the treated patients.[57] Thus, the objective levels of sleepiness improved in these patients with a short course of treatment, showing that treating the inflammatory cascade improved daytime sleepiness independently of the OSA treatment.

Sympathetic tone is increased in patients with OSA, and this is secondary to sympathetic nerve activity increasing in response to arousal from sleep, as well as hypoxemia, hypercapnia, and increased respiratory effort. This finding occurs not only with the acute apneic episode, but seems to carry over into the waking hours as well.[58] Sympathetic nervous system discharge occurring with apneas can cause vasoconstriction, which can be seen using peripheral arterial tonometry.[59,60] It must be assumed that the cerebral vascular bed is susceptible to the same vasoconstriction effects that occur in the throughout the body, and these can lead to a decrease in blood flow and the intermittent hypoxia to the tissue capillary beds.

The evidence shows that patients with OSA are more likely to have inflammation of the vascular bed, and there is evidence of this inflammation based on cytokine and inflammatory markers as well on measures of sympathetic tone. CPAP has been shown to reduce cytokines and inflammation. In a study that explored this relationship, patients were tested for TNF-a, IL-6, leukotriene B-4, and soluble TNF-a receptor (sTNFR), which is another marker of inflammation. The 2 arms of the study compared obese controls with obese patients with OSA. All markers except the sTNFR were similar between the two groups, but the sTNFR levels were higher in the OSA group. CPAP lowered circulating levels of the sTNFR after 3 months of therapy. The investigators of this study did not report whether overall TNF-a levels were affected by CPAP.[60] In terms of how this level of inflammation and endothelial function affects patients who have residual sleepiness after CPAP usage, one study showed that RDS does not represent a risk factor for cardiovascular disease. El-Solh and colleagues[61] found that CPAP-compliant patients with OSA with RDS did not have an increase in the inflammatory markers of C-reactive protein, TNF-a, or IL-6 compared with healthy controls. These studies show that TNF-a and IL-6 may be responsible for some of the sleepiness associated with untreated OSA, but it seems that CPAP alone improves the risk of endothelial injury, and that the RDS may have another cause, such as prior neuronal injury.

Orexin (also referred to as hypocretin) plays a major role in maintaining alertness and in narcolepsy with cataplexy, and shows normal levels in both treated and untreated patients with OSA.[62,63] Unlike narcoleptics with cataplexy, this does not seem to be a mechanism for the cause of residual sleepiness in OSA. However, orexin is inhibited by glucose and leptin. Leptin is an anorexogenic hormone that signals satiety in normal individuals. In patients with OSA, there is evidence of leptin resistance. In studies done in mice, orexin correlates negatively with leptin.[64] Although the relationship between leptin and orexin primarily relates to energy balance and food intake, leptin can inhibit orexin and so may play a role in the drowsiness associated with sleep apnea and in RDS. Although the exact nature of the relationship between OSA and chemical changes in the body and brain has been explored in animal models, the evaluation in human subjects does not have a clear picture at this time. From review of the literature, we suspect that improvement of daytime sleepiness in CPAP-compliant patients may not occur with CPAP alone in certain individuals. This subgroup may require stimulant medications in addition to PAP therapy to alleviate symptoms of somnolence.

Treatment of EDS in Patients with OSA

The bulk of the information concerning treatment of residual EDS in patients with OSA concerns the use of 2 medications: modafinil and the r-isomer, armodafinil. These medications are alerting agents that have US Food and Drug Administration approval for treatment of EDS associated with narcolepsy, shift work sleep disorder, and OSA syndrome. Modafinil was initially used to treat memory and EDS in OSA in 1997. The patients had a benefit in length of subjective daytime vigilance and improvement in memory without affecting nighttime sleep and respiration.[65] Pack and colleagues[66] examined the benefit that modafinil could have on patients with OSA with RDS. Patients were selected for the study if they had used CPAP for 2 months and had complaints of EDS with a concomitant ESS of 10 or more. Patient compliance was judged based on 4 or more hours of use per night on 5 of 7 nights per week over a 3-week period at home. The patients were randomized to placebo or modafinil and were evaluated with ESS and then with an overnight polysomnogram and MSLT. Patients who randomized to modafinil normalized their ESS scores at 4 weeks of therapy with the medication plus CPAP. Patients with placebo had improvement as well, but the difference between the two groups came when evaluating the MSLT. The patients given CPAP plus modafinil had improvement in their MSLs by 1.2 minutes, whereas the placebo patients showed worsening of their MSL.

Another study that examined the functional quality of life in patients with OSA who used CPAP found that the ESS score was lowered on average from 14 to approximately 8 in the patients receiving modafinil.[67] The benefit of modafinil to improve sleepiness in compliant patients with OSA was confirmed by a study done in Brazil that used the MWT instead of the MSLT to determine MSL. In this study, CPAP compliance was judged adequate if patients used their CPAP for 5 or more hours per night. ESS was measured, and there was a significant reduction in the ESS score of the modafinil treatment group. There was no difference in the MWT scores between the modafinil and placebo groups.[68] In a 12-month international study, modafinil was measured against placebo in patients with OSA. Patients were tested on functional quality of life with the Functional Outcomes of Sleep Questionnaire (FOSQ), the ESS, and the Short Form-36 Health Survey (SF-36). ESS scores improved at 3, 6, 9, and 12 months, but the FOSQ and SF-36 showed improvement at 6 and 12 months of therapy. This study was mainly designed to test the long-term efficacy and maintenance of alertness over time.[69]

Roth and colleagues[70,71] examined the benefit of armodafinil in the treatment of residual EDS in patients with OSA in a 12-week, double-blind, placebo-controlled trial. They collected data for the MWT, ESS, Clinical Global Impression of Change (CGI-C), and the Brief Fatigue Inventory. Three-hundred and ninety-five patients were enrolled and treated with armodafinil 150 mg, 250 mg, or placebo. There was no evidence of difference between treatment groups. The MSL in the MWT was significantly greater in the armodafinil groups,[70] and this was found again in patients with OSA and comorbid major depression. These patients were treated with armodafinil or placebo, and there was a significant improvement in MSL on the MWT as well as an improvement in the CGI-C test.

Adverse events associated with modafinil and armodafinil include headache, migraine, and dizziness. We found no head-to-head trials between either of these medications and other stimulants such as methylphenidate or dextroamphetamine. Modafinil and armodafinil seem to offer a safe and effective therapy for treatment of residual sleepiness in OSA. Patients should be evaluated with an ESS and the clinician should use judgment on when to proceed with an MWT or MSLT. It is not clear that the MWT or MSLT is superior to the ESS alone, but, when there is a question of malingering or when a patient does not tolerate modafinil or armodafinil, it is reasonable to use the MWT or MSLT in conjunction with an urine drug screen to confirm daytime sleepiness in a patient who claims to have RDS.

SUMMARY

There is evidence that patients with OSA, although treated adequately with CPAP, can have residual EDS. The data show that this may be related to other underlying sleep disorders such as insufficient sleep, narcolepsy, or RLS. When addressing patients with complaints of EDS, it is important to eliminate as many treatable causes of EDS as possible. This process should include a thorough evaluation of time spent sleeping each night either using an actigraph or the download data from the patient's CPAP to clarify the sleep duration, which may be the most common cause of continued EDS. Further areas of study concerning patients treated adequately for OSA include looking for a biomarker that can easily measure alertness or sleepiness. Radiological modalities may offer another means of assessing patients with EDS, but standards of care from national organizations are necessary. However, clinicians are responsible for treating patients within the confines of finite resources, and finding a modality that can provide data without costing too much is key. Some patients continue to have sleepiness after adequate treatment with CPAP, and until these patients can be better classified, it will be difficult to outline better treatment options. This area holds promise for future research and development.

REFERENCES

1. Gooneratne NS, Richards KC, Joffe M, et al. Sleep disordered breathing with excessive daytime sleepiness is a risk factor for mortality in older adults. Sleep 2011;34(4):435–42.
2. Pépin JL, Viot-Blanc V, Escourrou P, et al. Prevalence of residual excessive sleepiness in CPAP-treated sleep apnoea patients: the French multicentre study. Eur Respir J 2009;33(5):1062–7.
3. Jacobsen J, Shi L, Mokhlesi B. Factors associated with excessive daytime sleepiness in patients with severe obstructive sleep apnea. Sleep Breath 2013;17(2):629–35.
4. Nguyên XL, Rakotonanahary D, Chaskalovic J, et al. Residual subjective daytime sleepiness under CPAP treatment in initially somnolent apnea patients: a pilot study using data mining methods. Sleep Med 2008;9(5):511–6.
5. Santamaria J, Iranzo A, Ma Montserrat J, et al. Persistent sleepiness in CPAP treated obstructive

sleep apnea patients: evaluation and treatment. Sleep Med Rev 2007;11(3):195–207.

6. Kapur VK, Baldwin CM, Resnick HE, et al. Sleepiness in patients with moderate to severe sleep-disordered breathing. Sleep 2005;28(4):472–7.

7. Ye L. Factors influencing daytime sleepiness in Chinese patients with obstructive sleep apnea. Behav Sleep Med 2011;9(2):117–27.

8. Bixler EO, Vgontzas AN, Lin HM, et al. Excessive daytime sleepiness in a general population sample: the role of sleep apnea, age, obesity, diabetes, and depression. J Clin Endocrinol Metab 2005;90(8):4510–5.

9. Dement WC. Encyclopedia of sleep and dreaming. New York: Macmillan Publishing Company; 1993. p. 554–9.

10. TYoung T, Palta M, Dempsey J, et al. The occurrence of sleep-disordered breathing among middle-aged adults. N Engl J Med 1993;328(17):1230–5.

11. Barbé F, Mayoralas LR, Duran J, et al. Treatment with continuous positive airway pressure is not effective in patients with sleep apnea but no daytime sleepiness. A randomized, controlled trial. Ann Intern Med 2001;134(11):1015–23.

12. Chervin RD. Sleepiness, fatigue, tiredness, and lack of energy in obstructive sleep apnea. Chest 2000;118(2):372–9.

13. Hanly PJ, Shapiro CM. Excessive daytime sleepiness. In: Shapiro CM, editor. Sleep solutions manual. Quebec (Canada): Kommunicom Publications; 1995. p. 77–103.

14. Johns MW. A new method of measuring daytime sleepiness; the Epworth Sleepiness Scale. Sleep 1991;14:540–5.

15. Hoddes E, Zarcone V, Smythe H, et al. Quantification of sleepiness a new approach. Psychophysiology 1973;10(4):431–6.

16. Johns MW. Sensitivity and specificity of the Multiple Sleep Latency Test (MSLT), the Maintenance of Wakefulness Test (MWT), and the Epworth Sleepiness Scale: failure of the MSLT as gold standard. J Sleep Res 2000;9:5–11.

17. Littner MR, Kushida C, Wise M, et al. Practice parameters for clinical use of the multiple sleep latency test and the maintenance of wakefulness test. Sleep 2005;28(1):113–21.

18. Arand D, Bonnet M, Hurwitz T, et al. The clinical use of the multiple sleep latency test and maintenance of wakefulness test. Sleep 2005;28(1):123–44.

19. ESS website. Available at: www.epworthsleepinessscale.com. Accessed January, 2013.

20. Johns MW. Daytime sleepiness, snoring, and obstructive sleep apnea: the Epworth Sleepiness Scale. Chest 1993;103:30–6.

21. Antic NA, Catcheside P, Buchan C, et al. The effect of CPAP in normalizing daytime sleepiness, quality of life, and neurocognitive function in patients with moderate to severe OSA. Sleep 2011;34:111–9.

22. Feng J, Wu Q, Zhang D, et al. Hippocampal impairments are associated with intermittent hypoxia of obstructive sleep apnea. Chin Med J 2012;125(4):696–701.

23. Gozal D, Daniel JM, Dohanich GP. Behavioral and anatomical correlates of chronic episodic hypoxia during sleep in the rat. J Neurosci 2001;21(7):2442–50.

24. Medicare website. Available at: http://www.cms.gov/MLNGenInfo. Accessed January, 2013.

25. Dinges DF. An overview of sleepiness and accidents. J Sleep Res 1995;4(S2):4–14.

26. Kales A, Caldwell AB, Cadieux RJ, et al. Severe obstructive sleep apnea—II: associated psychopathology and psychosocial consequences. J Chronic Dis 1985;38(5):427–34.

27. Guilleminault C, Eldridge FL, Tilkian A, et al. Sleep apnea syndrome due to upper airway obstruction: a review of 25 cases. Arch Intern Med 1977;137(3):296–300.

28. Schwartz DJ, Kohler WC, Karatinos G. Symptoms of depression in individuals with obstructive sleep apnea may be amenable to treatment with continuous positive airway pressure. Chest 2005;128(3):1304–9.

29. Ohayon MM. The effects of breathing-related sleep disorders on mood disturbances in the general population. J Clin Psychiatry 2003;64(10):1195–200 [quiz: 1274–6].

30. Wheaton AG, Perry GS, Chapman DP. Sleep disordered breathing and depression among U.S. adults: National Health and Nutrition Examination Survey, 2005-2008. Sleep 2012;35(4):461–7.

31. Schröder CM, O'Hara R. Depression and obstructive sleep apnea OSA. Ann Gen Psychiatry 2005;4:13.

32. Sansa G, Iranzo A, Santamaria J. Obstructive sleep apnea in narcolepsy. Sleep Med 2010;11(1):93–5.

33. Rack M, Davis J, Roffwarg HP, et al. The multiple sleep latency test in the diagnosis of narcolepsy. Am J Psychiatry 2005;162(11):2198–9.

34. Ulfberg J, Nyström B, Carter N, et al. Prevalence of restless legs syndrome among men aged 18 to 64 years: an association with somatic disease and neuropsychiatric symptoms. Mov Disord 2001;16(6):1159–63.

35. Kallweit U, Siccoli MM, Poryazova R, et al. Excessive daytime sleepiness in idiopathic restless legs syndrome: characteristics and evolution under dopaminergic treatment. Eur Neurol 2009;62(3):176–9.

36. Guilleminault C, Raynal D, Takahashi S, et al. Evaluation of short-term and long-term treatment of the narcolepsy syndrome with clomipramine hydrochloride. Acta Neurol Scand 1976;54(1):71–87.

37. Ahmed I, Thorpy M. Clinical features, diagnosis and treatment of narcolepsy. Clin Chest Med 2010;31:371–81.

38. Quan SF. Proceedings of the conference: finding a research path for the identification of bio-markers of sleepiness. J Clin Sleep Med 2011; 7(5):S1–48.

39. Mignot E. Genetic and familial aspects of narco-lepsy. Neurology 1998;50(Suppl 1):S16–22.

40. Kapur VK, Resnick HE, Gottlieb DJ. Sleep Heart Health Study Group. Sleep disordered breathing and hypertension: does self-reported sleepiness modify the association? Sleep 2008;8:1127–32.

41. Feng J, He QY, Zhang XL, et al, Sleep Breath Disorder Group, Society of Respiratory Medicine. Epworth Sleepiness Scale may be an indicator for blood pressure profile and prevalence of coronary artery disease and cerebrovascular dis-ease in patients with obstructive sleep apnea. Sleep Breath 2012;16(1):31–40. http://dx.doi.org/10.1007/s11325-011-0481-5.

42. Barceló A, Barbé F, de la Peña M, et al. Insulin resistance and daytime sleepiness in patients with sleep apnoea. Thorax 2008;63(11):946–50.

43. Nena E, Steiropoulos P, Papanas N, et al. Sleepiness as a marker of glucose deregulation in obstructive sleep apnea. Sleep Breath 2012;16(1):181–6. http://dx.doi.org/10.1007/s11325-010-0472-y.

44. Javaheri S, Smith J, Chung E. The prevalence and natural history of complex sleep apnea. J Clin Sleep Med 2009;5(3):205–11.

45. O'Donoghue FJ, Wellard RM, Rochford PD, et al. Magnetic resonance spectroscopy and neurocogni-tive dysfunction in obstructive sleep apnea before and after CPAP treatment. Sleep 2012;35:41–8.

46. Row BW, Liu R, Xu W, et al. Intermittent hypoxia is associated with oxidative stress and spatial learning deficits in the rat. Am J Respir Crit Care Med 2003;167:1548–53.

47. Greenberg H, Ye X, Wilson D, et al. Chronic inter-mittent hypoxia activates nuclear factor-kB in car-diovascular tissues in vivo. Biochem Biophys Res Commun 2006;343:591–6.

48. Young T, Blustein J, Finn L, et al. Sleep-disordered breathing and motor vehicle accidents in a population-based sample of employed adults. Sleep 1997;20(8):608–13.

49. Pepperell JC, Ramdassingh-Dow S, Crosthwaite N, et al. Ambulatory blood pressure after therapeutic and subtherapeutic nasal continuous positive airway pressure for obstructive sleep apnoea: a randomised parallel trial. Lancet 2002;359(9302):204–10.

50. Mulgrew AT, Lawati NA, Ayas NT, et al. Residual sleep apnea on polysomnography after 3 months of CPAP therapy: clinical implications, predictors and patterns. Sleep Med 2010;11(2):119–25.

51. Morgenthaler TI, Kagramanov V, Hanak V, et al. Complex sleep apnea syndrome: is it a unique clin-ical syndrome? Sleep 2006;29:1203–9.

52. Malhotra A, Bertisch S, Wellman A. Complex sleep apnea: it isn't really. J Clin Sleep Med 2008;4(5):406–8.

53. Htoo AK, Greenberg H, Tongia S, et al. Activation of nuclear factor kB in obstructive sleep apnea: a pathway leading to systemic inflammation. Sleep Breath 2006;10:43–50.

54. Williams A, Scharf S. Obstructive sleep apnea, car-diovascular disease, and inflammation—is NF-kB the key? Sleep Breath 2007;11:69–76.

55. Krueger J. The role of cytokines in sleep regulation. Curr Pharm Des 2008;14(32):3408–16.

56. Vgontzas AN, Papanicolaou DA, Bixler EO, et al. Elevation of plasma cytokines in disorders of excessive daytime sleepiness: role of sleep distur-bance and obesity. J Clin Endocrinol Metab 1997; 82:1313–6.

57. Vgontzas AN, Zoumakis E, Lin HM, et al. Marked decrease in sleepiness in patients with sleep apnea by etanercept, a tumor necrosis factor-a antagonist. J Clin Endocrinol Metab 2004;89:4409–13.

58. Somers VK, Dyken ME, Clary MP, et al. Sympa-thetic neural mechanisms in obstructive sleep ap-nea. J Clin Invest 1995;96:1897–904.

59. Zou D, Grote L, Eder D, et al. Obstructive apneic events induce alpha-receptor mediated digital vasoconstriction. Sleep 2004;27(3):485–9.

60. Arias MA, Garcia-Rio F, Alonso-Fernandez A, et al. CPAP decreases plasma levels of soluble tumor necrosis factor-a receptor 1 in obstructive sleep apnea. Eur Respir J 2008;32:1009–15.

61. El-Solh AA, Akinnusi ME, Moitheennazima B, et al. Endothelial function in patients with post-CPAP resid-ual sleepiness. J Clin Sleep Med 2010;6(3):251–5.

62. Kanbayashi T. CSF hypocretin measures in pa-tients with obstructive sleep apnea. J Sleep Res 2003;12:339–41.

63. Mignot E, Lammers G, Ripley B, et al. The role of cerebrospinal fluid hypocretin measurement in the diagnosis of narcolepsy and other hypersomnias. Arch Neurol 2002;59:1553–62.

64. Yamanaka A, Beuckmann C, Willie JT, et al. Hypo-thalamic orexin neurons regulate arousal accord-ing to energy balance in mice. Neuron 2003;38:701–13.

65. Arnulf I, Homeyer P, Garma L, et al. Modafinil in obstructive sleep apnea-hypopnea syndrome: a pi-lot study in 6 patients. Respiration 1997;64:159–61.

66. Pack AI, Black JE, Schwartz JR, et al. Modafinil as adjunct therapy for daytime sleepiness in obstruc-tive sleep apnea. Am J Respir Crit Care Med 2001; 164:1675–81.

67. Schwartz JR, Hirshkowitz M, Erman MK, et al. Mod-afinil as adjunct therapy for daytime sleepiness in

obstructive sleep apnea: a 12-week, open-label study. Chest 2003;124:2192–9.

68. Bittencourt LR, Lucchesi LM, Rueda AD, et al. Placebo and modafinil effect on sleepiness in obstructive sleep apnea. Prog Neuropsychopharmacol Biol Psychiatry 2008;32:552–9.

69. Hirshkowitz M, Black J. Effect of adjunctive modafinil on wakefulness and quality of life in patients with excessive sleepiness-associated obstructive sleep apnea/hypopnea syndrome: a 12-month, open-label extension study. CNS Drugs 2007; 21(5):407–16.

70. Roth T, White D, Schmidt-Nowara W, et al. Effects of armodafinil in the treatment of residual excessive sleepiness associated with obstructive sleep apnea/hypopnea syndrome: a 12-week, multicenter, double-blind, randomized, placebo-controlled study in nCPAP-adherent adults. Clin Ther 2006; 28:689–705.

71. Krystal AD, Harsh JR, Yang R, et al. A double blind, placebo-controlled study of armodafinil for excessive sleepiness in patients with treated obstructive sleep apnea and comorbid depression. J Clin Psychiatry 2010;71(1):32–40.

Outcomes of Therapy for Hypersomnia for Obstructive Sleep Apnea

Pawan Sikka, MD, FACP, FAASM, CBSM[a],*,
Mary Aigner, PhD, RN, FNP-BC[b], Amit Mann, MD[c],
Archana Banerjee, RPh[d]

KEYWORDS

- Hypersomnia • Obstructive sleep apnea • Continuous positive airway pressure
- Excessive daytime sleepiness • Modafinil

KEY POINTS

- Some people with obstructive sleep apnea syndrome continue to experience and report hypersomnia despite routine use of positive airway pressure (PAP) therapy.
- Adequate compliance is defined as the use of PAP therapy for four hours or longer nightly, 70% of the time over a 30 day period.
- If compliance is considered to be adequate, then other common causes of sleepiness need to be ruled out.
- Treatment for the hypersomnia will depend on the cause or suspected cause. If other potential causes of hypersomnia are not found or believed to be the issue, then treatment with medication is warranted. Modafinil has been successfully utilized by many patients with improvement in the level of sleepiness they experience.
- For all patients who complain of hypersomnia, caution needs to be given about driving or operating heavy machinery.

Hypersomnia, or excessive daytime sleepiness, is common with obstructive sleep apnea (OSA) but normally improves with use of continuous positive airway pressure (CPAP) therapy. Rodenstein wrote, "the sleepiness of a normal human being after a long work day is very different from the sleepiness of a narcoleptic patient, or from that of an obstructive sleep apnea patient, or that of a paid student participating in his sleep restriction physiology study." He goes on to describe sleepiness as a sensation that is perceived by the individual, similar to the perception of pain or thirst, which varies from one person to another.[1]

OSA is well known for breathing disturbances associated with variations in heart rate, arousals, and resulting sleepiness in the daytime. Other common symptoms include nocturia, sweating, gastroesophageal reflux, and, on awakening, morning headache and complaints of dry mouth. Sleep architecture changes occur in patients with OSA. The light sleep stage (primarily stage I) increases, whereas the stages with slow waves (N3 sleep) decrease. Some have been found to have no slow wave sleep. Many patients, no matter the severity of their condition or how much time they spend in bed, wake up with the feeling of not being rested and not getting enough sleep.[2]

[a] Pulmonary, Critical Care & Sleep Medicine, Central Texas Veterans Health Care System, 1901 South 1st Street, Temple, TX 76504, USA; [b] Pulmonary, & Sleep Medicine, Central Texas Veterans Health Care System, 1901 South 1st Street, Temple, TX 76504, USA; [c] Pulmonary & Critical Care, Texas A&M University, Temple, TX, USA; [d] Department of Pharmacy, Central Texas Veterans Health Care System, 1901 South 1st Street, Temple, TX 76504, USA
* Corresponding author.
E-mail address: pawan.sikka@va.gov

Sleep Med Clin 8 (2013) 583–590
http://dx.doi.org/10.1016/j.jsmc.2013.07.005
1556-407X/13/$ – see front matter Published by Elsevier Inc.

There are also well-known risks for individuals with untreated OSA. One risk of excessive sleepiness is motor vehicle accidents (MVA). A study by Barbe and coworkers found a 2.6 higher risk of MVAs for patients with OSA than a control group. This risk decreased by more than half following treatment with CPAP therapy.[3(p46)] Other risks include impaired performance on tasks involving psychomotor performance or cognitive function (eg, memory, attention).[4]

CPAP or bilevel positive airway pressure therapy has long been considered the "gold standard for OSA treatment."[(p21)] It works by the use of pneumatic pressure to mechanically open the upper airway of the patient with OSA.[2] This therapy results in significant improvement of hypersomnia in most patients. It has been shown that even one night's use of CPAP therapy can improve daytime functioning.[5] Unfortunately, approximately 6%[(p1066)] of patients with OSA who use CPAP/bilevel positive airway pressure therapy continue to report excessive or residual daytime sleepiness (hypersomnia).[6] The criteria for good compliance with CPAP therapy has been defined for Medicare as "the use of PAP ≥4 hours per night on 70% of nights during a consecutive 30-day period, and the patient has objective clinical improvement in the symptoms of OSA."[7(pp542)]

In the authors' experience, patients with untreated OSA often report falling asleep at work, in classrooms, and sometimes, during a conversation with someone. These episodes can result in a negative impact on productivity, grades, safety, or even social relationships. Many report close calls or near accidents while driving as well because of their sleepiness.

WHAT IS HYPERSOMNIA?

Hypersomnia has also been termed excessive daytime sleepiness (EDS) or residual excessive sleepiness (RES). It can be a severe, disabling type of sleepiness that occurs despite a sleep period that is considered normal or even longer than normal (over 10 hours). The sensation of "sleep drunkenness (a prolonged and severe confusion upon awakening)"[(p98)] may be reported. There may be a decrease in executive functions and interference with usual daily activities. Sleep latency in the daytime may be decreased and this can be measured objectively through testing by a multiple sleep latency test or MSLT.[8]

The most common subjective complaints of people with hypersomnia associated with OSA is an impairment in their daytime ability to function. Other common complaints are that of being excessively sleepy in the daytime, feeling fatigued, a loss of memory or cognitive changes, and a negative impact on their mood and overall quality of life.[5] Hypersomnia that occurs with narcolepsy differs in that it also includes the objective measurement of early onset of REM (rapid eye movement) sleep episodes called SOREMPs (sleep onset REM periods). Idiopathic hypersomnia is different because the excessive daytime sleepiness occurs without apneic events and typically involves the symptom of sleep drunkenness. This symptom of sleep drunkenness is characterized by difficulty waking up after sleeping, automatic behavior, repeatedly falling back asleep, and confusion on awakening. Both narcolepsy and idiopathic hypersomnia are considered to be central hypersomnias.[8]

CAUSE AND EFFECTS OF HYPERSOMNIA IN PATIENTS WITH OSA

Hypersomnia, or EDS, is one of the most common symptoms associated with OSA. Sleep fragmentation and hypoxemia have both been theorized as possible causes. Sleep fragmentation, which disrupts sleep continuity, results in a loss of the restorative benefit of sleep to the patients. Even normal subjects in good health who are subjected to fragmentation of their sleep in studies have been found to have EDS. Apnea can cause a significant decrease in oxygenation in some individuals and thus hypoxemia has been hypothesized as one of the causes of EDS in the patient with OSA. One study in the late 1980s found evidence of brief arousals, sleep fragmentation that accompanied the apnea or hypopnea episodes, which then produced the hypersomnia. This same study found a correlation between EDS and hypoxemia. The researchers determined that both the quantity (length of sleep time) and the quality of the sleep period were the best predictors of sleepiness in the daytime.[9]

Roadway collisions are a major risk for patients with hypersomnia and OSA. Daytime sleepiness and reduced alertness have been shown to increase the risk of MVA in patients with OSA. Treatment with CPAP therapy has been shown to lower that risk. A study by George reported that the increased risk of an MVA was eliminated once patients were treated with CPAP therapy. The rates for MVA were compared for the subjects (n = 210) 3 years before and after initiation of CPAP therapy. During this time, the rates for accidents decreased to the normal level without a change in driving exposure/time. The subjects who refused CPAP therapy (n = 36) continued to have a higher rate of MVA.[10(pp509)]

Another study monitored 80 patients with OSA and 80 controls for 2 years before and after the initiation of CPAP therapy in the OSA group. Before CPAP use, those with OSA had a risk 2.6 times higher than the controls. Following 2 years of CPAP therapy, the collision rate was decreased by half.[p44] The authors of this study did identify several limitations, including "the so-called Hawthorne effect" and the possibility that participants changed their driving habits simply by being in the study or as a result of being in a MVA.[3] The Hawthorne effect simply states that participant behaviors or outcomes in any human study may alter if they are aware of being watched.[11]

One study reviewed health care data of more than four million veterans. A higher prevalence of mood disorders (eg, depression and bipolar disorder) was found in those who had sleep apnea, even when other chronic medical conditions were considered. A higher incidence of posttraumatic stress disorder, anxiety, and dementia were also found in patients diagnosed with sleep apnea than other veterans. Some researchers think hypoxemia as well as sleep fragmentation may contribute to the depressive symptoms.[12]

Lal and colleagues[13] wrote a recent review on neurocognitive impairment in patients with OSA. They stated OSA has a significant impact on reasoning, comprehension, and learning. Fine motor coordination is impaired in patients with OSA, although individual motor speed is unaffected.

MEASUREMENTS OF EXCESSIVE DAYTIME SLEEPINESS

The MSLT is an objective measurement of hypersomnia. It consists of a series of 4 to 5 opportunities to nap during the daytime spread 2 hours apart. Those with hypersomnia will exhibit a shortened sleep latency period, often less than 5 minutes but usually less than 10 minutes (normal is more than 10–15 minutes). Another sleep disorder, narcolepsy, will often have 2 or more events of sleep-onset REM periods or SOREMPs during these naps. Idiopathic hypersomnia findings from an MSLT will show the shortened sleep latency but without the SOREMPs found in an individual with narcolepsy.[14]

Actigraphy is an objective test that can be useful for examining the amount of time spent asleep versus awake in patients who use CPAP but still complain of EDS. Testing can be performed as an outpatient in the patient's home and consists of the use of an accelerometer with memory storage that is contained within a watchlike device. It is worn on the nondominant wrist during sleep. Actigraphy provides an estimate of the sleep/wake cycles based on movement differences during sleep and wakefulness. Actigraphy has been found to correlate well with sleep efficiency and total sleep time results when compared with measures from polysomnography (PSG). This test is less expensive than an MSLT, which is performed in a sleep laboratory and can be useful for patients using CPAP but still experiencing hypersomnia.[15]

When PSG is not available or practical, actigraphy is indicated as a method to estimate total sleep time in patients with OSA syndrome. Combined with a validated way of monitoring respiratory events, the use of actigraphy may improve accuracy in assessing the severity of OSA compared with the time spent in bed. The advantage of actigraphy over traditional PSG is that actigraphy can conveniently record continuously for 24 hours a day for days, weeks, or even longer.[15]

Another objective test that measures if the patient can stay awake during the day, after having slept at night, is the maintenance of wakefulness test (MWT). Typically, a PSG is not performed the night before. The MWT measures the ability to stay awake under soporific conditions for a defined period of time. It is based on the assumption that the volitional ability to stay awake is more important to know, in some instances, than the tendency to fall asleep (eg, pilots). Because there is no direct biologic measure of wakefulness available, this same phenomenon is calibrated indirectly by the inability or delayed tendency to fall asleep, as measured by the same electroencephalogram (EEG)-derived sleep latency used in the MSLT.[16]

Monitoring during the MWT includes use of EEG (both central and occipital), electro-oculography, mental or submental electromyography, and electrocardiography. A session is ended after unequivocal sleep or after 40 minutes if sleep does not occur. Sleep is considered unequivocal after 3 consecutive epochs of stage 1 sleep or one epoch of any other stage of sleep. For each session, the sleep latency is recorded. It is documented as being 40 minutes if the patient does not fall asleep. This routine is repeated every 2 hours, until the patient has completed 4 sessions. Staying awake for at least 40 minutes during all sleep sessions is strong objective evidence that the patient can stay awake. A mean sleep latency less than 8 minutes is considered abnormal. A mean sleep latency between 8 and 40 minutes is of unknown significance.[16]

Subjective measurement of EDS is most often obtained with use of the Epworth Sleepiness Scale or ESS. This tool was developed in 1991 and has been translated into at least 7 different languages. It consists of 8 questions and 4-point scales and is widely used in sleep facilities around the world as a convenient simple questionnaire patients can answer on their own. A cutoff rate of 10 (24 possible points) is usually used to separate normal from excessive daytime sleepiness.[17,18]

When using the ESS, it must be recognized that it is subjective and not an objective measurement of hypersomnia. Results can vary depending on personality traits, for instance. Patients scoring low on the ESS may still require a sleep study to determine if OSA is present. A study by Sil and colleagues found it to be only slightly useful in predicting the actual presence of OSA.[17] Another study by Lee and colleagues[18] found no correlation between the degree of sleep fragmentation and the score on the ESS tool. This study did find a significant correlation between the ESS score and the percentage of time spent snoring during sleep. Body mass index (BMI) was found to be related to the ESS rating as well in this study.

Despite the limitations of the ESS, it is widely used and a helpful tool in assessing the patient's perception of their daytime sleepiness. Researchers from another study found only a weak relationship between the objective MSLT measurement of hypersomnia and the subjective score of the ESS. Their recommendation was for additional research for the purpose of quantifying subjective sleepiness. There are other screening questionnaires available including the STOP-BANG tool, the Berlin questionnaire, and the Wisconsin Sleep questionnaire. These questionnaires are fairly easy to use in the outpatient setting but lack sensitivity and specificity as a predictor of OSA.[19] The Stanford Sleepiness Scale differs in that it measures subjective sleepiness at certain moments in time.[20]

HYPERSOMNIA WITH OSA DESPITE POSITIVE AIRWAY PRESSURE TREATMENT

First, patients with suspected OSA need to be followed up to evaluate treatment and make adjustments as indicated. Usually, symptoms including hypersomnia will resolve. Those with continued EDS will require a full assessment to rule out potential causes, such as, (1) not allowing enough time for sleep, (2) mask leakage or inadequate pressure level, (3) suboptimal adherence to treatment, (4) other potential sleep disorders (eg, narcolepsy), and medication usage, which can cause EDS including both prescription and over-the-counter medications. Should factors be determined, such as not having adequate sleep time, recommendations can be given and, once followed, the problem of hypersomnia should resolve. Similarly, often adjustments to the pressure, increased use of positive airway pressure (PAP) therapy, or changing to a different mask

with less leakage will result in resolution of the sleepiness. Other conditions, such as depression, restless leg syndrome, pain, or insomnia with poor sleep hygiene can also cause the daytime sleepiness and should be assessed[1,21] and treated as indicated.

Once other conditions have been ruled out, the next step would be to do a MSLT. This test is done by first performing an overnight PSG on PAP therapy the night before to be sure that the individual is indeed on the correct treatment. Then, the patient stays overnight in the sleep laboratory for the MSLT. A study on RES in patients with OSA by Vernet and coworkers that used the PSG followed by MSLT in the study found half of the patients with hypersomnia despite CPAP use awoke in the morning tired and had a headache. They did not exhibit hypnagogic hallucinations, cataplexy, or sleep drunkenness.[8]

This same study found patients with RES had less N3 sleep than controls or subjects with OSA but without RES. The daytime naps during the MSLT lasted twice as long in the RES group but total sleep time within 24 hours was no different from the controls or OSA patients without RES. The sleep latencies were lower in the subjects who had RES than the others and these subjects had more SOREMPs. However, none of them met the criteria for narcolepsy, despite the SOREMPs. Depression scores were found to be higher for all OSA patients in the study but no different between those with or without RES. The researchers found no significant relationship between the ESS score for the RES subjects and other measures of sleep, cognition, neuropsychology, or sleepiness.[8]

Other researchers have provided possible explanations for EDS in patients with OSA despite the use of PAP treatment. One of the explanations is the possibility of the patient having obesity hypoventilation syndrome or OHS. The other is if the patient also has chronic obstructive pulmonary disase and the "so-called overlap syndrome." Both OHS and overlap syndrome cause hypercapnia, which can lead to daytime sleepiness. Another possibility is the existence of "cardiovascular autonomic dysregulations induced by autonomic or 'subcortical' arousals."[(p226)] Thus, the regulation of arousals from brainstem neurons would be altered in some way. These researchers have reported a relationship between impaired autonomic cardiac regulation during the night and EDS, which they speculate could be related to brainstem dysfunction in the control of the cardiovascular system as well as alertness.[22]

Another study compared EEG results, in particular, slow wave measurements, of patients with

OSA before and after treatment with CPAP therapy. The level of EDS was also measured before and after treatment. Both results (and others) were compared with a control group without OSA. The study found slow wave sleep continued to have a low percentage even after treatment but, once treated, was not significantly different from the control group. Daytime sleepiness lessened with treatment but those with OSA continued to have a higher level of sleepiness than the control even with treatment. They found that the subjects with OSA "treated with CPAP remained significantly more somnolent than healthy control subjects."[p51] These researchers also concluded that persistent hypoxemia and persistent PLMS were probably not significantly related to having residual sleepiness. An elevated BMI and obesity were found to be significantly elevated in the patients with OSA and is often associated with EDS and fatigue even without OSA.[23]

POSSIBLE CAUSES OF EXCESSIVE DAYTIME SLEEPINESS AND CHANGES NOTED IN PATIENTS WITH OSA TREATED WITH PAP THERAPY

Several possible causes of EDS among patients with OSA who use PAP therapy have been suggested. The first cause to rule out includes noncompliance with therapy, which can include not understanding how to use the therapy, a need for improved CPAP titration, and other undiagnosed sleep disorders. Other possible effects include a lack of slow brain wave activity, dysfunction of brainstem neurons, hypoxemia, hypercapnia, autonomic arousals, catastrophizing, sleep fragmentation, OHS, depression, and sympathetic cardiac modulation. Some of these have been discussed in preceding paragraphs but some are reviewed in more detail herein.

A study by Roehrs and colleagues in 1989 (n = 466) found correlations between EDS and both sleep fragmentation and hypoxemia. The sleep fragmentation was related to brief electroencephalographic arousals along with the cessation of the hypopnea or apnea episode. This study found that the quality and quantity of the nocturnal sleep was the best predictor for daytime sleepiness, as measured by the Stanford Sleepiness Scale.[9]

A study reported in 2001 (n = 10) suggested that patients with OSA experience a lack of slow wave activity (SWA) during the first portion of the night resulting in EDS. These researchers concluded that the distribution of SWS during a night's sleep was important and that the peak of SWA, which normally occurs during the first part of sleep, is correlated to "daytime vigilance" or alertness.[p1812]

They speculated that as SWA decreases because of multiple microarousals, the level of EDS increases. However, they did not find a correlation with SWA and mean sleep latency on an MSLT with successful CPAP therapy.[24]

Vernet and colleagues[8] speculated that RES in patients with OSA is related to some form of "post-hypoxic hypersomnia."[p104] Sleep time has been found to be prolonged in animal models using intermittent hypoxemia even weeks afterward. Intermittent hypoxia can lead to injury in neuronal systems, including the wake-active neurons (catecholaminergic), cortex, serotonergic dorsal raphe nucleus, CA1 region of the hippocampus, and cholinergic lateral basal forebrain. However, the intermittent hypoxia seemed to have no effect on other arousal systems (eg, histamine and hypocretin neurons), which could be the explanation for why these patients do not meet the criteria for a diagnosis of narcolepsy. Before CPAP treatment, patients with OSA had similar exposure to intermittent hypoxia, suggesting that those with RES have a higher vulnerability to effects in their brain.

Patients with depression often complain of higher levels of fatigue and daytime sleepiness. It has been estimated that 20% of subjects with either depression or OSA will have the other disorder as well. The existence of both hypoxia and sleep fragmentation are thought to be main factors for the depressive symptoms in a patient with OSA. Higher ESS scoring has been correlated to higher levels of depression, suggesting that "OSA-related hypoxemia affects mood."[p20] Disturbed serotonin activity in depression may contribute to lower dilator tone of the upper airway during sleep as well, which could be another factor in OSA.[2]

Sampaioand coworkers wrote that "the perception and interpretation of symptoms arise from the relationship between external and internal stimuli and from individuals' beliefs."[p138] People who have depression tend to be more pessimistic about actions taken (such as use of CPAP therapy) than those who are not depressed. These researchers found patients who perceive the disease of OSA as threatening reported an impaired quality of life. This, in turn, could lead to higher reported levels of somnolence despite treatment of the OSA.[25]

Finally, several studies and articles have discussed a correlation between obesity, BMI, OHS, and higher levels of EDS. Patients with OHS tend to have periods of sustained hypoxemia with resulting hypercapnia. These patients usually have higher scores on the ESS than patients with OSA even when matched for BMI, apnea hypopnea index, and age.[26]

TREATMENTS FOR HYPERSOMNIA WITH OBSTRUCTIVE SLEEP APNEA IN PATIENTS TREATED WITH PAP THERAPY

Stimulant medication is the most common treatment for EDS in patients using CPAP therapy once other possible causes of the hypersomnia have been eliminated. Modafinil is described as a wake-promoting agent chemically different from central nervous system stimulants with a different pharmacologic profile. It has been shown to be an effective and well-tolerated treatment for narcolepsy.[27]

Modafinil is usually the first choice and one study found 6 (30%) of 20 subjects to respond well to this drug. Of those who did not respond to Modafinil, 7 then tried methylphenidate, of which 2 (29%) then responded well. Two other medications were used, mazindol for one subject, and sodium oxybate for 2 subjects, with no effect or benefit to them.[8]

A larger multicenter study (n = 125) using Modafinil or placebo along with CPAP therapy reported significant clinical improvement. This study involved 12 weeks of open-label testing after subjects had completed double-blind, placebo-controlled study over 4 weeks. During the open-label portion of the research, all patients received 200 mg daily of Modafinil during the first week and then 400 mg daily during the second week. At the end of the second week, the researcher determined what dose was most effective for the individual subject based on tolerability and efficacy. The subjects were then given either 200 mg, 300 mg, or 400 mg for the next 10 weeks of the study.[27]

The researchers for the combined studies reported wakefulness remained improved through the 16 weeks of the study for those using Modafinil and ESS scores stayed less than 10. The most common side effects in this study were reported as headache, anxiety, and nervousness. To a lesser degree, insomnia, nausea, rhinitis, infection and dizziness occurred in some of the subjects using Modafinil. To a lesser extent, all of these side effects were also reported by those who used the placebo during the double-blind 4-week portion of the study.[27]

Caution is needed with Modafinil treatment in patients with a history of heart disease, arrhythmias, or mitral valve prolapse because the side effects of tachycardia, hypertension, palpitations, and chest pain have been noted. However, these cardiovascular side effects are thought to be less common with Modafinil than with methylphenidate and the amphetamines that have also been used to treat excessive daytime sleepiness. "Patients should be observed for signs of misuse or abuse (e.g., incrementation of dosage or drug seeking behavior). The abuse potential of modafinil (200, 400, and 800 mg) was assessed relative to methylphenidate (45 and 90 mg) in an inpatient study in individuals experienced with drugs of abuse. Results from this clinical study demonstrated that modafinil produced psychoactive and euphoric effects and feelings consistent with other scheduled CNS stimulants (methylphenidate)."[28(pp14)]

Nonpharmacologic treatment must be considered for patients with EDS as well. One study examined the effect of exercise on daytime functioning of individuals with OSA (n = 43). The study found exercise training to be of help in reducing sleepiness and symptoms of fatigue, with improved vigor reported. Exercise was also found to improve symptoms of depression and had some impact on quality-of-life scores. A drop of approximately 2.5 points on the ESS was found in this study that was comparable to the use of CPAP therapy but was not found to be a significant reduction. The researchers did not study the effect of exercise training specifically on individuals with EDS despite CPAP therapy but speculated that improvements in daytime functioning would occur for anyone. Thus, their recommendation was to combine CPAP therapy with exercise training to augment improvements in levels of fatigue, sleepiness, and quality of life.[5]

Another type of PAP therapy has been studied as a method of reducing residual sleepiness in patients with OSA who use CPAP therapy. Adaptive servoventilation using a more technologically advanced machine was studied in 42 patients with severe OSA. Some patients with severe OSA also have some central sleep apnea (CSA) events resulting in a condition referred to as complex sleep apnea. Although complex sleep apnea is not well defined at present, it is suspected that CPAP therapy or even a change of position while asleep can change OSA events into CSA events. These new CSA events can then lead to fragmentation of sleep and EDS. Results of this study using adaptive servoventilation found a significant decrease in the ESS score, which normalized by day 7, as well as decreases in apnea hypopnea index and other measurements.[29]

SUMMARY

CPAP therapy has long been recognized as the best treatment for OSA and, for most individuals, symptoms will resolve and the individual wakes feeling well rested for the remainder of the day. However, some people continue to experience and report hypersomnia despite routine use of CPAP therapy. Excessive sleepiness can be dangerous for the individual when driving or operating heavy equipment, can lead to mistakes and problems in the workplace or school, result in memory loss, and cause a general decline in the quality of life.

Assessment of patients with OSA who continue to complain of excessive sleepiness despite CPAP use must include an initial assessment of therapy compliance. Medicare has defined compliance as the use of PAP therapy for 4 hours or longer nightly, 70% of the time over a 30-day period.[7] If compliance is considered to be adequate, then other common causes need to be ruled out. Some patients simply do not allow themselves enough time to obtain adequate sleep, perhaps working 2 or 3 jobs, or working and also being a full-time student. Air leakage from a mask can interrupt sleep, causing inadequate treatment as can inadequate pressure. Medications are a common cause of sleepiness, both prescription and over-the-counter medications. Obesity and OHS can lead to hypersomnia as well. Finally, other sleep disorders should be ruled out, such as narcolepsy, or a type of complex sleep apnea.

Treatment for the hypersomnia will depend on the cause or suspected cause. In many cases, correcting the cause is somewhat simple. Instruction can be given on sleep hygiene techniques with allowance for adequate sleep time. Adjustments of CPAP pressure or refitting of a mask may resolve the problem. Medications for pain, muscle spasms, mental health problems, and other disorders can be evaluated and, when possible, adjusted to decrease the effect of sleepiness on the individual. Sometimes, it is discovered that patients take one medication to help them sleep and then complain of residual sleepiness throughout the day. Weight loss for the morbidly obese with OHS can aid in reducing the sense of hypersomnia. Treatment with special equipment can resolve central apneas that are present in complex sleep apnea.

If other potential causes of hypersomnia are not found or thought to be the issue, then treatment with medication is warranted. Modafinil has been successfully used by many patients with improvement in the level of sleepiness they experience. Other stimulants are available but may have more potential side effects. Instructions on dosing and the time of dosing need to be given carefully as secondary insomnia could occur.

For all patients who complain of hypersomnia, caution needs to be given about driving or operating heavy machinery. Having someone else drive is ideal but, when not possible, pulling over to either take a quick nap or walk outside the vehicle can restore the sense of wakefulness.

Further research is needed to better define adequate compliance and to address the question, "should we be aiming for close to 100% usage and will that lead to better outcomes?" There is also a need for an ideal tool for assessing EDS. The question, "Do we need to do an MSLT in all patients with OSA with RES despite adequate CPAP compliance?," still remains as well.

REFERENCES

1. Rodenstein D. What is this thing called somnolence? Eur Respir J 2011;38(2):7–8.
2. Bilyukov RO, Georgiev OB, Petrova DS, et al. Obstructive sleep apnea syndrome and depressive symptoms. Folia Med (Plovdiv) 2009;51(3):18–24.
3. Barbe F, Sunyer J, de la Pena A, et al. Effect of continuous positive airway pressure on the risk of road accidents in sleep apnea patients. Respiration 2007;74:44–9. http://dx.doi.org/10.1159/000094237.
4. Creizler CA, Walsh JK, Wesnes KA, et al. Armodafinil for treatment of excessive sleepiness associated with shift work disorder: a randomized controlled study. Mayo Clin Proc 2009;84(11):958–72.
5. Kline CE, Ewing GB, Burch JB, et al. Exercise training improves selected aspects of daytime functioning in adults with obstructive sleep apnea. J Clin Sleep Med 2012;8(4):357–65.
6. Pepin JL, Viot-Blanc V, Escourrou P, et al. Prevalence of residual excessive sleepiness in CPAP-treated sleep apnoea patients: the French multicentre study. Eur Respir J 2009;33:1062–7. http://dx.doi.org/10.1183/09031936.00016808.
7. Nelson ME. Coding and billing for home (out-of-center) sleep testing. Chest 2013;143(2):539–43. http://dx.doi.org/10.1378/chest.12-0425.
8. Vernet C, Redolfi S, Attali V, et al. Residual sleepiness in obstructive sleep apnoea: phenotype and related symptoms. Eur Respir J 2011;38(1):98–105. http://dx.doi.org/10.1183/09031936.00040410.
9. Roehrs T, Zorick F, Wittig R, et al. Predictors of objective level of daytime sleepiness in patients with sleep-related breathing disorders. Chest 1989;95(6):1202–6.
10. George CF. Reduction in motor vehicle collisions following treatment of sleep apnoea with nasal CPAP. Thorax 2001;56:508–12. http://dx.doi.org/10.1136/thorax.56.7.508.
11. Mangione-Smith R, Elliott MN, McDonald L, et al. An observational study of antibiotic prescribing behavior and the Hawthorne Effect. Health Serv Res 2002;37(6):1603–23.
12. Sharafkhaneh A, Giray N, Richardson P, et al. Association of psychiatric disorders and sleep apnea in a large cohort. Sleep 2005;28(11):1405–11.
13. Lal C, Strange C, Bachman D. Neurocognitive impairment in obstructive sleep apnea. Chest 2012;141(6):1601–10. http://dx.doi.org/10.1378/chest.11-2214.

14. Black JE, Brooks SN, Nishino S. Conditions of primary excessive daytime sleepiness. Neurol Clin 2005;23:1025–44. http://dx.doi.org/10.1016/j.ncl.2005.08.002.

15. Otake M, Miyata S, Noda A, et al. Monitoring sleep-wake rhythm with actigraphy in patients on continuous positive airway pressure therapy. Respiration 2011;82:136–41. http://dx.doi.org/10.1159/000321238.

16. Littner MR, Kushida C, Wise M, et al. Practice parameters for clinical use of the multiple sleep latency test and the maintenance of wakefulness test. Sleep 2005;28(1):113–21.

17. Sil A, Barr G. Assessment of predictive ability of Epworth scoring in screening of patients with sleep apnoea. J Laryngol Otol 2012;126:372–9. http://dx.doi.org/10.1017/S0022215111003082.

18. Lee SJ, Kan HW, Lee LH. The relationship between the Epworth Sleepiness Scale and polysomnographic parameters in obstructive sleep apnea patients. Eur Arch Otorhinolaryngol 2012;269:1143–7. http://dx.doi.org/10.1007/s00405-011-1808-3.

19. Eiseman NA, Westover MB, Mietus JE, et al. Classification algorithms for predicting sleepiness and sleep apnea severity. J Sleep Res 2012;21:101–12. http://dx.doi.org/10.1111/j.1365-2869.2011.00935.x.

20. Shahid A, Wilkinson K, Marcu S, et al, editors. Standford sleepiness scale (SSS), chapter 91, in STOP, THAT and one hundred other sleep scales. Science+Business Media, LLC; 2012. http://dx.doi.org/10.1007/978-1-4419-9893-4_91.

21. Epstein LJ, Kristo D, Strollo PJ, et al. Clinical guidelines for the evaluation, management and long-term care of obstructive sleep apnea in adults. J Clin Sleep Med 2009;5(3):263–76.

22. Castiglioni P, Lombardi D, Cortelli P, et al. Why excessive sleepiness may persist in OSA patients receiving adequate CPAP treatment [letter to the editor]. Eur Respir J 2012;39(1):226–8.

23. Morisson F, Decary A, Petit D, et al. Daytime sleepiness and EEG spectral analysis in apneic patients before and after treatment with continuous positive airway pressure. Chest 2001;119(1):45–52.

24. Heinzer R, Gaudreau H, Decary A, et al. Slow-wave activity in sleep apnea patients before and after continuous positive airway pressure treatment. Chest 2001;119(6):1807–13.

25. Sampaio R, Pereira MG, Winck JC. Psychological morbidity, illness representations, and quality of life in female and male patients with obstructive sleep apnea syndrome. Psychol Health Med 2012;17(2):136–49.

26. BaHamman A. Excessive daytime sleepiness in patients with sleep-disordered breathing [letter to editor]. Eur Respir J 2004;31(3):685–6.

27. Schwartz JR, Hirshkowitz M, Erman MK, et al. Modafinil as adjunct therapy for daytime sleepiness in obstructive sleep apnea. Chest 2003;124(6):2192–9.

28. Circa Pharmaceuticals. Modafinil (Provigil): product information. 2012. Available at: http://www.modafinil.com/prescribe/index.html.

29. Mei S, Xilong Z, Mao H, et al. Adaptive pressure support servoventilation: a novel treatment for residual sleepiness associated with central sleep apnea events. Sleep Breath 2011;15:695–9. http://dx.doi.org/10.1007/s11325-010-0424-6.

Obstructive Sleep Apnea and Transportation: Medicolegal Issues

Vidya Krishnan, MD, MHS[a], Susheel P. Patil, MD, PhD[b],*

KEYWORDS

- Obstructive sleep apnea • Automobile driving • Medical legal issues • Legal issues
- Neurocognitive impairment • Drivers

KEY POINTS

- Obstructive sleep apnea (OSA) is associated with neurocognitive deficits, particularly in the domains of attention/vigilance, delayed long-term visual and verbal memory, visuospatial/constructional abilities, and executive function.
- Patients with OSA with sleep restriction have further impairments in neurocognitive function and driving ability.
- Subjective and objective testing have been used to assess daytime functioning. Limitations of these tests preclude definitive policies based solely on testing to identify those patients at risk for driving accidents.
- Legal culpability for an accident depends on the level of consciousness of the individual as well as the degree of understanding that an action will result in harm. Thus, education of the patient and public on the risk of OSA on driving ability is a critical role of the clinician.
- Laws and regulations regarding OSA and driving vary by region, and physicians are responsible for familiarizing themselves with policies that govern their jurisdiction.

INTRODUCTION

Excessive sleepiness and neurocognitive impairments from sleep restriction or other sleep disorders are a public health issue that has resulted in industrial accidents, reduced worker productivity, motor vehicle accidents (MVAs), and work-related injuries.[1] Several high-profile catastrophes such as the Exxon Valdez oil spill, the chemical plant disaster in Bhopal, India, and the Chernobyl nuclear power plant accident implicated sleep loss as an important factor leading to errors by workplace personnel. These events serve as stark reminders that humans require healthy sleep for optimal performance and safety.

Obstructive sleep apnea (OSA) is perhaps the best understood sleep disorder that results in excessive sleepiness and neurocognitive impairment. Impairments in cognition range from subtle to more overt manifestations and can affect vigilance, executive functioning, delayed long-term visual and verbal memory, and visuospatial abilities. Whether or not these impairments are the consequences of the chronic sleep restriction from recurrent arousals or the effects of the associated intermittent hypoxia on neural substrate, or both, remains to be delineated. Regardless of the mechanisms, the resulting sleep loss and neurocognitive impairment in patients with untreated OSA places them at higher risk for accidents than the general

Disclosures: None.
a Case Western Reserve University, MetroHealth Medical Center, Division of Pulmonary, Critical Care, and Sleep Medicine, 2500 MetroHealth Drive, BG3-38, Cleveland, OH 44113, USA; b Johns Hopkins School of Medicine, Division of Pulmonary and Critical Care Medicine, Johns Hopkins Sleep Disorders Center, 5501 Hopkins Bayview Circle, Room 4B.50, Baltimore, MD 21224, USA
* Corresponding author.
E-mail address: spatil@jhmi.edu

Sleep Med Clin 8 (2013) 591–605
http://dx.doi.org/10.1016/j.jsmc.2013.07.014
1556-407X/13/$ – see front matter Crown Copyright © 2013 Published by Elsevier Inc. All rights reserved.

population, and is of particular concern if the patient is in the mass transportation industry (eg, buses, trucks, railroad, airplanes) or commercial motor vehicle driving. Medical providers are often called on to evaluate the potential fitness for duty of the patient with OSA if they are in these areas of work or even for renewal/issuance of standard driving licenses. Clinicians, therefore, have an ethical and sometimes a legal responsibility to discuss with their patients with untreated OSA about the risks of sleepiness and neurocognitive impairment and to discourage driving or placing others at risk in the workplace when sleepy.

In this article, the consequences of OSA on neurocognitive function, alertness, and performance are reviewed. Common objective and subjective tools are then reviewed that clinicians use to assess impairments with a particular focus on driving. Current laws and regulations that may affect patients with OSA, particularly patients in certain occupations, and the role of the clinician and sleep physician in educating patients and the community of the effects of sleepiness are also reviewed.

CONSEQUENCES OF OSA ON NEUROCOGNITIVE PERFORMANCE

OSA is implicated as a causal factor in thousands of sleep-related work accidents and MVAs annually.[1] Although patients with OSA can manifest overt daytime sleepiness, resulting in drowsy driving or drowsiness during activities that require vigilance, in contrast the effects of OSA on neurocognitive performance can be more subtle. Impairment of restorative processes in the central nervous system with sleep fragmentation and intermittent hypoxia has been shown to directly affect cognition.[2,3] Cognitive domains, including executive function, verbal and visual memory, attention and vigilance, and global cognitive function, can affect driving capacity. As a result, the impact of OSA on driving ability and safety has been an area of public health interest.

Neurocognitive Function and OSA

Neurocognitive dysfunction as a result of OSA has several postulated pathophysiologic mechanisms: (1) sleep fragmentation resulting in sleep deprivation and excessive daytime sleepiness; (2) incomplete restoration of neuronal functioning in the prefrontal cortex, leading to cellular and biochemical stress; (3) hormonal imbalances; (4) intermittent hypoxia; and (5) systemic inflammation. There have been 2 recent thorough reviews of this topic.[4,5] The complex interactions of fixed and modifiable risk factors for OSA result in hypoxia, inflammation, and hormonal imbalance exposures,

which contribute to neurocognitive impairment (Fig. 1). Many of the risk factors for OSA are independently associated with neurocognitive decline. For example, fixed risk factors, including increasing age, male sex, and certain genetic profiles (such as Down syndrome) have associations with cognitive decline. Furthermore, modifiable OSA risk factors, such as obesity, cigarette and alcohol abuse, and psychoactive medication (including first-generation antidepressants and antipsychotics like imipramine, amitriptyline, clozapine, and thioridazine; and anticonvulsants such as clonazepam, primidone, and phenytoin), which are common in populations with OSA, can result in cognitive decline. Disentangling neurocognitive deficits that are attributable to OSA or risk factors common to OSA and neurocognitive decline remains challenging.

Most studies have shown an association between OSA and deficits in attention/vigilance, delayed long-term visual and verbal memory, visuospatial/constructional abilities, and executive function.[4–7] For example, 1 study investigated the dose-response relation between OSA severity and cognitive function. The investigators found that attention/vigilance and global cognitive function were linearly and inversely related to OSA severity; whereas language ability, delayed long-term visuospatial memory, and psychomotor function were not.[4] Attention and vigilance were associated with the degree of sleep fragmentation, whereas global cognitive function correlated with hypoxemia, suggesting differential intermediate mechanisms by which OSA leads to neurocognitive impairments. Treatment studies have shown conflicting results on cognitive function. Although some studies have reported improvements in executive function, delayed long-term memory, and global cognitive function with continuous positive airway pressure (CPAP) therapy, 1 recent study reported persistent reduction in working memory, complex attention, executive function, and psychomotor speed despite CPAP treatment of OSA.[7,8]

Sleep Loss: Consequences and Perception

The relative balance and interaction between the homeostatic drive for sleep, the counteracting circadian drive, and internal and external stimuli determine whether the individual is sleepy or alert. Sleep loss, whether acute or chronic, has consequences that are diverse. More is understood about acute sleep loss compared with chronic sleep loss. Performance decrements based on the psychomotor vigilance test (PVT) have been reported to occur after more than 16 hours of

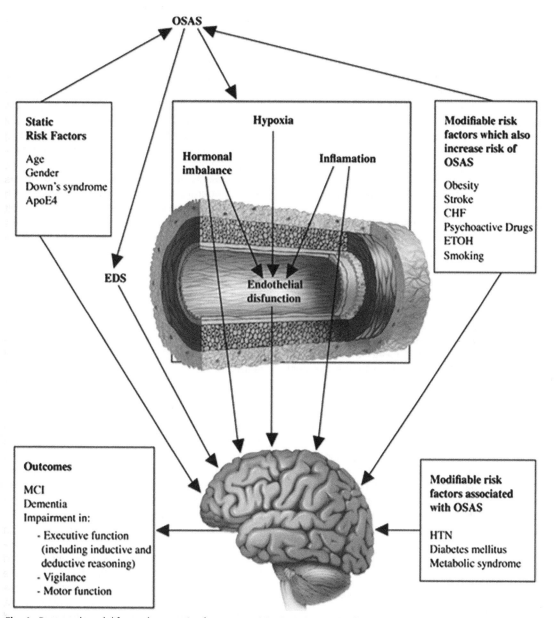

Fig. 1. Proposed model for pathogenesis of neurocognitive impairment in obstructive sleep apnea syndrome. ApoE4, apolipoprotein E ε4 allele; CHF, congestive heart failure; EDS, excessive daytime sleepiness; ETOH, ethanol; HTN, hypertension; MCI, mild cognitive impairment; OSAS, obstructive sleep apnea syndrome. (*From* Lal C, Strange C, Bachman D. Neurocognitive impairment in obstructive sleep apnea. Chest 2012;141(6):1603; with permission.)

cumulative wakefulness, regardless of the nightly sleep duration.[9] Young adults show impairments in cognitive performance when subjected to 5 hours of sleep per night for 1 week. Milder levels of sleep restriction to 6 hours per night for 2 weeks result in similar levels of cognitive impairment seen with 24 hours of complete sleep deprivation. In addition to cognitive impairment, sleep loss is recognized to result in impairments in short-term memory consolidation, information processing, executive functioning, and visuospatial abilities.

This situation results in reduced performance on attention tasks and impaired motor skills, such as driving. Sleep loss can also result in variable moods, irritability, and low energy, which contribute to fatigue and sleepiness, which could result in injury on the road or in the workplace.

What is perhaps most remarkable is the observation that individuals report subjective adaptation to chronic sleep loss despite objective evidence of impairment on cognitive performance measures. For example, in the experiments performed by

Van Dongen and colleagues,[9] subjective reports of sleepiness in groups randomized to 4 or 6 hours of sleep per night for 2 weeks increased over the first several days and stabilized over the remainder of the 2 weeks. This adaptation has often been compared with individuals who drive while intoxicated. Individuals with blood alcohol levels exceeding the legal limit subjectively report that their performance is better than what is objectively recorded. This inability to judge the level of impairment has been attributed both to a scarcity of physiologic warning signs in some sleepy individuals and lack of recognition of these warning signs in others.[10,11]

In patients with OSA, absolute bed time may be preserved or increased, but reductions in total sleep time, sleep efficiency, sleep quality, and rapid eye movement (REM) sleep result in deranged sleep architecture. Persons with untreated OSA may be particularly susceptible to the neurocognitive impairments of sleep restriction when the underlying sleep quality is impaired. Results of a meta-analysis of studies of CPAP treatment of OSA have suggested that CPAP treatment can reduce subjective sleepiness, with the greatest benefit observed in patients with more severe sleep apnea and baseline sleepiness.[12,13] In addition, CPAP treatment of OSA for 3 weeks resulted in a significant reduction in patient-reported fatigue and an increase in vigor/energy, as measured by 2 validated fatigue and vigor questionnaires.[14] Despite optimal treatment of OSA with CPAP, about 5% of patients have residual daytime sleepiness (and another subset of patients with residual fatigue), which can result in persistent daytime functional impairment.[15]

ASSESSMENT OF EXCESSIVE SLEEPINESS AND ALERTNESS
Subjective Assessments of Excessive Sleepiness

Both subjective and objective tools are used to quantify sleepiness (**Table 1**). Two common subjective metrics that have been used to assess excessive sleepiness with driving include the Epworth Sleepiness Scale (ESS) and the reporting of near-miss accidents.

The ESS is an 8-question survey designed to assess the propensity for falling asleep in different situations. The score ranges from 0 (no propensity to fall asleep) to 24 (a very high propensity to fall asleep). A score of 11 or more is typically used to define excessive sleepiness. In another common interpretation, an ESS of 0 to 8 is normal, 9 to 12 represents mild sleepiness, 13 to 16 represents moderate excessive sleepiness, and more than 16 represents severe sleepiness.[16] The ESS has been compared with objective measures of sleepiness, such as the multiple sleep latency test (MSLT). After adjustments for age, sex, race, education level, marital status, and body mass index (BMI, calculated as weight in kilograms divided by the square of height in meters), the hazards ratio progressively increased between increasing quartiles of the ESS (<9, 10–13, 14–17, and ≥18) and reduced mean sleep latency on the MSLT (1.0, 1.3, 1.9, and 2.5, respectively).[17]

The use of the ESS within 2 to 6 weeks of the automobile accidents has been examined in a case-control study sponsored by the AAA Foundation for Traffic Safety.[10] In the study, 1000 individuals involved in an accident (crashers) were compared with 400 control participants (noncrashers). Car crashes were further subdivided into sleep-related, fatigue-related, or neither. Sleep-related crashers had a slightly higher prevalence of a diagnosed sleep disorder compared with noncrashers (3.2% vs 1.7%, respectively). The prevalence of diagnosed sleep disorders was low, given that 25% of sleep-related crashers reported more than 10 drowsy driving episodes and 91% reported haven fallen asleep while driving at least once. Sleep-related crashers had a higher ESS (mean ± SD), compared with those in non–sleep-related crashers, and noncrashers (7.6 ± 4.4, 5.6 ± 3.4, and 5.1 ± 3.4, respectively).

Table 1	
Common subjective and objective measurements of daytime sleepiness	
Subjective Measures of Sleepiness	**Objective Measures of Sleepiness**
Epworth Sleepiness Scale	Multiple sleep latency test
Reporting of MVAs and near-miss MVAs	Maintenance of wakefulness test
Sleep diaries (reported sleep hours/duration)	Driving simulators
Stanford Sleepiness Scale	Real-world driving testing
Karolinska Sleepiness Scale	Psychomotor vigilance test (PVT)
	Oxford Sleep Resistance Test

Progressive sleepiness by ESS groups (<5, 6–11, 11–15, >16) was associated with increasing odds of a sleep-related crash (odds ratio: 1.0, 1.4, 3.0, 5.8). Although the ESS initially seems to be a good predictor of sleep-related crashes, it has a high false-negative rate, with 40% of sleep-related crashers reporting an ESS less than 5. In another study of habitually sleepy drivers (fear of falling asleep 1 of 3 times while driving), only 50% reported an ESS greater than 9.[18] In contrast to the study by Stutts and colleagues, the ESS did not explain the increase in sleep-related auto accidents, despite these individuals performing poorly in driving simulators. Furthermore, other studies that have used state government databases for MVAs have not reported an association between the ESS and MVAs.[19,20]

Another self-reported metric that has been reported is the number of near-miss accidents. Investigators have reported a correlation between near-miss automobile accidents and automobile accidents. In their Internet survey of 35,217 respondents, the risk of an accident, in unadjusted analyses, increased from 23% of respondents reporting no near-miss accidents to 45% in those reporting 4 or more near-accidents. After adjusting for alcohol intake, night driving, driving distance, age, sex, and family income, participants with at least 1 near-miss accident were 13% more likely to report an accident compared with participants reporting no near-miss accidents. Furthermore, participants with 4 or more near-miss accidents were 87% more likely to report an accident compared with those not reporting any near-miss accidents, after the same adjustments. The best predictive factor for near-misses is the occurrence of at least 1 severe sleepiness episode while driving in the last year. with an odds ratio of 6.50 (95% confidence interval [CI]: 5.20–8.12).[21] These data suggest that asking about near-miss accidents may be useful in determining the future risk of automobile accident when evaluating driving safety.

However, patients may not be forthcoming about their own assessment of their sleepiness if they fear the loss of driving privileges or employment. For example, 70% of patients under evaluation for OSA indicated that they would avoid medical evaluation if there was mandatory reporting by the physician to the local motor vehicle administration.[22] In another study, 25% of individuals who initially denied any driving impairment of sleepiness, subsequently admitted experiencing difficulties.[23] Thus, self-reported measures of sleepiness can be subject to patient's concerns about the impact on their livelihood and personal mobility.

Objective Assessments of Excessive Sleepiness and Alertness

Several objective tests of excessive sleepiness or alertness have been evaluated for their usefulness in making clinical judgments about safety with driving and other tasks that require vigilance and coordination. These tests include the MSLT, the maintenance of wakefulness test (MWT), driving simulators, and real-world driving courses.

MSLT

The MSLT is an objective measure of an individual's physiologic drive for sleep. The test consists of 4 or 5, 20-minute nap opportunities, each separated by 2 hours, during which the patient is asked to try to fall asleep. From the test, the mean sleep latency is determined, with a mean sleep latency less than 10 minutes indicating sleepiness.[24] The test is traditionally used for clinical purposes in the evaluation of disorders of excessive sleepiness such as narcolepsy or idiopathic hypersomnolence. The mean sleep latency from the MSLT does not strongly correlate with the ESS score.[19,25,26] However, individuals with an ESS greater than 12, compared with those with an ESS less than 5, have a 69% increased likelihood of sleep onset during the 20-minute opportunities.[27]

The MSLT is of limited usefulness in the prediction of MVAs. In 1 study, the MSLT was evaluated in a clinic sample of patients with sleep disorders as a predictor of self-reported MVA.[28] Although patients with narcolepsy or OSA accounted for 71% of self-reported, sleep-related MVAs, the MSLT was not different in patients involved in an MVA compared with patients not in an MVA. However, the use of a clinic-based sample and self-reported MVAs may have limited the detection of a possible association. In a population-based study in Wisconsin using a state government accident database to examine the association between OSA and MVA over a 5-year period, the mean sleep latency on the MSLT was not associated with an MVA,[20] although the study may have lacked power. Men involved in multiple MVAs trended toward lower sleep latency, whereas women had no differences in sleep architecture based on involvement in multiple MVAs. In contrast, in a population-based study in Michigan in which MVAs were ascertained from the state police database, participants with excessive sleepiness (MSLT<5 minutes) were 26% more likely to be involved in a crash compared with alert participants (MSLT>10 minutes), although the MVAs may not necessarily have been sleep related.[19]

Several considerations may limit the usefulness of the MSLT as the singular determinant of sleepiness in an individual.[24] First, the MSLT is a physiologic measure of sleepiness rather than alertness and, therefore, may not accurately reflect an individual's ability to stay awake during important tasks. Second, the MSLT may not accurately reflect an individual's safety risk because it is conducted in the absence of multiple external stimuli found in real-world environments. Third, although an MSLT less than 10 minutes suggests sleepiness, the normative range (based on the mean ± 2 standard deviations [SDs]) for the MSLT would span 1.2 to 20 minutes. Motivation, such as fear of job loss, can increase sleep latency (ie, appear less sleepy) on the MSLT.[29] These issues and the mixed results of the studies described earlier make it difficult to provide specific guidelines on the use of the MSLT in determining safety, particularly when driving. Given this finding, current guidelines suggest that the MSLT should not be used in isolation and should be interpreted in the context of the patient's history.[24]

MWT

The MWT is an objective test of an individual's ability to stay awake. The test involves 4 40-minute sessions spaced 2 hours apart during which individuals are asked to stay awake in a quiet, dimly lit room while sitting comfortably in bed. From the test, the mean sleep latency is reported in minutes. Normative data that are reported suggest that the mean sleep latency in normal individuals is 30.4 ± 11.2 minutes.[24] In patients with disorders of sleepiness such as severe OSA, the MWT is reduced at 20.2 minutes, although there is a broad range of values (7.6–40 minutes).[30]

Several studies have examined the usefulness of the MWT in the assessment of driving safety, also with mixed results. In 1 cross-sectional study,[31] drivers involved in a car crash (cases) in New Zealand were compared with individuals matched on age, sex, height, weight, and BMI (controls). The prevalence of OSA was similar in both groups, and the mean MWT sleep latency was 17 ± 4 minutes in cases versus 18 ± 4 minutes for controls ($P = .06$). A limitation of this study was the use of a 20-minute MWT, when the 40-minute MWT has been shown to be more sensitive to the detection of impaired alertness. In another study,[32] the mean MWT sleep latency after a 5-hour period of sleep restriction did not correlate well with driving simulator performance and explained only 20% to 30% of driving performance after sleep restriction. Only when sleep restriction was combined with alcohol ingestion (0.004 g/dL) was there a correlation between the MWT and the number of crashes in a driving

simulator. In contrast, a French study of 38 patients with untreated OSA (mean apnea-hypopnea index (AHI) ± SD: 41 ± 25 events/h) versus 14 healthy individuals[33] reported a correlation between MWT results and the number of inappropriate line crossings (Spearman $r = -0.3339$) during a 90-minute real-life driving session. Individuals with a mean MWT sleep latency less than 33 minutes had significantly more inappropriate line crossings than control drivers. In another study of 24 patients with severe OSA (mean AHI ± SD: 54 ± 16 events/h),[34] the mean MWT sleep latency was inversely correlated with the number of crashes during a driving simulation (Spearman $r = -0.836$; $P<.005$). In this small sample, a mean MWT sleep latency less than 8 minutes was predictive of crashes in a driving simulator based on receiver operating characteristic (ROC) values (area under the curve [AUC]: 0.87 ± 0.08; $P = .005$) and a mean MWT sleep latency greater than 30 minutes was predictive of no crashes (ROC AUC: 0.92 ± 0.06; $P = .001$). Taken together, these studies suggest that the MWT may be most beneficial when the sleep latency is clearly reduced (<8 minutes) or when it is only slightly reduced (>33 minutes) and when a physiologic challenge such as sleep restriction is combined with alcohol ingestion. More difficult is determining what to do with results that are intermediate.

The MWT has had an appeal in the evaluation of safety risk, given that it measures the individual's capacity to remain awake. The test has been used in licensing for commercial motor vehicle drivers, aviation pilots, coastguard personnel, and railroad workers; areas in which public safety is a particular issue. Nevertheless, the MWT has inherent limitations that may limit its usefulness and must be interpreted in the context of the patient's history. First, the body of normative data compared with the MSLT is limited. Second, the normative range from available data (based on the mean ± 2 SDs) for the MWT spans 8 to 40 minutes.[24] Third, although the MWT measures the ability to stay awake, it is performed under dim light settings while the individual is seated in bed and may not be predictive of maintaining alertness in more complex environments such as flying.[29]

Simulated driving performance

The use of driving simulators has been examined in predicting MVAs in individuals with and without sleep disorders, under conditions of sleep restriction, after alcohol ingestion, or a combination of exposures. Driving simulations are timed tests in which individuals are asked to engage in a variety of tasks that occur with real-world driving, such as maintaining a certain speed, keeping in their lane, or stopping when appropriate. The task is performed for at least 30 minutes, although longer durations (90–120 minutes) may be more sensitive in detecting poor performance.

The link between OSA and accidents has been investigated via simulated scenarios. Although it seems intuitive that neurocognitive impairment or sleep loss can directly contribute to MVAs, 1 study showed no association with any neuropsychological test and driving ability.[35] The same study showed that 6 weeks of CPAP treatment of patients with OSA improved 1-hour monotonous driving accuracy, suggesting a mechanism other than neurocognitive impairment for the increased MVA risk. No control group was used, to know whether simulated driving accuracy returned to normal with CPAP use.

Furthermore, poor performance on a driving simulator has also not been shown to correlate strongly with MVAs in patients with untreated OSA.[36,37] However, studies have shown differences in performance when OSA is treated. In 1 investigation from the United Kingdom using a monotonous 2-hour afternoon driving simulator, patients with OSA treated with CPAP had no difference in driving accuracy, in terms of driving performance or self-assessment of sleepiness, compared with age-matched healthy control patients.[38] This finding suggests that CPAP therapy can return driving accuracy and sleepiness perception to normal. When the OSA and control groups were subjected to a single night of 5-hour sleep restriction, patients with OSA had significantly shorter safe driving time compared with the healthy controls (65 minutes vs 91 minutes), and their ability to perceive their sleepiness was worse, suggesting that patients with OSA remain vulnerable to sleep alterations despite successful treatment. In another study using the same simulator model, patients with OSA treated with CPAP adherent to therapy were studied after normal sleep with CPAP and after 1 night without CPAP.[39] Neglecting CPAP therapy even for a single night was shown to result in significantly more road lane drifts, shorter safe driving duration, and greater subjective sleepiness. This study suggested that nightly adherence with CPAP therapy is crucial to safe driving, as tested in this driving simulator setting. Investigators have also examined the use of wake-promoting medications to offset the effects of acute withdrawal of CPAP on daytime function. In 1 study,[40] modafinil was given in the morning for 2 days after acute withdrawal of CPAP therapy for 2 nights. Driving performance, as tested with a driving simulator, as well as PVT and subjective sleepiness, all improved with modafinil use, suggesting that the effects of acute CPAP withdrawal can be overcome acutely.

However, some have called into question the validity of simulated driving performance in predicting real-world driving. Depending on the realism of the simulator, the graphics, and the size of the visualization, it may be difficult to extrapolate results from simulators to real-word driving performance. Motivation, risks of injury, and financial and legal consequences are also different between the 2 situations. Experimental conditions, including driving duration and monotony of the driving environment affect driving performance and are more difficult to vary in the simulator environment. For example, drivers who were tested under rested and sleep-restricted condition had a 10-fold increase in inappropriate line crossings when in the simulator compared with an on-the-road driving condition, independent of the testing conditions.[41] In the DROWSI project,[42] healthy individuals reported a high level of subjective sleepiness during day driving with a simulator. The simulation may have facilitated the reports of sleepiness given the absence of real-world external stimuli. For these reasons, driving simulators, may therefore not be a valid reflection of real driving situations.

Real-world driving performance

Research studies have attempted to overcome the limitations of driving simulators by using real-world driving courses to examine the propensity of an individual for an MVA. Study participants are typically asked to drive a highway course at a standard speed with a professional driving instructor ready to take control of the car if needed for safety. This approach has been used to assess the effects of sleep disorders such as OSA, extended driving, or the influence of the circadian system on alertness during driving. In 1 study examining the effects of extended driving on nighttime performance,[43] participants were asked to drive a control condition (9–10 PM) and were compared against their driving from 3 to 5 AM (short), 1 to 5 AM (intermediate), and 9 PM to 5 AM (long). Compared with the control condition, drivers in the last hour of driving had markedly higher incidence rate ratio (IRR) for inappropriate line crossings than the short (IRR: 6.0), intermediate (IRR: 15.4), and long sessions (IRR: 24.3). The study suggested that the interaction between night driving and the circadian drive markedly impairs nocturnal driving.

Another study by the same investigators examined subjective and objective measures of sleepiness using the real-world driving course in patients with untreated OSA compared with healthy control participants.[33] Subjective measures of sleepiness (ESS and Karolinska Sleepiness Scale) and objective measurement (MWT) were found to be associated with the number of inappropriate line crossings during a 90-minute real-life driving session. However, this study did not assess the effect of OSA treatment on the predictive abilities of the factors assessed.

Although a wide array of subjective and objective tests exist to assess excessive sleepiness or alertness, their correlation with MVAs has not been fully validated. Each also has inherent strengths and weaknesses. These tests should not be used in isolation and must be fully integrated with the patient's clinical history if used to assess driving risk.

OSA AND MVAS

Although tools are available to assess alertness, sleepiness, and neurocognitive function, the question remains as to whether patients with OSA are at higher risk of an MVA. The current balance of data suggests that patients with OSA are at higher risk of an MVA, although predicting which patients will have an MVA is difficult and remains controversial. The association between OSA and MVAs is likely related to the sleep loss and subsequent neurocognitive impairments experienced by patients with OSA, rather than being specific to OSA.

Risk and Costs of Accidents in Patients with OSA

The association between OSA and MVAs is supported by a recent meta-analysis performed for the Federal Motor Carrier Safety Administration (FMCSA), which showed that the risk of an MVA was 2.4 times higher in drivers with OSA.[48] The risk of driving accidents has been reported to range 2 to 10 times higher in patients with untreated OSA, compared with controls.[44–50] The absolute risk of an MVA in 1 study using MVA data from the Ontario Ministry of Transportation database was 0.18 versus 0.06 MVA/driver/y over a 3-year period in patients with untreated OSA compared with randomly selected control drivers matched on age, gender, and type of driver's license.[47]

Although the overall literature supports an association between OSA and MVAs, not all studies have the same results. For example, in a longitudinal study of older drivers using self-reported driving patterns and sleep questionnaires (insomnia severity index, ESS, and Sleep Apnea Clinical Score),[49] investigators found sleep disturbances to be mild and not associated with adverse driving events. The investigators speculated that the

absence of an association may have been caused by self-regulation of driving that occurs in this population when they are aware of potential impairments that pose a driving risk. In another study, Philip and colleagues[50] surveyed more than 35,000 highway drivers in France for sleep symptoms and disorders. In this study population, 5.2% reported the OSA syndrome and 7.2% reported a driving accident in the past year. Risk of accidents was associated with narcolepsy and hypersomnia, multiple sleep disorders, age 18 to 30 years, and single status, but not with the diagnosis of OSA. In a study conducted in Spain of 60 patients with OSA and 60 control individuals,[36] the investigators determined that patients with OSA were 2.3 times more likely to be in at least 1 MVA over a 3-year period. However, when potential predictors of an MVA risk were assessed in this study, such as the ESS, anxiety and depression scores, driving simulator performance, and OSA metrics, the investigators found no association between these metrics and the risk of an MVA in these patients with OSA. Thus, predicting which patients with OSA will have an MVA is difficult and most likely explains why all patients with untreated OSA are not restricted from driving.

The consequences of OSA-related MVAs are not limited to psychomotor performance and MVA-related bodily injury to self and others but also involve significant financial burden. Using data from the National Safety Council and from published studies, Sassani and colleagues[51] estimated that 810,000 MVAs and 1400 fatalities were directly attributable to untreated OSA, with a total cost of $15.9 billion.

Effects of Therapy for OSA on Accidents

As discussed in the previous section, drivers with OSA carry a higher risk of MVAs than drivers without OSA. The next logical question is whether treatment of OSA reduces the risk of MVA. In the study using the Ontario Ministry of Transportation database,[47] patients with OSA treated with CPAP for 3 years had a reduction in MVAs to levels seen in non-OSA controls, whereas patients with untreated OSA had no change in the rate of MVAs over time. When 9 studies examining MVA in patients with OSA were aggregated for a meta-analysis, Tregear and colleagues[52] reported a substantial risk reduction (risk ratio = 0.278; 95% CI: 0.22–0.35). These results should be applied with caution for at least several reasons. First, the quality of the studies is considered to be low and susceptible to bias. For example, many of the studies use a historical control approach, rather than a concurrent control, which can affect how participants behave after an intervention. Second, because of the nature of the studies, control for confounding factors such as CPAP adherence or distance driven was not possible. Third, other behavioral and health modifications, such as improved sleep hygiene and adherence to overall medical care, may have also changed during the period and contributed to the improvement in driving risk in the treated OSA group.

In addition to reducing MVAs rates, OSA treatment with CPAP may reduce direct and indirect costs observed with OSA and MVAs. Sassani and colleagues[51] cost-analyses estimated that treatment of OSA could reduce MVAs by 567,000, reduce fatalities by 1000, and save $7.9 billion, after accounting for the cost of treatment of OSA. In addition, indirect economic costs of OSA-related MVAs would include costs of injuries, lost productivity, increased insurance premiums, and increased health care use. Schneider National, a trucking company, acknowledged these exorbitant and avoidable costs by implementing a commercial driver sleep apnea program to screen and treat for OSA. Eighty percent of the 547 drivers screened had a sleep disorder. With treatment, monthly medical costs were cut in half, preventable driving accidents were reduced by 74%, and driver retention rates were increased 2.29-fold, all contributing to the financial betterment of the company.[53]

The evidence base suggests that OSA is associated with a higher risk of MVAs and that therapy may normalize the MVA risk. Furthermore, the direct and indirect costs of untreated OSA support the need to identify OSA in drivers as a risk factor for MVA and support the justification to enforce treatment of OSA in drivers.

LAWS AND REGULATIONS REGARDING OSA SCREENING

Laws and regulations are developed based on the needs of a society, and vary by country and region. Although a comprehensive review of all laws related to sleep medicine is beyond the scope of this review, a physician is still expected to know the regulations in the jurisdiction in which they practice. The risk management departments within health care systems, State Medical Boards, or the FindLaw Web site[54] are good resources to understand the particular aspects of both federal and state law. In addition, state medical boards and medical societies[55,56] may offer position statements to guide practitioners on recommended conduct and obligations. Medicolegal aspects of sleep medicine in general have increasingly become a topic of interest, and were recently reviewed elsewhere.[57]

Foundation of Laws and Regulations

Criminal liability for a sleep-related incident depends on the presence of culpability, or blameworthiness of an individual for a behavior. The US justice system categorizes culpability by degrees of mental state: (1) purposeful; (2) knowing; (3) reckless, or (4) negligent behaviors (**Table 2**).[58] The definitions of these terms depend on whether a behavior can result in substantial but unjustifiable risk, intention of the individual to perform an act, and the awareness of the individual that a behavior will result in harm. Given the established link between untreated OSA and driving performance, patients with OSA should be counseled on the risk of driving drowsy if untreated, nonadherent to therapy, or if their sleep is restricted.

The issue of awareness in culpability depends on a sound mental state, or *mens rea*. The standard test of criminal liability is expressed in the Latin phrase *actus non facit reum nisi mens sit rea*, which translates as "the act does not make a person guilty unless the mind is also guilty." This requires the action to have occurred in a conscious state, but in cases of sleepiness-related accidents, can be extended to include actions that begin in a conscious state. Driving while drowsy is a decision made by the driver in a conscious state, but an accident may have occurred during a state of sleep. The state of awareness before and during the sleepiness-related accident is often the central point when determining criminal liability.

The preponderance of literature concerning sleep-related incidents addresses driving regulations and OSA. Policies and regulations are in place that address both personal driving and commercial driving liability in the context of OSA. Other professions with OSA-specific regulations include airline pilots, railroad engineers, and construction workers.

OSA and Commercial Driver's Licenses

Commercial motor vehicle (CMV) driving accidents in the United States account for 12% of all worker deaths, with 4932 fatal crashes involving a large truck in 2005.[59] The Commercial Motor Vehicle Safety Act of 1986 was enacted to improve highway safety by ensuring that drivers of large trucks and buses were qualified to operate the vehicles. Although states retained the authorization to issue driver's licenses, the act provided minimum standards for commercial driver's license (CDL) holders. These minimum standards applied primarily to driving knowledge and skills. The CDL in the United States is regulated by the FMCSA.

CDL holders must have medical qualification examinations every 2 years. A CDL may be denied

Table 2
Basis for determination of culpability by degree of mental state

Term	Definition
Purposely	1. The element involves the nature of his conduct or a result thereof, it is his conscious object to engage in conduct of that nature or to cause such a result; and 2. The element involves the attendant circumstances, he is aware of the existence of such circumstances or he believes or hopes that they exist • Subset of knowing • Equivalent to intentional in non-MPC statutes
Knowingly	1. If the element involves the nature of his conduct or the attendant circumstances, he is aware that his conduct is of that nature or that such circumstances exist; and 2. If the element involves a result of his conduct, he is aware that it is practically certain that his conduct will cause such a result • Subset of reckless • Equivalent to willfully in non-MPC statutes
Recklessly	1. He consciously disregards a substantial and unjustifiable risk that the material element exists or will result from his conduct 2. The risk must be of such a nature and degree that, considering the nature and intent of the actor's conduct and the circumstances known to him, its disregard involves a gross deviation from the standard of conduct that a reasonable person would observe in the actor's situation • Minimum standard if no culpability is stated by statue
Negligently	1. He should be aware of a substantial and unjustifiable risk that the material element exists or will result from his conduct 2. The risk must be of such a nature and degree that the actor's failure to perceive it, considering the nature and intent of his conduct and the circumstances known to him, involves a gross deviation from the standard of care that a reasonable person would observe in the actor's situation

Abbreviation: MPC, model penal code.
Model Penal Code copyright © 1985 by The American Law Institute. Reproduced with permission. All rights reserved.
Adapted from Dubber M. Criminal law: model penal code. New York: Foundation Press; 2002.

for certain medical conditions such as OSA, with an opportunity for a waiver under specific conditions. To obtain a waiver, CMV drivers with OSA must undergo an annual recertification process to maintain their CDL. Federal qualification standards for medical issues related to OSA, as addressed in Section 391.41 (b) Title 49 CFR (Federal Motor Carrier Regulations),[60] include only "respiratory dysfunction likely to interfere with his/her ability" to drive safely. In 1991, the FMCSA specifically recommended that patients with OSA undergo a yearly MSLT or MWT as part of a safety evaluation. Medical societies and patient advocacy organizations recognized the limited usefulness of the MWT in assessing accident risk in CMV drivers. This situation led to the development of suggested guidelines for screening CDL holders for OSA by a joint task force of the American College of Chest Physicians, the American College of Occupational and Environmental Medicine, and the National Sleep Foundation (NSF). Recommendations were provided for determining criteria for in-service versus out-of-service evaluation and for fitness for duty once the diagnosis of OSA is

established.[55] Major differences of the task force recommendations compared with previous guidelines were the reliance on objective risk factors for OSA (eg, BMI, neck circumference, hypertension), reporting of adequate CPAP adherence, and no need for the MWT. The validity of the recommendations in identifying at-risk CMV drivers was studied. In 1 clinic evaluating 1443 CDL holders, 13% met criteria for a 3-month limited certification. Of the 190 at-risk CMV drivers identified, 56 declined further assessment for OSA. Of the remaining drivers, 94.8% had OSA, with 65.3% having moderate to severe OSA.[61] Although many of the task force recommendations were adopted by occupational medicine clinics and some trucking companies, the recommendations have not been adopted by the FMCSA.

In 2007, the Medical Review Board (MRB) for the FMCSA requested that a Medical Expert Panel (MEP) be convened to re-evaluate current FMCSA regulations regarding OSA in CDL holders.[62] The MEP conducted an evidence-based review of the literature and presented their recommendation to the MRB in January, 2008. These recommendations were mostly adopted by the MRB (**Table 3**). Many CDL medical examiners and trucking companies have adopted these recommendations in anticipation of their acceptance by the FMCSA; however, as of this publication, the FMCSA has yet to formally adopt the MRB/MEP recommendations. Whether or not these driving regulations result in reduced accidents remains to be determined.

Table 3
Summary of recommendations from the MEP/MRB of the FMCSA for CMV drivers

Category	Specific Recommendations
Conditions for certification of driver	No OSA: unconditional certification possible With OSA a. Untreated OSA with AHI <20 b. No daytime sleepiness c. OSA is effectively treated
Conditions for disqualification or denial of certification for driver	Daytime sleepiness experienced with driving Crash experience associated with falling asleep AHI >20 until PAP compliance established (conditional certification possible) Any OSA-related surgery pending 3 mo postoperative evaluation Noncompliance with PAP therapy
Conditional certification	BMI ≥30 kg/m² certified for 1 mo pending evaluation for OSA Diagnosis of OSA, 1 mo pending treatment If PAP compliant at 1 mo, then 3 mo certification If compliant at 3 mo, then 1 y certification
Identification of individuals with undiagnosed OSA	Obstructive breathing symptoms Daytime sleepiness Age, BMI ≥28 kg/m², small jaw, large neck, small airway, family history Presence of hypertension, DM2, hypothyroidism
Method of diagnosis	Overnight polysomnography preferred Portable monitor with oxygen saturation, nasal pressure, sleep/wake time
Treatment of OSA with PAP	PAP is the preferred therapy Adequate titration in laboratory or autotitration Certification after 1 wk if sleepiness resolved and compliance demonstrated
Treatment alternatives	Oral appliances are not acceptable because of inability to monitor compliance Surgery is acceptable
Bariatric surgery	Can be recertified if compliant with CPAP or if 6 mo postoperative check with clearance by physician, AHI <10, and not sleepy
Oropharyngeal, tracheostomy, and facial bone surgery	Can be recertified >1 mo postoperatively if cleared by physician, AHI <10, and not sleepy
Patient education	Education on importance of adequate sleep, lifestyle changes, including a. Weight loss b. Exercise c. Reduced alcohol intake d. Importance of treatment compliance e. Consequences of untreated OSA

Abbreviations: DM2, type 2 diabetes mellitus; PAP, positive airway pressure.
Adapted from Federal Motor Carrier Safety Administration. Expert panel recommendations on obstructive sleep apnea and commercial motor vehicle driver safety. Washington DC: US Department of Transportation; 2008.

OSA and Personal/Noncommercial Driving

As of 2008, the NSF reported that no state had a law that addressed nonfatal, sleep-related motor-vehicle crashes.[63] The only state with a specific law under which a sleep-deprived driver who killed another driver could be charged is New Jersey (Maggie's law).[64] However, each state treats sleep disorders such as OSA differently, often on a case-by-case basis. Some US states, including Texas and California, have mandatory reporting laws, which protect the physicians but may discourage patients from revealing their full medical information with their physician. Other states take action only after a sleepiness-related driving accident. Voluntary reporting programs exist in most states, but may place the physician at risk of litigation if individual privacy rights outweigh the benefits to society. The American Thoracic Society provides recommendations for reporting sleepy drivers, but these guidelines are not legally enforceable and are limited by lack of support from the scientific literature.[56]

The variability in reporting rules and driving restriction guidelines is an area that needs attention from the national and international sleep and safety councils to provide better guidelines to establish the rights of patients to drive versus the right of the public safety.

OSA and Other Professions

Significantly less is known about pilot fatigue and OSA, but the lessons learned from research in driving fatigue and OSA have been applied to aeronautics and railroad engineering.

In 2008 and 2009, 2 high-profile air incidents occurred near destination airports in Hawaii and Minnesota, when the crews overflew the airport after falling asleep. The investigations included evaluations for common causes of daytime sleepiness, including sleep deprivation before work, jet lag, and long duty hours but also recognized OSA as a potential contributor to sleepiness. The Federal Aviation Administration (FAA) requires medical certification of pilots, which includes screening for clinical evaluation of OSA and restless legs syndrome. However, there do not seem to be any standardized criteria for referring a pilot for formal polysomnography testing. A diagnosis of OSA of any severity should result in disqualification for the aviation license. A medical waiver under the Special Issuance provisions of 14 CFR 67.401 can be granted if the pilot undergoes sufficient testing and treatment.[65] This strategy includes a split-study or second sleep study after treatment, a normal MWT or MSLT, and documentation that the pilot/controller no longer experiences any daytime sleepiness. Despite the limitations of the MWT in assessing driving fatigue, it is still used as the standard of testing by the FAA.[66]

Even less regulation seems to be applicable to train engineers and merchant sailors. The US National Transportation Safety Board recommended in 2009 that truck and bus drivers, commercial pilots, train engineers and merchant sailors should all be screened for sleep apnea. However, further laws and regulations seem to be in their infancy in these fields.

ROLE OF THE SLEEP PHYSICIAN

The physician's first role is to diagnose and manage the patient's medical condition. Furthermore, the physician needs to educate the patient and the community of the potential consequences of OSA. Once a patient is identified as having OSA, or even if OSA is suspected, then the role of the physician expands beyond the care of the patient. A fundamental tenet of a criminal act is whether an individual is culpable, or blameworthy, for a behavior. As discussed earlier, the level of criminal liability rests on whether a reasonable person would be aware of a substantial and unjustifiable risk. A reasonable person may be expected to know the consequences of OSA only if a concerted effort is made to educate the patient and the public. Therefore, a fundamental role of the sleep physician is to educate the patient about OSA and its possible consequences. Educating the local community raises awareness of self-identified sleep-related impairments in others and may facilitate early referral, screening, and treatment.

Another role of the sleep physician is to provide medical screening and treatment of OSA in patients in high-risk professions. When the profession requires OSA screening for public safety, such as truck drivers with CDLs and pilots, the physician becomes an advocate for the public over the individual patient. Thus, screening examinations are often performed by independent physicians, rather than the patient's primary physician.

SUMMARY

The medicolegal implications of OSA and driving are complex. The effects of OSA on driving, and other high-risk situations, results in sleep-loss–related or intermittent hypoxia-related neurocognitive impairments in domains vital to performance, such as attention/vigilance, delayed long-term visual and verbal memory, visuospatial/constructional abilities, and executive function. Identifying the subset of the population with driving impairments remains challenging given that subjective and objective tests to test drowsiness and driving ability are limited in their accuracy. To complicate matters, not all patients with OSA or abnormal testing show impaired driving ability, and restricting their driving privilege based on imperfect testing could violate their rights. Professions that require high-level functioning, such as commercial drivers, pilots, and railroad engineers, may restrict credentialing based on qualifications of the person. Laws and policies that regulate driving for both public and professional reasons vary by region, in part because of local needs and in part because of the uncertainty in medical testing. The development of more accurate testing for driving accident risk would aid in developing more uniform regulations and in educating the patient and public of the importance of sleep and safety. The clinician must, therefore, integrate all available information both subjective and objective to help patients with OSA recognize when they might be impaired and how best to manage symptoms to promote safe driving and other transportation-related activities.

REFERENCES

1. Colten HR, Altevogt BM, Institute of Medicine (US). Committee on sleep medicine and research., sleep disorders and sleep deprivation: an unmet public health problem. Washington, DC: Institute of Medicine: National Academies Press; 2006. p. 404.

2. Veasey SC, Davis CW, Fenik P, et al. Long-term intermittent hypoxia in mice: protracted hypersomnolence with oxidative injury to sleep-wake brain regions. Sleep 2004;27(2):194–201.

3. Zhan G, Serrano F, Fenik P, et al. NADPH oxidase mediates hypersomnolence and brain oxidative injury in a murine model of sleep apnea. Am J Respir Crit Care Med 2005;172(7):921–9.

4. Bucks RS, Olaithe M, Eastwood P. Neurocognitive function in obstructive sleep apnoea: a meta-review. Respirology 2012;18(1):61–70.

5. Lal C, Strange C, Bachman D. Neurocognitive impairment in obstructive sleep apnea. Chest 2007;141(6):1601–10.

6. Aloia MS, Arnedt JT, Davis JD, et al. Neuropsychological sequelae of obstructive sleep apnea-hypopnea syndrome: a critical review. J Int Neuropsychol Soc 2004;10(5):772–85.

7. Lau EY, Eskes GA, Morrison DL, et al. Executive function in patients with obstructive sleep apnea treated with continuous positive airway pressure. J Int Neuropsychol Soc 2010;16(6):1077–88.

8. Canessa N, Castronovo V, Cappa SF, et al. Obstructive sleep apnea: brain structural changes and neurocognitive function before and after

treatment. Am J Respir Crit Care Med 2011; 183(10):1419–26.

9. Van Dongen HP, Maislin G, Mullington JM, et al. The cumulative cost of additional wakefulness: dose-response effects on neurobehavioral functions and sleep physiology from chronic sleep restriction and total sleep deprivation. Sleep 2003; 26(2):117–26.

10. Stutts JC, Wilkins JW, Vaughn BV. Why do people have drowsy driving crashes? Input from drivers who just did. Washington, DC: AAA Foundation for Traffic Safety; 1999. p. 1–81.

11. Itoi A, Cilveta R, Voth M, et al. Can drivers avoid falling asleep at the wheel? Washington, DC: AAA Foundation for Traffic Safety; 1993.

12. Marshall NS, Barnes M, Travier N, et al. Continuous positive airway pressure reduces daytime sleepiness in mild to moderate obstructive sleep apnoea: a meta-analysis. Thorax 2006;61(5): 430–4.

13. Patel SR, White DP, Malhotra A, et al. Continuous positive airway pressure therapy for treating sleepiness in a diverse population with obstructive sleep apnea: results of a meta-analysis. Arch Intern Med 2003;163(5):565–71.

14. Tomfohr LM, Ancoli-Israel S, Loredo JS, et al. Effects of continuous positive airway pressure on fatigue and sleepiness in patients with obstructive sleep apnea: data from a randomized controlled trial. Sleep 2011;34(1):121–6.

15. Guilleminault C, Philip P. Tiredness and somnolence despite initial treatment of obstructive sleep apnea syndrome (what to do when an OSAS patient stays hypersomnolent despite treatment). Sleep 1996;19(Suppl 9):S117–22.

16. Mitler MM, Carskadon MA, Hirshkowitz M. Chronic sleep deprivation. In: Kryger MH, Roth T, Dement WC, editors. Principles and practice of sleep medicine. Philadelphia: Elsevier/Saunders; 2005. p. 1417–23.

17. Aurora RN, Caffo B, Crainiceanu C, et al. Correlating subjective and objective sleepiness: revisiting the association using survival analysis. Sleep 2011;34(12):1707–14.

18. Masa JF, Rubio M, Findley LJ. Habitually sleepy drivers have a high frequency of automobile crashes associated with respiratory disorders during sleep. Am J Respir Crit Care Med 2000;162(4 Pt 1):1407–12.

19. Drake C, Roehrs T, Breslau N, et al. The 10-year risk of verified motor vehicle crashes in relation to physiologic sleepiness. Sleep 2010;33(6): 745–52.

20. Young T, Blustein J, Finn L, et al. Sleep-disordered breathing and motor vehicle accidents in a population-based sample of employed adults. Sleep 1997;20(8):608–13.

21. Sagaspe P, Taillard J, Bayon V, et al. Sleepiness, near-misses and driving accidents among a representative population of French drivers. J Sleep Res 2010;19(4):578–84.

22. Findley LJ, Suratt PM. Serious motor vehicle crashes: the cost of untreated sleep apnoea. Thorax 2001;56(7):505.

23. Philip P, Taillard J, Klein E, et al. Effect of fatigue on performance measured by a driving simulator in automobile drivers. J Psychosom Res 2003;55(3): 197–200.

24. Littner MR, Kushida C, Wise M, et al. Practice parameters for clinical use of the multiple sleep latency test and the maintenance of wakefulness test. Sleep 2005;28(1):113–21.

25. Benbadis SR, Mascha E, Perry MC, et al. Association between the Epworth sleepiness scale and the multiple sleep latency test in a clinical population. Ann Intern Med 1999;130(4 Pt 1):289–92.

26. Chervin RD, Aldrich MS. The Epworth Sleepiness Scale may not reflect objective measures of sleepiness or sleep apnea. Neurology 1999;52(1):125–31.

27. Punjabi NM, Bandeen-Roche K, Young T. Predictors of objective sleep tendency in the general population. Sleep 2003;26(6):678–83.

28. Aldrich MS. Automobile accidents in patients with sleep disorders. Sleep 1989;12(6):487–94.

29. Bonnet MH. The MSLT and MWT should not be used for the assessment of workplace safety. J Clin Sleep Med 2006;2(2):128–31.

30. Hack M, Davies RJ, Mullins R, et al. Randomised prospective parallel trial of therapeutic versus subtherapeutic nasal continuous positive airway pressure on simulated steering performance in patients with obstructive sleep apnoea. Thorax 2000;55(3):224–31.

31. Arzi L, Shreter R, El-Ad B, et al. Forty- versus 20-minute trials of the maintenance of wakefulness test regimen for licensing of drivers. J Clin Sleep Med 2009;5(1):57–62.

32. Banks S, Catcheside P, Lack LC, et al. The maintenance of wakefulness test and driving simulator performance. Sleep 2005;28(11):1381–5.

33. Philip P, Sagaspe P, Taillard J, et al. Maintenance of wakefulness test, obstructive sleep apnea syndrome, and driving risk. Ann Neurol 2008;64(4):410–6.

34. Pizza F, Contardi S, Mondini S, et al. Daytime sleepiness and driving performance in patients with obstructive sleep apnea: comparison of the MSLT, the MWT, and a simulated driving task. Sleep 2009;32(3):382–91.

35. Orth M, Duchna HW, Leidag M, et al. Driving simulator and neuropsychological [corrected] testing in OSAS before and under CPAP therapy. Eur Respir J 2005;26(5):898–903.

36. Barbé, Pericás J, Muñoz A, et al. Automobile accidents in patients with sleep apnea syndrome. An epidemiological and mechanistic study. Am J Respir Crit Care Med 1998;158(1):18–22.

37. Turkington PM, Sircar M, Allgar V, et al. Relationship between obstructive sleep apnoea, driving simulator performance, and risk of road traffic accidents. Thorax 2001;56(10):800–5.

38. Filtness AJ, Reyner LA, Horne JA. Moderate sleep restriction in treated older male OSA participants: greater impairment during monotonous driving compared with controls. Sleep Med 2011;12(9): 838–43.

39. Filtness AJ, Reyner LA, Horne JA. One night's CPAP withdrawal in otherwise compliant OSA patients: marked driving impairment but good awareness of increased sleepiness. Sleep Breath 2012; 16(3):865–71.

40. Williams SC, Marshall NS, Kennerson M, et al. Modafinil effects during acute continuous positive airway pressure withdrawal: a randomized crossover double-blind placebo-controlled trial. Am J Respir Crit Care Med 2010;181(8):825–31.

41. Philip P, Sagaspe P, Taillard J, et al. Fatigue, sleepiness, and performance in simulated versus real driving conditions. Sleep 2005;28(12):1511–6.

42. Akerstedt T, Ingre M, Kecklund G, et al. Reaction of sleepiness indicators to partial sleep deprivation, time of day and time on task in a driving simulator–the DROWSI project. J Sleep Res 2010; 19(2):298–309.

43. Sagaspe P, Taillard J, Akerstedt T, et al. Extended driving impairs nocturnal driving performances. PLoS One 2008;3(10):e3493.

44. Horstmann S, Hess CW, Bassetti C, et al. Sleepiness-related accidents in sleep apnea patients. Sleep 2000;23(3):383–9.

45. Haraldsson PO, Carenfelt C, Diderichsen F, et al. Clinical symptoms of sleep apnea syndrome and automobile accidents. ORL J Otorhinolaryngol Relat Spec 1990;52(1):57–62.

46. Haraldsson PO, Akerstedt T. Drowsiness–greater traffic hazard than alcohol. Causes, risks and treatment. Lakartidningen 2001;98(25):3018–23.

47. George CF. Reduction in motor vehicle collisions following treatment of sleep apnoea with nasal CPAP. Thorax 2001;56(7):508–12.

48. Tregear S, Reston J, Schoelles K, et al. Obstructive sleep apnea and risk of motor vehicle crash: systematic review and meta-analysis. J Clin Sleep Med 2009;5(6):573–81.

49. Vaz Fragoso CA, Araujo KL, Van Ness PH, et al. Sleep disturbances and adverse driving events in a predominantly male cohort of active older drivers. J Am Geriatr Soc 2010;58(10):1878–84.

50. Philip P, Sagaspe P, Lagarde E, et al. Sleep disorders and accidental risk in a large group of regular registered highway drivers. Sleep Med 2010; 11(10):973–9.

51. Sassani A, Findley LJ, Kryger M, et al. Reducing motor-vehicle collisions, costs, and fatalities by treating obstructive sleep apnea syndrome. Sleep 2004;27(3):453–8.

52. Tregear S, Reston J, Schoelles K, et al. Continuous positive airway pressure reduces risk of motor vehicle crash among drivers with obstructive sleep apnea: systematic review and meta-analysis. Sleep 2010;33(10):1373–80.

53. Schneider: sleep apnea treatment pays off. FleetOwner; 2006. Available at: http://fleetowner. com/management/news/sleep_apnea_treatment. Accessed April 9, 2013.

54. FindLaw. 2009. Available at: http://www.findlaw. com/. Accessed April 9, 2013.

55. Hartenbaum N, Collop N, Rosen IM, et al. Sleep apnea and commercial motor vehicle operators: statement from the joint task force of the American College of Chest Physicians, the American College of Occupational and Environmental Medicine, and the National Sleep Foundation. Chest 2006; 130(3):902–5.

56. Sleep apnea, sleepiness, and driving risk. American Thoracic Society. Am J Respir Crit Care Med 1994;150(5 Pt 1):1463–73.

57. Krishnan V, Shaman Z. Legal issues encountered when treating the patient with a sleep disorder. Chest 2011;139(1):200–7.

58. Dubber M. Criminal law: model penal code. Turning point series. New York, NY: Foundation Press; 2002.

59. Tregear SJ, Tiller M, Fontarrosa J, et al. Executive summary: obstructive sleep apnea and commercial motor vehicle driver safety. ECRI Institute. Plymouth Meeting, PA; Federal Motor Carrier Safety Administration; 2007.

60. U.S Department of Transportation Federal Motor Carrier Safety Administration. Physical qualifications for drivers. § 391.41. Published July 16, 2013. Available at: http://www.fmcsa.dot.gov/rules-regulations/administration/fmcsr/fmcsrruletext. aspx?reg=391.41. Accessed August 30, 2013.

61. Talmage JB, Hudson TB, Hegmann KT, et al. Consensus criteria for screening commercial drivers for obstructive sleep apnea: evidence of efficacy. J Occup Environ Med 2008;50(3):324–9.

62. Ancoli-Israel S, et al. Obstructive sleep apnea and commercial motor vehicle driver safety. ECRI Institute. Plymouth Meeting, PA; Federal Motor Carrier Safety Administration; 2008.

63. NSF, state of the states report on drowsy driving: summary of findings. Washington, DC: National Sleep Foundation; 2008.

64. H.R. 968—108th Congress: Maggie's Law: National Drowsy Driving Act of 2003. (2003). In www.Gov Track.us. Retrieved August 30, 2013, from http://www.govtrack.us/congress/bills/108/hr968.

65. U.S. Government Printing Office. Code of Federal Regulations. 14 CFR 67.401 - Special issuance of medical certificates. Published January 1, 2012. Available at: http://www.ecfr.gov/cgi-bin/text-idx?c=ecfr& sid=5c12e1df62f1c4ac9b50bbb0eb923875&rgn= div8&view=text&node=14:2.0.1.1.5.5.1.1&idno=14. Accessed August 30, 2013.

66. AMAS. Medical articles. 2013. Available at: http://aviationmedicine.com/articles/index.cfm?fuseaction= displayArticle&articleID=54. Accessed March 12, 2013.

Index

Note: Page numbers of article titles are in **boldface** type.

A

Accidents. See Motor vehicle accidents.

Acetazolamide, in OSA therapy, 531

Acetylcholinesterase inhibitors, in OSA therapy, 532–533

Acromegaly, OSA and, 534

Acupuncture, for OSA therapy, 549–550

Adaptive servoventilation (ASV), treatment of complex OSA with, 470–471

Adenoidectomy, for OSA therapy, 496–497

Adenotonsillectomy, for OSA therapy in children, 484–486, 498

Age, effect on pathophysiology of OSA, 429

Airway collapsibility, in OSA pathophysiology, 427

Alternative therapies, for OSA, **543–556**
    acupuncture, 549–550
    diaphragmatic pacing, 553
    hypoglossal nerve stimulation, 547–549
    musical instruments, 550–551
    nasal cannulas, 551–552
    nasal resistive devices, 543–545
    nasal strips, 552–553
    positional therapy, 545–547
    snore pillows, 547
    speech exercises, 550

Amphetamines, use in CPAP users with residual sleepiness, 529–530

Anatomy, influence on pathophysiology of OSA, 425–427

Anesthetic agents, to avoid or monitor in OSA patients, 537

Apnea. See Obstructive sleep apnea.

Appliances, oral. See Oral appliance therapy.

Armodafinil. See Modafinil.

Arousal response, in OSA pathophysiology, 428

Arrhythmias, effects of OSA therapy on, 456–457

Atherosclerosis, subclinical, effects of OSA therapy on, 454–456

Automobile driving, by patients with OSA. See Transportation.

B

Barbiturates, to avoid or monitor in OSA patients, 536

Bariatric surgery, to treat OSA in children, 488

Benzodiazepines, to avoid or monitor in OSA patients, 536

Bilevel positive airway pressure (BPAP), mask interfaces for, **477–481**

treatment of complex OSA with, 470

Biomarkers, for EDS in OSA patients, 576–578

C

Caffeine, use in CPAP users with residual sleepiness, 529–530

Cannulas, nasal, for OSA therapy, 551–552

Cardiac arrhythmias, effects of OSA therapy on, 456–457

Cardiovascular disease, effects of OSA therapy on, **453–461**
    arrhythmias, 456–457
    coronary heart disease, 457–458
    overview, 453–454
    stroke, 458–460
    subclinical atherosclerosis, 454–456

Central sleep apnea, as part of complex OSA, 463–467

Cheyne-Stokes respiration, in complex OSA, 464–465

Children. See Pediatrics.

Commercial driver's licenses, OSA and, 599–601

Comorbid conditions, with OSA, medications for, 535–536

Complex obstructive sleep apnea, **463–475**
    clinical characteristics, 468–469
    natural history, 469–470
    pathophysiology, 464–467
        primary, 467
        treatment-emergent, 464–467
    prevalence, 467–468
    treatment, 470–472
        ASV, 470–471
        BPAP and APAP, 470
        CPAP, 470
        dead space, 471–472
        oxygen, 472
        pharmacotherapy, 471

Compliance, costs of inadequate adherence to CPAP, 564–566
    with OSA treatment, mask interfaces for, **477–481**

Continuous positive airway pressure (CPAP), as means of weight loss in OSA therapy, 522
    cost -effectiveness of, *versus* oral appliances, 561–562
    costs of inadequate adherence to, 564–566
    mask interfaces for, **477–481**
    residual sleepiness in OSA patients treated with, **571–582**

Sleep Med Clin 8 (2013) 607–613
http://dx.doi.org/10.1016/S1556-407X(13)00114-8
1556-407X/13/$ – see front matter © 2013 Elsevier Inc. All rights reserved.

United States Postal Service
Statement of Ownership, Management, and Circulation
(All Periodicals Publications Except Requestor Publications)

1. Publication Title
Sleep Medicine Clinics

2. Publication Number
0 2 5 - 0 5 3

3. Filing Date
9/14/13

4. Issue Frequency
Mar, Jun, Sep, Dec

5. Number of Issues Published Annually
4

6. Annual Subscription Price
$184.00

7. Complete Mailing Address of Known Office of Publication (*Not printer*) (*Street, city, county, state, and ZIP+4®*)

Elsevier Inc.
360 Park Avenue South
New York, NY 10010-1710

Contact Person
Stephen R. Bushing

Telephone (*Include area code*)
215-239-3688

8. Complete Mailing Address of Headquarters or General Business Office of Publisher (*Not printer*)
Elsevier Inc., 360 Park Avenue South, New York, NY 10010-1710

9. Full Names and Complete Mailing Addresses of Publisher, Editor, and Managing Editor (*Do not leave blank*)

Publisher (*Name and complete mailing address*)
Linda Belfus, Elsevier, Inc., 1600 John F. Kennedy Blvd. Suite 1800, Philadelphia, PA 19103-2899

Editor (*Name and complete mailing address*)
Katie Saunders, Elsevier, Inc., 1600 John F. Kennedy Blvd. Suite 1800, Philadelphia, PA 19103-2899

Managing Editor (*Name and complete mailing address*)
Adrianne Brigido, Elsevier, Inc., 1600 John F. Kennedy Blvd. Suite 1800, Philadelphia, PA 19103-2899

10. Owner (*Do not leave blank. If the publication is owned by a corporation, give the name and address of the corporation immediately followed by the names and addresses of all stockholders owning or holding 1 percent or more of the total amount of stock. If not owned by a corporation, give the names and addresses of the individual owners. If owned by a partnership or other unincorporated firm, give its name and address as well as those of each individual owner. If the publication is published by a nonprofit organization, give its name and address.*)

Full Name	Complete Mailing Address
Wholly owned subsidiary of	1600 John F. Kennedy Blvd., Ste. 1800
Reed/Elsevier, US holdings	Philadelphia, PA 19103-2899

11. Known Bondholders, Mortgagees, and Other Security Holders Owning or Holding 1 Percent or More of Total Amount of Bonds, Mortgages, or Other Securities. If none, check box ▶ ☐ None

Full Name	Complete Mailing Address
N/A	

12. Tax Status (*For completion by nonprofit organizations authorized to mail at nonprofit rates*) (*Check one*)
The purpose, function, and nonprofit status of this organization and the exempt status for federal income tax purposes:
☐ Has Not Changed During Preceding 12 Months
☐ Has Changed During Preceding 12 Months (*Publisher must submit explanation of change with this statement*)

PS Form 3526, September 2007 (Page 1 of 3 (Instructions Page 3)) PSN 7530-01-000-9931 PRIVACY NOTICE: See our Privacy policy in www.usps.com

---

13. Publication Title
Sleep Medicine Clinics

14. Issue Date for Circulation Data Below
September 2013

15. Extent and Nature of Circulation

		Average No. Copies Each Issue During Preceding 12 Months	No. Copies of Single Issue Published Nearest to Filing Date
a. Total Number of Copies (*Net press run*)		536	510
b. Paid Circulation (By Mail and Outside the Mail)	(1) Mailed Outside-County Paid Subscriptions Stated on PS Form 3541. (*Include paid distribution above nominal rate, advertiser's proof copies, and exchange copies*)	366	360
	(2) Mailed In-County Paid Subscriptions Stated on PS Form 3541 (*Include paid distribution above nominal rate, advertiser's proof copies, and exchange copies*)		
	(3) Paid Distribution Outside the Mails Including Sales Through Dealers and Carriers, Street Vendors, Counter Sales, and Other Paid Distribution Outside USPS®	27	28
	(4) Paid Distribution by Other Classes Mailed Through the USPS (e.g. First-Class Mail®)		
c. Total Paid Distribution (*Sum of 15b (1), (2), (3), and (4)*)	▶	393	388
d. Free or Nominal Rate Distribution (By Mail and Outside the Mail)	(1) Free or Nominal Rate Outside-County Copies Included on PS Form 3541	57	57
	(2) Free or Nominal Rate In-County Copies Included on PS Form 3541		
	(3) Free or Nominal Rate Copies Mailed at Other Classes Through the USPS (e.g. First-Class Mail)		
	(4) Free or Nominal Rate Distribution Outside the Mail (Carriers or other means)		
e. Total Free or Nominal Rate Distribution (Sum of 15d (1), (2), (3) and (4))	▶	57	57
f. Total Distribution (Sum of 15c and 15e)	▶	450	445
g. Copies not Distributed (See instructions to publishers #4 (page #3))	▶	86	65
h. Total (Sum of 15f and g)	▶	536	510
i. Percent Paid (15c divided by 15f times 100)		87.33%	87.19%

16. Publication of Statement of Ownership
☐ If the publication is a general publication, publication of this statement is required. Will be printed in the December 2013 issue of this publication. ☐ Publication not required.

17. Signature and Title of Editor, Publisher, Business Manager, or Owner

Stephen R. Bushing

Stephen R. Bushing – Inventory Distribution Coordinator

Date
September 14, 2013

I certify that all information furnished on this form is true and complete. I understand that anyone who furnishes false or misleading information on this form or who omits material or information requested on the form may be subject to criminal sanctions (including fines and imprisonment) and/or civil sanctions (including civil penalties).

PS Form 3526, September 2007 (Page 2 of 3)

Moving?

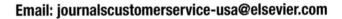

Make sure your subscription moves with you!

To notify us of your new address, find your **Clinics Account Number** (located on your mailing label above your name), and contact customer service at:

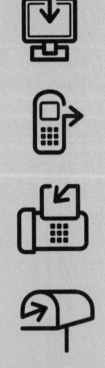

Email: journalscustomerservice-usa@elsevier.com

800-654-2452 (subscribers in the U.S. & Canada)
314-447-8871 (subscribers outside of the U.S. & Canada)

Fax number: 314-447-8029

Elsevier Health Sciences Division
Subscription Customer Service
3251 Riverport Lane
Maryland Heights, MO 63043

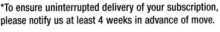

Printed and bound by CPI Group (UK) Ltd, Croydon, CR0 4YY

03/10/2024

01040309-0016